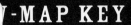

T0151045

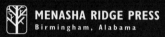

MENASHA RIDGE PRESS
Birmingham, Alabama

60 HIKES WITHIN 60 MILES

ATLANTA

Including MARIETTA, LAWRENCEVILLE, and PEACHTREE CITY

THIRD EDITION

RANDY AND PAM GOLDEN

60 HIKES WITHIN 60 MILES: ATLANTA

Copyright © 2013 by Randy and Pam Golden
All rights reserved
Printed in the United States of America
Published by Menasha Ridge Press
Distributed by Publishers Group West
Third edition, fifth printing 2022

Library of Congress Cataloging-in-Publication Data
  Golden, Randy, 1953–
    60 hikes within 60 miles : Atlanta including Marietta, Lawrenceville,
  and Peachtree city / Randy and Pam Golden. — Third edition.
      pages cm
    Includes index.
    ISBN-13: 978-0-89732-709-1 (pbk); eISBN 978-0-89732-713-8;
    978-1-63404-158-4 (hardcover). ISBN-10: 0-89732-709-8
    1. Hiking—Georgia—Atlanta Region—Guidebooks. 2. Atlanta Region
  (Ga.)—Guidebooks. I. Golden, Pam. II. Title. III. Title: Sixty hikes
  within sixty miles.
    GV199.42.G462A855 2013
    917.5804'44—dc23

                                                          2013003870

Editors: Ritchey Halphen and Amber Kaye Henderson
Cover design and cartography: Scott McGrew
Text design: Steveco International
Cover and interior photos: Randy and Pam Golden
Indexer: Ann Cassar / Cassar Technical Services

MENASHA RIDGE PRESS
An imprint of AdventureKEEN
2204 First Avenue South, Suite 102
Birmingham, Alabama 35233
menasharidge.com

DISCLAIMER

This book is meant only as a guide to select trails in the Atlanta area and does not guarantee hiker safety—you hike at your own risk. Neither Menasha Ridge Press nor Randy and Pam Golden are liable for property loss or damage, personal injury, or death that may result from accessing or hiking the trails described in this guide. Be especially cautious when walking in potentially hazardous terrains with, for example, steep inclines or drop-offs. Do not attempt to explore terrain that may be beyond your abilities. Please read carefully the introduction to this book, as well as safety information from other sources. Familiarize yourself with current weather reports and maps of the area you plan to visit (in addition to the maps provided in this guidebook). Be cognizant of park regulations, and always follow them. While every effort has been made to ensure the accuracy of the information in this guidebook, land and road conditions, phone numbers and websites, and other information can change from year to year.

TABLE OF CONTENTS

ACKNOWLEDGMENTS

FIRST AND FOREMOST, we'd like to thank the dedicated individuals whose hard work created and maintains these trails. Without them this book would not be possible. We also owe a debt of gratitude to the many park rangers, hikers, and local historians who freely shared their time and knowledge of their areas' history, flora and fauna, and interesting trivia. Other people who made a significant contribution include Steve Storey, an outdoor enthusiast who works for the state of Georgia and gave us a number of ideas for hikes to include, as well as our friends Rick and Denise Kearney and Harm and Ev Garrin, who joined us on many of these hikes. Finally, a heartfelt thanks to the folks at Menasha Ridge Press.

—Randy and Pam Golden

FOREWORD

WELCOME TO MENASHA RIDGE PRESS'S 60 Hikes within 60 Miles, a series designed to provide hikers with the information they need to find and hike the very best trails surrounding metropolitan areas.

Our strategy is simple: First, find a hiker who knows the area and loves to hike. Second, ask that person to spend a year researching the most popular and very best trails around. And third, have that person describe each trail in terms of difficulty, scenery, condition, elevation change, and other categories of information that are important to hikers. "Pretend you've just completed a hike and met up with other hikers at the trailhead," we told each author. "Imagine their questions, and be clear in your answers."

Experienced hikers and writers, Randy and Pam Golden have selected 60 of the best hikes in and around the Atlanta metropolitan area. From greenways and urban hikes to flora- and fauna-rich treks in state and national parks, the Goldens provide hikers (and walkers) with a great variety of outings— and all within roughly 60 miles of Atlanta.

You'll get the most from this book if you take a moment to read the Introduction, which explains how to read the trail listings. The "Topographic Maps" section will help you understand how useful topos are on a hike, and will also tell you where to get them. And though this is a where-to rather than a how-to guide, readers who haven't hiked extensively will find the Introduction of particular value.

As much to free the spirit as to free the body, let these hikes elevate you above the urban fray.

All the best,
The Editors at Menasha Ridge Press

ABOUT THE AUTHORS

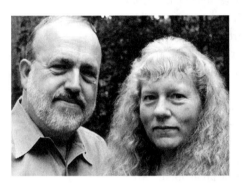

RANDY AND PAM GOLDEN have shared their lifelong love of hiking since they met at college in Florida in 1975. After marrying in 1977, they began hiking across the United States and into Canada. Among their favorite foreign destinations are Puerto Rico's El Yunque and Australia's Dandenong Ranges. They began writing about their adventures at the website **About North Georgia** (ngeorgia.com) in 1995. In 1998 they spun off that site's hiking section into a site of its own, **Georgia Trails** (georgiatrails.com).

PREFACE

WHEN WE WERE FIRST WRITING *60 Hikes within 60 Miles: Atlanta,* Pam and I frequently heard, "There are 60 trails in the Atlanta area?" To the contrary, our problem wasn't finding trails but deciding which ones best represented the region's tremendous variety. In addition to Atlanta proper, Lawrenceville, Marietta, and Peachtree City, our area included a portion of the North Georgia mountains—a well-known hiking destination—and hiking-oriented towns such as Roswell and Cartersville. The most difficult region for finding representative trails was south of the city, but that's changing: great additions such as Sprewell Bluff Wildlife Management Area, Charlie Elliott Wildlife Center, and Cochran Mill Nature Center have increased the number of hiking trails there.

ATLANTA: AMERICA'S FIRST GREAT INLAND CITY

According to tradition, Stephen Long rode a horse to Hardy Ivy's cabin, placed a marker at the site of the zero-mile post of the Western and Atlantic Railroad, and then returned to his office in Marietta. Although Long didn't actually place the marker at what today is the heart of downtown Atlanta, he did write in his journal that the area would never amount to much. Even the man charged with building the railroad didn't understand the importance of this revolutionary mode of transportation.

Farmers and businessmen, though, learned quickly, and by the time the Western and Atlantic was completed in 1850, Atlanta was a thriving rail hub that had already undergone two name changes (it was first called Terminus, then Marthasville). Formerly a hard ride of two days—or more, depending on what you were carrying—Chattanooga was now just 10 hours away by train, at the astounding speed of

10 miles per hour. Soon it became apparent that for a railroad to survive, it had to come to Atlanta.

Unscathed by the Civil War until 1864, the railroads brought Atlanta its utter destruction. Union General William Tecumseh Sherman followed the Western and Atlantic to Atlanta, where he earned two sobriquets, "The Father of Modern Warfare" and "The Father of Urban Renewal." He ordered the central city burned before leaving it. Yet with less than $2 in the city treasury, Atlanta began to rebuild.

Opportunity in the burgeoning city attracted a wide variety of people, including former slaves. The freedmen formed a community centered on the African American churches on Auburn Avenue, just east of downtown. John Wesley Dobbs, a noted black civic leader, anointed the neighborhood "Sweet Auburn" and, referencing its economic potential, proclaimed the streets "paved with gold." That community formed the nucleus of the civil-rights movement in the South and was the birthplace of many of the movement's early leaders, including Martin Luther King Jr. Sadly, with each door opened by integration, one closed on Sweet Auburn, but the district began to revive in the 1990s.

Farmers and farmhands were attracted to higher-paying industrial jobs in the growing city, and what was a trickle of new people at the start of the 20th century became a flood in the 1920s, helped by the boll weevil, falling cotton prices, and a historic drought. Well-to-do Atlantans, meanwhile, moved north to Ansley Park and Druid Hills.

When airplanes began to take over mail routes from the railroads, Atlanta built an airport to once again become a hub in Southeastern transportation. Although the first airmail route—between Atlanta and Miami—lasted less than a year, more followed, and by 1930 planes were a common sight in the skies over the capital of the Peach State.

After trying for many years, in the 1960s Atlanta became a major-league town with the Braves and Falcons, and later the Hawks. Jimmy Carter built the first presidential library here amid much controversy, and a memorial to Dr. King and the civil-rights movement was completed in the 1980s. In 1996 Atlanta hosted the Summer Olympics, building Centennial Park in a blighted area of downtown, now the site of the Georgia Aquarium and the World of Coca-Cola.

THE TRAILS

These hikes are diverse in terms of location, configuration, and length, but a few places within the scope of this book boast a particularly high concentration of trails. Leading the pack is the **Chattahoochee River National Recreation Area (CRNRA).** Other trail-rich areas include the **Georgia State Parks** in all four regions represented by this guide; **Chattahoochee National Forest,** which forms the northern rim of the CRNRA; and **Kennesaw Mountain National Battlefield Park,** which commemorates the men who fought and died in the bloodiest battle of the Atlanta Campaign and at other Civil War sites.

CHATTAHOOCHEE RIVER NATIONAL RECREATION AREA

In 1978 President Jimmy Carter signed into law a bill creating the CRNRA (678-538-1200; **nps.gov/chat**). It comprises 16 named parks covering 9,359 acres and offering a wide range of outdoor fun: hiking, biking, walking, canoeing, kayaking, and rafting. The CRNRA is headquartered at the Island Ford Unit, where you can buy an annual pass covering the entire area for $25. Otherwise, each visit will cost you $3, paid at the trail kiosks in the parking lots. The most popular park in the system is **Cochran Shoals,** just north of I-285. The most scenic, in our opinion, is **East Palisades,** and the most remote is **Bowmans Island,** just south of Lake Sidney Lanier. Fulton, Cobb, Forsyth, and Gwinnett Counties each have park areas within the boundaries of the CRNRA.

Although not part of the recreation area, **Chattahoochee Nature Center** (770-992-2055; **chattnaturecenter.org**) is adjacent to the river and offers an enjoyable hike, along with informative displays and creatures from the wild. The raptor aviary is home to two American bald eagles as well as assorted hawks and owls.

The river flows northwest of downtown Atlanta, and you'll find great places not far off its route to shop, eat, and sleep, including the **Cumberland Mall–Galleria** area in Cobb County, and **Sandy Springs** and **Roswell** in Fulton County.

CHATTAHOOCHEE NATIONAL FOREST

The northern rim of our 60-mile area is covered by this national forest (770-297-3000; **fs.usda.gov/conf**). Originally part of the Cherokee National Forest, the area was reorganized along state lines in the 1930s, and the Chattahoochee National Forest was created. Within its bounds are Georgia's high point, **Brasstown Bald,** and the evocatively named **Blood Mountain,** site of a battle between the area's first inhabitants, Creek and Cherokee natives. Hiking trails here number in the hundreds; most lie outside this book's 60-mile radius from Atlanta. We've chosen three hikes that represent why we love the Georgia mountains so much. If you're intrigued by our choices and you'd like to continue your exploration, we recommend Tim Homan's excellent book *The Hiking Trails of North Georgia.*

Unlike the sharp, tall peaks farther north in the Appalachian Mountains, Georgia's Blue Ridge Mountains are somewhat softer but not easy by any stretch. The remote nature of these mountain trails makes them great for solitude, but be careful—if you get injured on a hike, it will be difficult to contact rescue personnel, much less get them to your location. We don't want you to be afraid of hiking in the mountains; after all, we've been doing it for years. Just follow a few obvious safety tips: don't hike alone, make sure somebody knows where you're going and when you'll be back, be cautious when hiking in wildlife-management areas during hunting season, and bring a map and compass, even if you have a GPS unit.

When you're done traipsing through the woods, Georgia's mountain towns have some great places to eat. Check out **Poole's Bar-B-Q** in East Ellijay (706-635-4100; **www.poolesbarbq.com**) or, for expansive family dining, **The Smith House** in Dahlonega (800-852-9577 or 706-867-7000; **smithhouse.com**) or **The Dillard House** north of Clayton (706-746-5348; **dillardhouse.com**).

Excellent accommodations greatly improve any hike. **Enota Mountain Retreat** (706-896-9966; **enota.com**), near Brasstown Bald, is our favorite place for a cabin or camping experience; for something more upscale, try **Brasstown Valley Resort & Spa** in Young Harris (800-201-3205; **brasstownvalley.com**) or **The Ridges Resort & Marina** in Hiawassee (888-834-4409; **theridgesresort.com**).

STONE MOUNTAIN PARK

We have two hikes from this park (770-498-5690; **stonemountainpark.com**) in the book, but you'll find that the fun is practically endless at this destination, from the Summit Skyride to Crossroads, the re-creation of an 1870s Georgia town.

GEORGIA STATE PARKS

One of the best things about Georgia is its park system (800-864-7275; **gastateparks .org**). Within it you'll find a huge array of entertainment, and we don't mean just hiking. From Civil War sites such as **Pickett's Mill** to the highest waterfall in Georgia (**Amicalola**), Georgia's state parks form a nucleus of excellent hiking and other fun pursuits. Other state parks whose hiking trails we've included in the book are **High Falls, Sweetwater,** and **Hard Labor Creek.**

KENNESAW MOUNTAIN NATIONAL BATTLEFIELD PARK AND OTHER CIVIL WAR SITES

When Ulysses S. Grant took over command of the Union Army in 1864, he initiated a coordinated effort to end the Confederacy. While the Army of the Potomac marched against Robert E. Lee and his Army of Northern Virginia, General William Tecumseh Sherman marched against Joe Johnston's Army of Tennessee, which defended Georgia. Sherman engaged the Confederates at Dalton, Resaca, New Hope Church, Pickett's Mill, Dallas, Kolb's Farm, Kennesaw Mountain, Peachtree Creek, Atlanta, Ezra Church, and Jonesboro before claiming the city of Atlanta as "ours, and fairly won." In the middle of these battles, Confederate President Jefferson Davis replaced Johnston with John Bell Hood, a more aggressive but less capable general. Following the loss of Atlanta, Hood moved into North Georgia, where he engaged Union forces at Allatoona Pass before moving north into Tennessee.

Hikes that visit battlefields include **Kolb's Farm Loop, Burnt Hickory Loop,** and **Cheatham Hill Trail,** in Kennesaw Mountain National Battlefield Park (770-427-4686; **nps.gov/kemo**); **Allatoona Pass Trail; Miss Daisy's Atlanta** (Freedom Parkway passes through the site of Confederate and Union lines; the site of Sherman's headquarters during the Battle of Atlanta is at The Carter Presidential Center); and **Pickett's Mill Trail.**

60 HIKES BY CATEGORY

HIKE CATEGORIES

✓ < 3 miles	✓ > 6 miles	✓ urban hike
✓ 3–6 miles	✓ kid-friendly	✓ busy trail

DIFFICULTY: ıll = easy ıIl = moderate ıII = hard

REGION — Hike Number/Hike Name	page	< 3 miles	3–6 miles	> 6 miles	kid-friendly	urban hike	busy trail
ATLANTA							
1 Atlanta Ramble	18		moderate			✓	✓
2 Big Trees Forest Preserve Trail	23	easy			✓		
3 Grant Park Loop (Includes Zoo Atlanta)	27		easy		✓	✓	✓
4 Island Ford Trail	32		moderate*				
5 Johnson Ferry Trail	36	easy					
6 Midtown Romp	40			moderate		✓	
7 Miss Daisy's Atlanta	45			moderate		✓	✓
8 Palisades East Trail	50		moderate				
9 Palisades West Trail	54			moderate			
10 Paper Mill Trail	58		moderate*				
11 Powers Landing Trail	62	moderate*					
12 Reynolds Nature Preserve	66	easy			✓		
13 Silver Comet Trail: Mavell Road to Floyd Road	70		easy	moderate			✓
NORTHWEST OF ATLANTA							
14 Allatoona Pass Trail	76		moderate				
15 Chattahoochee Nature Center Trail	81	easy			✓		
16 Cheatham Hill Trail	85		easy				
17 Heritage Park Trail	90		easy				

Mixed difficulty (for example, mostly easy with moderate sections)

REGION / Hike Number / Hike Name	page	< 3 miles	3–6 miles	> 6 miles	kid-friendly	urban hike	busy trail
NORTHWEST OF ATLANTA (continued)							
18 Iron Hill Loop	94		▪		✓		
19 Kennesaw Mountain: Burnt Hickory Loop	98		▪				✓
20 Kolb's Farm Loop	103		▪				
21 Pickett's Mill Trail	108		▪				
22 Pine Mountain Trail: East Loop	113	▪					
23 Poole's Mill Covered Bridge	116	▪					
24 Rome Heritage Trail	120			▪	✓	✓	
25 Silver Comet Trail: Rockmart	124			▪			
26 Springer Mountain Loop	129		▪				
27 Talking Rock Nature Trail	133	▪					
28 Three Forks Loop	137			▪			
29 Vickery Creek Trail	142			▪			
30 Wildcat Creek Trail	147		▪*				
NORTHEAST OF ATLANTA							
31 Amicalola Falls Loop	152	▪					
32 Big Creek Greenway: North Point	156			▪			
33 Bowmans Island Trail	160	▪					
34 Cook's Greenway Trail	164			▪			
35 DeSoto Falls Trail	169	▪*					
36 East and West Lake Trails	174		▪				
37 Gwinnett Environmental and Heritage Center Trail	179		▪				
38 Hard Labor Creek Trail	183	▪					
39 Indian Seats Trail	187		▪*			✓	
40 Jones Bridge Trail	190		▪				
41 Little Mulberry Trail	195		▪*		✓		
42 McDaniel Farm Park Trail	199		▪		✓		✓
43 Stone Mountain Loop	204		▪				
44 Stone Mountain Walk Up Trail	209	▪					✓

*Mixed difficulty

REGION Hike Number/Hike Name	page	< 3 miles	3–6 miles	> 6 miles	kid-friendly	urban hike	busy trail
NORTHEAST OF ATLANTA (continued)							
45 Suwanee Greenway	214			▁▃▅			✓
46 Tribble Mill Trail	219	▁▃▅			✓		
SOUTH OF ATLANTA							
47 Arabia Mountain Trail	226	▁▃▅			✓	✓	
48 Charlie Elliott Wildlife Center Trails	232	▁▃▅				✓	
49 Cochran Mill Trail	237	▁▃▅					
50 High Falls Trail	241	▁▃▅					
51 McIntosh Reserve Trail	246		▁▃▅				
52 Ocmulgee River Trail	250		▁▃▅				
53 Panola Mountain Trail	254		▁▃▅		✓		
54 Peachtree City Cart Path	258			▁▃▅	✓	✓	
55 Piedmont National Wildlife Refuge Trails	263		▁▃▅		✓		
56 Pine Mountain Trail: Wolfden Loop	268			▁▃▅			✓
57 Sprewell Bluff Trail	273	▁▃▅*					✓
58 Starr's Mill Trail	277	▁▃▅					
59 Sweetwater History (Red) and East Side (Yellow) Trails	281	▁▃▅*					
60 Sweetwater Nongame Wildlife Trails	286	▁▃▅					

Mixed difficulty

60 HIKES BY CATEGORY (CONT'D.)

HIKE CATEGORIES

- ✓ solitude
- ✓ steep terrain
- ✓ waterfalls
- ✓ wildflowers
- ✓ wildlife
- ✓ historical trail
- ✓ scenic hike

REGION Hike Number/Hike Name		page	solitude	steep terrain	waterfalls	wildflowers	wildlife	historical trail	scenic hike
ATLANTA									
1	Atlanta Ramble	18							
2	Big Trees Forest Preserve Trail	23							
3	Grant Park Loop (includes Zoo Atlanta)	27							
4	Island Ford Trail	32							
5	Johnson Ferry Trail	36							
6	Midtown Romp	40				✓			
7	Miss Daisy's Atlanta	45						✓	
8	Palisades East Trail	50							✓
9	Palisades West Trail	54		✓					
10	Paper Mill Trail	58						✓	
11	Powers Landing Trail	62							
12	Reynolds Nature Preserve	66				✓			
13	Silver Comet Trail: Mavell Road to Floyd Road	70							
NORTHWEST OF ATLANTA									
14	Allatoona Pass Trail	76						✓	
15	Chattahoochee Nature Center Trail	81				✓	✓		
16	Cheatham Hill Trail	85						✓	
17	Heritage Park Trail	90						✓	

REGION Hike Number/Hike Name	page	solitude	steep terrain	waterfalls	wildflowers	wildlife	historical trail	scenic hike
NORTHWEST OF ATLANTA (continued)								
18 Iron Hill Loop	94						✓	
19 Kennesaw Mountain: Burnt Hickory Loop	98	✓					✓	✓
20 Kolb's Farm Loop	103						✓	
21 Pickett's Mill Trail	108						✓	
22 Pine Mountain Trail: East Loop	113	✓						
23 Poole's Mill Covered Bridge	116						✓	
24 Rome Heritage Trail	120						✓	
25 Silver Comet Trail: Rockmart	124						✓	
26 Springer Mountain Loop	129	✓						✓
27 Talking Rock Nature Trail	133		✓					✓
28 Three Forks Loop	137	✓						
29 Vickery Creek Trail	142						✓	
30 Wildcat Creek Trail	147	✓		✓				
NORTHEAST OF ATLANTA								
31 Amicalola Falls Loop	152		✓	✓				✓
32 Big Creek Greenway: North Point	156							
33 Bowmans Island Trail	160							
34 Cook's Greenway Trail	164					✓		
35 DeSoto Falls Trail	169			✓				
36 East and West Lake Trails	174		✓					
37 Gwinnett Environmental and Heritage Center Trail	179						✓	
38 Hard Labor Creek Trail	183	✓						
39 Indian Seats Trail	187		✓					✓
40 Jones Bridge Trail	190						✓	
41 Little Mulberry Trail	195			✓				✓

REGION Hike Number/Hike Name	page	solitude	steep terrain	waterfalls	wildflowers	wildlife	historical trail	scenic hike
NORTHEAST OF ATLANTA *(continued)*								
42 McDaniel Farm Park Trail	199				✓		✓	
43 Stone Mountain Loop	204						✓	✓
44 Stone Mountain Walk Up Trail	209	✓					✓	✓
45 Suwanee Greenway	214							
46 Tribble Mill Trail	219							
SOUTH OF ATLANTA								
47 Arabia Mountain Trail	226				✓			
48 Charlie Elliott Wildlife Center Trails	232	✓		✓	✓	✓		
49 Cochran Mill Trail	237			✓			✓	
50 High Falls Trail	241			✓				
51 McIntosh Reserve Trail	246						✓	
52 Ocmulgee River Trail	250	✓						
53 Panola Mountain Trail	254							
54 Peachtree City Cart Path	258							
55 Piedmont National Wildlife Refuge Trails	263	✓			✓	✓		
56 Pine Mountain Trail: Wolfden Loop	268			✓				✓
57 Sprewell Bluff Trail	273	✓						✓
58 Starr's Mill Trail	277						✓	
59 Sweetwater History (Red) and East Side (Yellow) Trails	281			✓		✓	✓	
60 Sweetwater Nongame Wildlife Trails	286			✓		✓		✓

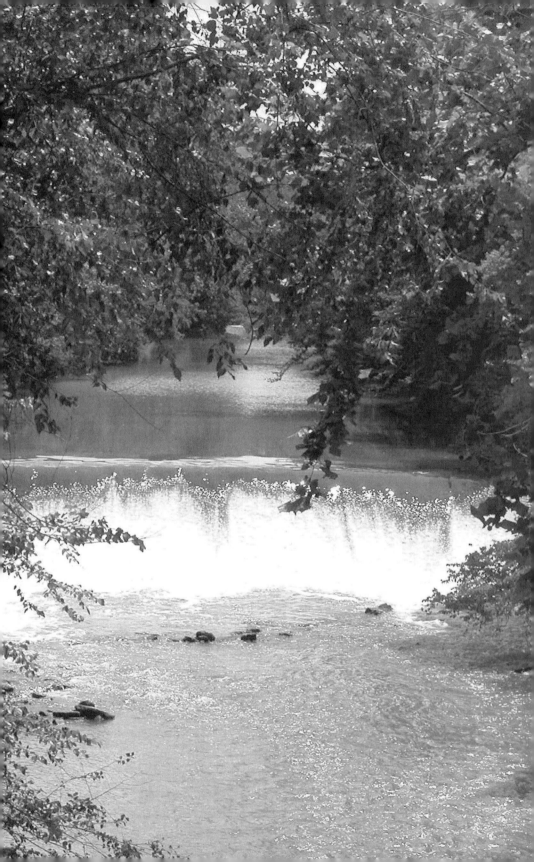

INTRODUCTION

HOW TO USE THIS GUIDEBOOK

OVERVIEW MAP, MAP KEY, AND MAP LEGEND

The overview map on the inside front cover shows the primary trailheads for all 60 hikes. The numbers on the overview map pair with the key on the facing page. A legend explaining the map symbols used throughout the book appears on the inside back cover.

REGIONAL MAPS

The book is divided into regions, and prefacing each regional section is an overview map. The regional maps provide more detail than the overview map, bringing you closer to the hikes.

TRAIL MAPS

In addition to the overview map on the inside cover, a detailed map of each hike's route appears with its profile. On each of these maps, symbols indicate the trailhead, the complete route, significant features, facilities, and topographic landmarks such as creeks, overlooks, and peaks.

To produce the highly accurate maps in this book, we used a handheld GPS unit to gather data while hiking each route, then sent that data to Menasha Ridge Press's expert cartographers. Be aware, though, that your GPS device is no substitute for sound, sensible navigation that takes into account the conditions that you observe while hiking.

Further, despite the high quality of the maps in this guidebook, we strongly recommend that you always carry an additional map, such as the ones noted in "Maps" in each hike's Key At-a-Glance Information.

ELEVATION PROFILES

Each hike contains a detailed elevation profile that corresponds directly to the trail map. This graphical element provides a quick look at the trail from the side, enabling you to visualize how the trail rises and falls. On the diagram's vertical axis, or height scale, the number of feet indicated between each tick mark lets you visualize the climb. To avoid making flat hikes look steep and steep hikes appear flat, varying height scales provide an accurate image of each hike's climbing challenge.

GPS INFORMATION

As noted in "Trail Maps," on the previous page, we used a handheld GPS unit to obtain geographic data and sent the information to the cartographers at Menasha Ridge. Provided for each hike profile, the GPS coordinates—the intersection of latitude (north) and longitude (west)—will orient you from the trailhead. In some cases, you can drive within viewing distance of a trailhead. Other hiking routes require a short walk to the trailhead from a parking area. As a complementary aid to navigation, we've also provided street addresses where available.

The latitude–longitude grid system is likely quite familiar to you, but here's a refresher, pertinent to visualizing the coordinates:

Imaginary lines of latitude—called *parallels* and approximately 69 miles apart from each other—run horizontally around the globe. The equator is established to be 0°, and each parallel is indicated by degrees from the equator: up to 90°N at the North Pole, and down to 90°S at the South Pole.

Imaginary lines of longitude—called *meridians*—run perpendicular to lines of latitude and are likewise indicated by degrees. Starting from 0° at the Prime Meridian in Greenwich, England, they continue to the east and west until they meet 180° later at the International Date Line in the Pacific Ocean. At the equator, longitude lines also are approximately 69 miles apart, but that distance narrows as the meridians converge toward the North and South Poles.

In this book, latitude and longitude are expressed in degree–decimal minute format. For example, the coordinates for Hike 1, Atlanta Ramble (page 18), are as follows:

N33° 44.227' W84° 23.441'

To convert GPS coordinates given in degrees, minutes, and seconds to degrees and decimal minutes, divide the seconds by 60. For more on GPS technology, visit **usgs.gov**.

HIKE PROFILES

Each hike contains seven key items: an In Brief description of the trail, a Key At-a-Glance Information box, directions to the trail, GPS coordinates, a trail map, an elevation profile, and a trail description; many hikes also include notes on things to see and do nearby. Combined, the maps and information provide a clear method to assess each trail from the comfort of your favorite reading chair.

IN BRIEF

A taste of the trail. Think of this section as a snapshot focused on the historic landmarks, beautiful vistas, and other sights you may encounter on the hike.

KEY AT-A-GLANCE INFORMATION

This gives you a quick idea of the statistics and specifics of each hike:

LENGTH How long the trail is from start to finish. There may be options to shorten or extend the hikes, but the mileage corresponds to the described hike. Use the Description as a guide to customizing the hike for your ability or time constraints.

CONFIGURATION A description of what the trail might look like from overhead. Trails can be loops, balloons, out-and-backs (trails on which one enters and leaves along the same path), point-to-points, figure eights, or a combination of shapes.

DIFFICULTY The degree of effort an average hiker should expect on a given hike. For simplicity, the trails are rated as *easy, moderate,* or *hard.*

SCENERY A short summary of the hike's attractions and what to expect in terms of plant life, wildlife, natural wonders, and historical features.

EXPOSURE A quick check of how much sun you can expect on your shoulders during the hike.

TRAFFIC Indicates how busy the trail might be on an average day. Trail traffic, of course, varies from day to day and season to season. Weekend days typically see the most visitors. Multiuse trails are also noted and can include bikes, skaters, and/or horses. Horses hooves can impact trail surfaces, especially in heavy-use areas or under wet conditions, so if the trail can be used by horses, we make a note of it.

TRAIL SURFACE Indicates whether the path is paved, rocky, gravel, dirt, board-walk, or a mixture of elements.

WHEELCHAIR ACCESS Notes whether the trail described (or trails nearby) can be used by persons with disabilities.

HIKING TIME How long it takes to hike the trail. A slow but steady hiker will average 2–3 miles an hour, depending on the terrain.

ACCESS Tells you when the trail is open, as well as any required fees or permits.

MAPS Resources for maps, in addition to those in this guidebook, are listed here. As noted earlier, we recommend that you carry more than one map—and that you consult those maps before you hit the trail in order to resolve any confusion or discrepancy.

MORE INFO Listed here are phone numbers and/or websites for checking trail conditions and gleaning other basic information.

FACILITIES Includes restrooms, phones, water, picnic tables, and other basics at or near the trailhead.

SPECIAL COMMENTS These may include insider information or special considerations about the trail, access, warnings, or ideas for enhancing your hiking experience.

DISTANCE These hikes lie within a circle with a radius of 60 miles—or 60 miles as the crow flies—extending from either the Georgia State Capitol, in downtown Atlanta, or from the I-285 beltway, known locally as the Perimeter. We say "as the crow flies" because we humans are limited to driving along established roads, which means travel distances sometimes exceed 60 miles. For this reason, we provide distances in miles from a fixed location. For trails inside the Perimeter, these distances are measured from the capitol; for trails outside the Perimeter, they're measured from a point on I-285. We used mapping software to determine the most efficient directions for each hike.

DIRECTIONS

Used in conjunction with the overview map, the driving directions will help you locate each trailhead from nearby interstate highway exits. Once you arrive at the trailhead, park only in designated areas.

GPS INFORMATION

Trailhead coordinates and/or street addresses can be used in addition to the driving directions if you enter the data into your GPS unit before you set out. See page 2 for more information.

DESCRIPTION

The heart of each hike. Here, we summarize the trail's essence and highlight any special traits the hike has to offer. The route is clearly outlined, including any landmarks, side trips, and possible alternate routes along the way. Ultimately, the Description will help you choose which hikes are best for you.

NEARBY ACTIVITIES

Look here for information on appealing attractions in the vicinity of the trail—parks, historic sites, museums, restaurants, and the like. Note that not every hike has a listing.

WEATHER

One of Atlanta's best-kept secrets is its weather. During the winter, warm days and cool evenings are the norm, although there are usually at least a couple of cold spells, rarely lasting more than two or three days. As the mercury slides up the thermometer in summer, average temperatures spend two months near the 90°F mark, which is when many hikers head for North Georgia, where temps can average 3°–5°F less. Extremes aside, summer and winter are full of mild days that provide excellent opportunities for hiking. For those who like to watch leaves change, flowers bloom, and birds migrate, spring and fall are prime times for a ramble.

Although the seasons provide a bounty of possible weather conditions, you'll sometimes encounter major variations within the regions in this book. When local forecasters talk about "a wedge of [cooler/warmer/drier] air," they're referring to a phenomenon created by the unique geography of the area. The Blue Ridge Mountains and the Atlantic Ocean create a weather system between them that frequently extends past the city to the Alabama–Georgia border. This phenomenon is most noticeable when the air in Georgia is drier than the air in Alabama and a rain shower evaporates as it reaches the state line.

With all these variations in Atlanta weather, the word to remember is *adaptability*. If you want to hike all year, it helps to have apparel that's appropriate for a range of conditions. Especially in winter and early spring, consider bringing an extra layer of clothing. Even on a warm spring or fall day, a trip to the mountains may require a light windbreaker. Adaptability, however, isn't just a question of wearing sandals or snowshoes, hiking shorts or insulated pants—it's also an attitude. Being adaptable means thinking less about how the weather ought to be and thinking more about ways to find pleasure in a variety of conditions.

AVERAGE TEMPERATURES BY MONTH: ATLANTA					
	JAN	FEB	MAR	APR	MAY	JUN
HIGH	52°	57°	65°	73°	80°	86°
LOW	34°	38°	44°	52°	60°	68°
	JUL	AUG	SEP	OCT	NOV	DEC
HIGH	89°	88°	82°	73°	64°	54°
LOW	71°	71°	65°	54°	45°	37°

WATER

How much is enough? Well, one simple physiological fact should convince you to err on the side of excess when deciding how much water to pack: a hiker walking steadily in 90° heat needs about 10 quarts of fluid per day—that's 2.5 gallons. A good rule of thumb is to hydrate prior to your hike, carry (and drink) 6 ounces of water for every mile you plan to hike, and hydrate again after the hike. For most people, the pleasures of hiking make carrying water a relatively minor price to pay to remain safe and healthy, so pack more water than you anticipate needing, even for short hikes.

If you find yourself tempted to drink "found water," proceed with extreme caution. Many ponds and lakes you'll encounter are fairly stagnant, and the water tastes terrible. Drinking such water presents inherent risks for thirsty trekkers. Giardia parasites contaminate many water sources and cause the absolutely awful intestinal ailment giardiasis, which can last for weeks after onset. For more information, visit the Centers for Disease Control and Prevention website: **cdc.gov/parasites/giardia.**

Effective treatment is essential before you use any water source found along the trail. Boiling water for 2–3 minutes is always a safe measure for camping, but day hikers can consider iodine tablets, approved chemical mixes, filtration units rated for giardia, and ultraviolet filtration. Some of these methods (for example, filtration with an added carbon filter) remove bad tastes typical in stagnant water, while others add their own taste. Even if you've brought your own water, consider bringing along a means of water purification in case you've underestimated your consumption needs.

CLOTHING

The most important thing to remember is that you want to be comfortable on the trail, and being comfortable means keeping cool in summer and warm in winter. For warmer weather, **Under Armour** (888-727-6687; **underarmour.com**) makes T-shirts that wick moisture away from your skin, helping you stay cool and dry; its shorts are popular for their loose, comfortable fit. If you'll be hiking in the grasslands or woodlands, a pair of hiking pants will help protect your legs from the ticks and snakes commonly found in these areas. At many outdoors shops you can find lightweight, quick-drying, UV-protective pants that will keep you suitably cool. Consider a pair that converts into shorts so you can unzip them when you're done with the trail.

Hiking in cooler weather brings its own set of problems, because even though it might be cold out, you'll find yourself sweating after a little exertion. Layering is a good solution, and an important part of staying comfortable. Wear an Under Armour winter T-shirt as a base—again, for the incredible wicking—and top it with a lightweight fleece or sweater. (Cotton not only hangs on to sweat but can even lead to hypothermia if the temperature drops quickly.) In winter, add an outer jacket. More than likely you'll find yourself taking off and putting on layers throughout the hike.

You'll need a good pair of hiking shoes year-round. Day hikers are a great choice for most Atlanta-area trails. They come in both low-top and high-top styles, are lightweight, and have good tread and support. Workout shoes are fine for paved trails but aren't the best choice for dirt paths. A hat, essential at any time of year, not only keeps the Georgia sun from burning your face but also doubles as protection against insects and low-hanging limbs. Another useful item is a rain jacket that can be compressed small enough to stuff in your pack—if you get caught in the rain, you'll be thankful for it.

THE 10 ESSENTIALS

One of the first rules of hiking is to be prepared for anything. The simplest way to be prepared is to carry the 10 essentials. In addition to carrying the items listed below, you need to know how to use them, especially navigation items. Always consider worst-case scenarios such as getting lost, hiking back in the dark, broken gear (for example, a broken hip strap on your pack or a water filter that gets plugged), twisting an ankle, or a brutal thunderstorm. The listed items don't cost a lot of money, don't take up much room in a pack, and don't weigh much—but they might just save your life.

EXTRA FOOD: trail mix, granola bars, or other high-energy snacks.

EXTRA CLOTHES: raingear, a change of socks, and depending on the season, a warm hat and gloves.

FLASHLIGHT OR HEADLAMP with extra bulb and batteries.

INSECT REPELLENT: For some areas and seasons, this is vital.

MAPS AND A HIGH-QUALITY COMPASS: Don't leave home without them, even if you know the terrain well from previous hikes. As previously noted, bring maps in addition to those in this guidebook, and consult them before you hike. If you're GPS-savvy, bring that device too, but don't rely on it as your sole navigational tool—battery life is limited, after all—and be sure to check its accuracy against that of your maps and compass.

POCKETKNIFE AND/OR MULTITOOL.

SUN PROTECTION: Sunglasses, lip balm, sunscreen (check the expiration date), and sun hat.

WATER: Again, bring more than you think you'll drink. Depending on your destination, you may want to bring a container and iodine or a filter for purifying water in case you run out.

WHISTLE: It could become your best friend in an emergency.

WINDPROOF MATCHES AND/OR A LIGHTER, as well as a fire starter.

FIRST-AID KIT

In addition to the preceding items, those that follow may seem daunting to carry along for a day hike. But any paramedic will tell you that the products listed here are just the basics. The reality of hiking is that you can be out for a week of backpacking and acquire only a mosquito bite. Or you can hike for an hour, slip, and suffer a cut or broken bone. Fortunately, the items listed pack into a very small space. Convenient prepackaged kits are available at your pharmacy or online.

Ace bandages or Spenco joint wraps

Adhesive bandages

Antibiotic ointment (such as Neosporin)

Aspirin, acetaminophen (Tylenol), or ibuprofen (Advil)

Athletic tape

Blister kit (such as Moleskin or Spenco 2nd Skin)

Butterfly-closure bandages

Diphenhydramine (Benadryl), in case of allergic reactions

Epinephrine in a prefilled syringe (EpiPen), typically available by prescription only, for people known to have severe allergic reactions to hiking mishaps such as bee stings

Gauze (one roll and a half-dozen 4-by-4-inch pads)

Hydrogen peroxide or iodine

HIKING WITH CHILDREN

No one is too young for a hike in the outdoors. Be mindful, though. Flat, short, and shaded trails are best with an infant. Toddlers who haven't quite mastered walking can still tag along, riding on an adult's back in a child carrier. Use common sense to judge a youngster's capacity to hike a particular trail, and be ready for the child to tire quickly and need to be carried.

When packing for the hike, remember the child's needs as well as your own. Make sure children are adequately clothed for the weather, have proper shoes, and are protected from the sun with sunscreen. Kids dehydrate quickly, so make sure you have plenty of fluids for everyone. Hikes suitable for children are noted in the chart on pages xiv–xvi.

GENERAL SAFETY

While many folks hit the trail full of enthusiasm and energy, others may find themselves feeling apprehensive about potential outdoor hazards. Although potentially dangerous situations can occur anywhere, your hike can be as safe and enjoyable as you hoped, as long as you use sound judgment and prepare yourself before hitting the trail. Here are a few tips to make your trip safer and easier:

- Hike with a buddy. Not only is there safety in numbers, but a hiking companion can help you if you twist an ankle on the trail or if you get lost, can assist in carrying food and water, and can be a partner in discovery. A buddy is good to bring along not only to infrequently traveled or remote areas but also to urban areas.

- If you're hiking alone, leave your hiking itinerary with someone you trust, and let him or her know when you return.

- If you plan to hike in a state or national park, forest, or wildlife-management area, check to see if there will be hunting going on. If so, outfit everyone in your group in hunter's orange—pets included.

- Sign in and out of any trail registers provided. Comment on the trail condition if space is provided; that's your opportunity to alert others to any problems you encounter.

- Don't count on a mobile phone for your safety. Reception may be spotty or nonexistent on the trail, even on an urban walk—especially one embraced by towering trees.

- Always carry food and water, even on short hikes. Food will give you energy, help keep you warm, and sustain you in an emergency until help arrives. Bring more water than you think you'll need—we can't emphasize this enough. Georgia heat and humidity can be brutal, and a little exertion can quickly have you sweating. Hydrate throughout your hike and at regular intervals; don't wait until you feel thirsty. Treat water from a stream or other source before drinking it.

- Ask questions. Public-land employees are on hand to help. It's a lot easier to solicit advice before a problem occurs, and it will help you avoid a mishap away from civilization when it's too late to amend an error.

- Stay on designated trails. Most hikers get lost when they leave the path. Even on the most clearly marked trails, you usually reach a point where you have to stop and consider the direction in which to head. If you become disoriented, don't panic. As soon as you think you may be off-track, stop, assess your current direction, and then retrace your steps back to the point where you went awry. Using a map, a compass, and this book—and keeping in mind what you've passed thus far—reorient yourself and trust your judgment about which way to continue. If you become absolutely unsure of how to continue, return to your vehicle the way you came in. Should you become completely lost and have no idea how to return to the trailhead, remaining in place along the trail and waiting for help is most often the best option for adults and always the best option for children.

- Always carry a whistle. It may become a lifesaver if you get lost or hurt.

- Be especially careful when crossing streams. Whether you are fording the stream or crossing on a log, make every step count. If you have any doubt about maintaining your balance on a foot log, go ahead and ford the stream instead. When fording a stream, use a trekking pole or stout stick for balance and *face upstream as you cross.* If a stream seems too deep to ford, turn back. Whatever is on the other side isn't worth risking your life for.

- Be careful at overlooks. While these areas may provide spectacular views, they are potentially hazardous. Stay back from the edge of outcrops, and be absolutely sure of your footing.

- Standing dead trees and storm-damaged living trees pose a hazard to hikers and tent campers. These trees may have loose or broken limbs that could fall at any time. When choosing a spot to rest, camp, or snack, *look up.*

- Know the symptoms of heat exhaustion, or hyperthermia. Light-headedness and loss of energy are the first two indicators. If you feel these symptoms coming on, find some shade, drink your water, remove as many layers of clothing as practical, and stay put until you cool down. Marching through heat exhaustion leads to heatstroke—which can be deadly. If you should be sweating and you're not, that's the signature warning sign. If you or a companion reaches this point, your hike is over: do whatever you can to cool down, and seek medical help immediately.

- Likewise, know the symptoms of subnormal body temperature, or hypothermia. Shivering and forgetfulness are the two most common indicators of this stealthy killer. Hypothermia can occur at any elevation, even in the summer—especially if you're wearing lightweight cotton clothing. If symptoms develop, get to shelter, hot liquids, and dry clothes ASAP.

- Most important, take along your brain. A cool, calculating mind is the single most important asset on the trail. Think before you act. Watch your step. Plan ahead. Avoiding accidents before they happen is the best way to ensure a rewarding and relaxing hike.

ANIMAL AND PLANT HAZARDS

Hikers should be aware of the following concerns regarding plant life and wild-life, described in alphabetical order.

MOSQUITOES In Atlanta the summer months bring mosquitoes, and with them the highest risk periods for West Nile virus. These pests are especially prolific on trails with tall grasses, in marshy or swampy areas, and at sunrise and sunset. Culex mosquitoes, the primary variety that transmits the virus to humans, thrive in urban rather than natural areas. They lay their eggs in stagnant water and can breed in any standing water that remains for more than five days. Thankfully, contracting West Nile from a mosquito bite isn't a common occurrence. Among those who do get infected, most people have no symptoms of illness, although some may become ill 3–15 days after being bitten.

Any time you expect mosquitoes to be buzzing around, wear loose-fitting, light-colored pants and long-sleeved shirts, and wear socks with your shoes. Spray clothing with insect repellent, or check outdoor retailers for clothes that come preinfused with repellent. According to the U.S. Centers for Disease Control and Prevention, repellents containing the active ingredients DEET or picaridin offer the best protection; follow the instructions on the container, and take extra care with children. Oil of lemon eucalyptus is an effective natural alternative.

POISON IVY, OAK, AND SUMAC Recognizing and avoiding poison ivy, oak, and sumac are the most effective ways to prevent the painful, itchy rashes associated with these plants. Poison ivy occurs as a vine or ground cover, three leaflets to a leaf; poison oak occurs as either a vine or shrub, also with three leaflets; and poison sumac flourishes in swampland, each leaf having 7–13 leaflets. Urushiol, the oil in the sap of these plants, is responsible for the rash. Within 14 hours of exposure, raised lines and/or blisters will appear on your skin, accompanied by a terrible itch. Try to refrain from scratching, though, because bacteria under your fingernails can cause an infection. Wash and dry the affected area thoroughly, applying cala-mine lotion to help dry out the rash. If the itching or blistering is severe, seek medical attention. To keep from spreading the misery to someone else, wash not only any exposed parts of your body but also any oil-contaminated clothes, hiking gear, and pets. Again, long pants and a long-sleeved shirt may offer the best protection.

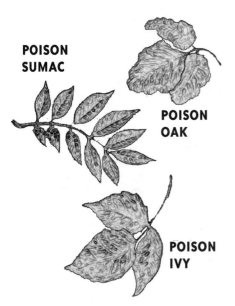

POISON
SUMAC

POISON
OAK

POISON
IVY

SNAKES Spend some time hiking in Atlanta, and you may be surprised by the variety of snakes in the area. Most encounters will be with nonvenomous species, such as Eastern garter and king snakes. Atlanta does have its share of venomous snakes, but the only ones we've seen on the trail are the diamondback rattlesnake and the copperhead. Coral snakes are surprisingly common in lakes, though sightings of this smaller rattler are rare. You might spend a few minutes studying snakes before heading into the woods, but a good rule of thumb is to give whatever animal you encounter a wide berth and leave it alone.

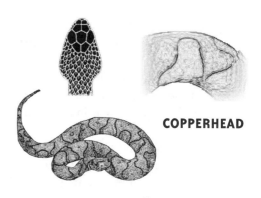

COPPERHEAD

TICKS These arachnids are often found on brush and tall grass, where they seem to be waiting to hitch a ride on warm-blooded passersby. They become more common in the warm spring in the Atlanta area, and are a problem throughout the summer. Their numbers dwindle in the fall, but in Atlanta it's possible to get infected with a tick-borne disease any month of the year. Among the local varieties of ticks, the ones that carry diseases are the American dog tick, the Lone Star tick, and the black-legged (deer) tick. Deer ticks are the primary carriers of Lyme disease; other kinds carry Rocky Mountain spotted fever and tick-related monocytic ehrlichiosis. All ticks need to attach for several hours before they can transmit disease.

A few precautions: Use insect repellent that contains DEET. Wear light-colored clothing, which will make it easy for you to spot ticks before they migrate to your skin. When your hike is done, inspect your hair, the back of your neck, your armpits, and your socks. During your posthike shower, take a moment to do a more complete body check. To remove a tick that is already embedded, use tweezers made especially for this purpose. Treat the bite with disinfectant solution.

TOPOGRAPHIC MAPS

The maps in this book have been produced with great care and, used with the hiking directions, will direct you to the trail and help you stay on course. However, you'll find superior detail and valuable information in the U.S. Geological Survey's 7.5-minute-series topographic maps. One well-known free topo service on the Web is **Microsoft Research Maps (msrmaps.com)**, which also offers satellite imagery. Online services such as **Trails.com** charge annual fees for additional features such as shaded relief, which makes the topography stand out more. If you expect to print out many topo maps each year, it might be worth paying for such extras. The downside to USGS maps is that most are outdated, having been created 20–30 years ago; nevertheless, they provide excellent topographic detail.

Digital programs such as DeLorme's **Topo North America** enable you to review topo maps on your computer. Data gathered while hiking with a GPS unit can be downloaded into the software, letting you plot your own hikes. Of course, **Google Earth** (**earth.google.com**) does away with topo maps and their inaccuracies . . . replacing them with satellite imagery and its inaccuracies. Regardless, what one lacks, the other augments. Google Earth is an excellent tool whether you have difficulty with topos or not.

If you're new to hiking, you might be wondering, "What's a topographic map?" In short, a topo indicates not only linear distance but elevation as well, using contour lines. These lines spread across the map like dozens of intricate spiderwebs. Each line represents a particular elevation, and at the base of each topo a contour's interval designation is given. If the contour interval is 20 feet, then the distance between each contour line is 20 feet. Follow five contour lines up on the same map, and the elevation has increased by 100 feet.

Let's assume that the 7.5-minute-series topo reads "contour interval 40 feet," that the short trail we'll be hiking is 2 inches in length on the map, and that it crosses five contour lines from beginning to end. What do we know? Well, because the linear scale of this series is 2,000 feet to the inch (roughly 2.75 inches representing 1 mile), we know that our trail is about 0.75 mile long (2 inches equals 4,000 feet). But we also know that we'll be climbing or descending 200 vertical feet (five contour lines are 40 feet each) over that distance. And the elevation designations written on occasional contour lines will tell us if we're heading up or down.

In addition to the outdoors shops listed in Appendix A, you'll find topos at major universities and some public libraries. If you want your own and can't find them locally, visit **nationalmap.gov** or **store.usgs.gov**.

BACKCOUNTRY-CAMPING ADVICE

Backcountry, or primitive, camping is available in Chattahoochee National Forest and in many state parks and wildlife-management areas. Always practice low-impact camping: adhere to the adages "Pack it in; pack it out," and "Take only pictures; leave only footprints." **Leave No Trace** ethics make hiking and camping more fun for others (see **lnt.org** for more information).

Some backcountry sites are also public game areas. As we've recommended earlier, find out whether it's hunting season before you set out, and wear hunter's orange during these periods.

Bury solid human waste in a hole at least 3 inches deep and at least 200 feet away from trails and water sources; a trowel is basic backpacking equipment.

Rules about open fires vary depending on where you go, so check before your visit; when collecting firewood, you may be required to collect downed wood instead of chopping branches. In addition, Georgia State Parks allow fires only in fire rings, fireplaces, and campsite grills. Burn bans, especially during drought periods, can restrict fires—including those at campsite grills. Double-check before your trip, because a state park may or may not be affected by a countywide burn ban.

If you plan on fishing, you'll need a license. You can get one online (**georgia wildlife.com/licenses-permits-passes**), by phone (800-366-2661), or from outdoor retailers, sporting-goods stores, and bait-and-tackle shops.

Following the guidelines above will help ensure a pleasant, safe, and low-impact interaction between you and the rest of nature. Regulations can change over time, so contact the appropriate park office before you enter the backcountry.

TRAIL ETIQUETTE

Whether you're hiking in a city, county, state, or national park, always remember that great care and resources (from nature as well as from your tax dollars) have gone into creating these spaces. Treat the trail, wildlife, and fellow hikers with respect.

- **HIKE ON OPEN TRAILS ONLY.** Respect trail and road closures (ask if you're not sure), avoid possible trespassing on private land, and obtain all permits and authorization as required. Also, leave gates as you found them or as marked.

- **BE SENSITIVE TO THE GROUND BENEATH YOU.** This also means staying on the existing trail and not blazing any new trails. Pack out what you pack in. No one likes to see the trash that someone else has left behind.

- **NEVER SPOOK ANIMALS.** An unannounced approach, a sudden movement, or a loud noise can startle them. A surprised animal can be dangerous to you, others, and itself. Give animals plenty of space.

- **PLAN AHEAD.** Know your equipment, your ability, and the area in which you are hiking—and prepare accordingly. Be self-sufficient at all times; carry necessary supplies for changes in weather or other conditions. Get online or on the phone to check things such as park hours, trail closings, and hunting seasons. A well-executed trip is a satisfaction to you and to others.

- **BE COURTEOUS TO OTHER HIKERS, BIKERS, EQUESTRIANS, AND OTHERS** you encounter on the trails. Hikers and bikers should yield to equestrians, bikers should yield to hikers, and, whenever safe, everyone should yield to uphill hikers, bikers, or equestrians. In the last case, it's very helpful to move off-trail to the downhill side and greet the equestrian. This helps the horse understand that you aren't a threat.

TIPS FOR ENJOYING ATLANTA HIKES

If you plan to hike in a state park or national forest, visit its website for information that will familiarize you with your destination's roads, features, and attractions. General and detailed maps of specific wilderness areas are often available online or at a park office (check "Maps" and "More Info" in Key At-a-Glance Information). In addition, the tips on the next page will make your visit enjoyable and rewarding:

- Hike smart when it's hot outside. If there's a hike that you just don't want to miss out on in the dead of summer, do it early in the morning—at dawn, temperatures will likely be 10°–20°F cooler than they'll be later in the day. And there's no better way to start your day than by listening to the cheerful singing of birds as you hike.

- Take your time on the trail. Atlanta is filled with wonders both big, such as Amicalola Falls, and small, such as an antebellum shed now used as a garage. Don't rush past a tiny lizard to get to that overlook. Pace yourself. Stop and smell the wildflowers. Peer into a clear creek for minnows. Don't miss the trees for the forest. Shorter hikes allow you to stop and linger more than long hikes do. Something about staring at the front end of a 10-mile trek naturally pushes you to speed up. That said, take close notice of the elevation profiles that accompany each hike. If you see lots of ups and downs, you'll obviously need more time. Inevitably, you'll finish some of the hikes long before (or after) the estimated hiking time. Nevertheless, leave yourself plenty of time for those moments when you simply feel like stopping and taking it all in.

- Time your hike to avoid crowds. We can't always schedule time off when we want it, but try to hike during the week and avoid the traditional holidays, if possible. Trails that are packed in the spring and fall are often clear during the hotter or colder months. If you're hiking on a busy day, go early in the morning; it will enhance your chances of seeing wildlife. The trails really clear out during rainy times (of course, you shouldn't hike during a thunderstorm). After a heavy rain, hike a trail with a waterfall to enjoy the rushing water at full volume.

- Investigate different areas around Atlanta. The scenery you'll find hiking through meadows and grasslands is pleasantly different from that in the riparian forest along a fork of the Chattahoochee River, and different still from lakeside views. Sample a few hikes in each area to see what it has to offer and what appeals most to you.

- Hike during different seasons. Trails change dramatically from spring to winter, sometimes transforming themselves into something you might not even recognize. If you've found a trail you particularly liked—or didn't—try it at another time of year.

- Hike a loop trail backward for a different perspective. Watch for scenic views that may not have been obvious when you hiked the path as outlined in this book. Be aware, though, that the hike can be harder.

Right: The Illinois Monument, honoring a Union brigade from Illinois that perished in the Battle of Cheatham Hill, was the first Civil War memorial built in Kennesaw Mountain National Battlefield Park. *(See Hike 16, Cheatham Hill Trail, page 85.)*

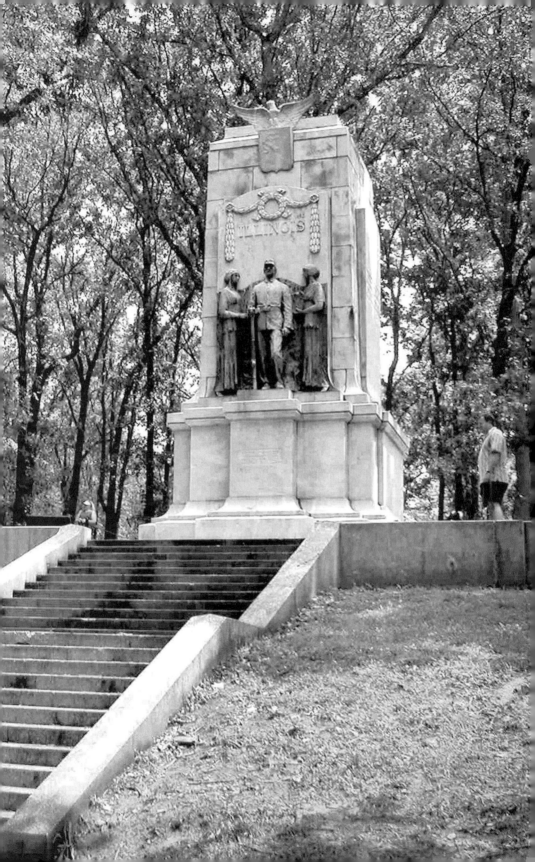

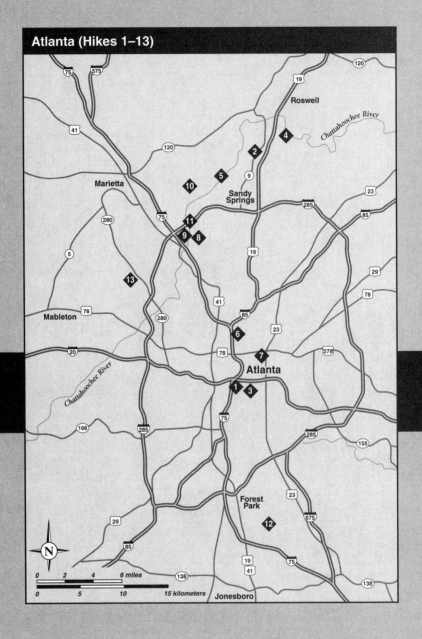

Atlanta (Hikes 1–13)

ATLANTA

1 ATLANTA RAMBLE

KEY AT-A-GLANCE INFORMATION

LENGTH: 5.4 miles

CONFIGURATION: Loop

DIFFICULTY: Easy

SCENERY: Urban scenes, including high-rise buildings

EXPOSURE: Full sun

TRAFFIC: Heavy

TRAIL SURFACE: Concrete sidewalks

WHEELCHAIR ACCESS: Yes

HIKING TIME: 5 hours

ACCESS: Daily, year-round, 24/7 (but see Special Comments); see Description for access to specific attractions.

MAPS: Atlanta Convention and Visitors Bureau; Metro Atlanta Chamber of Commerce; USGS *Northwest Atlanta, Southwest Atlanta*

MORE INFO: 404-521-6600; atlanta.net

FACILITIES: Restrooms, water, and other facilities plentiful throughout the hike

SPECIAL COMMENTS: We recommend walking this route during daylight hours.

DISTANCE: 0.4 mile from the state capitol

GPS INFORMATION

N33° 44.227' W84° 23.441'

755 Hank Aaron Dr. SE
Atlanta, GA 30315

IN BRIEF

From Turner Field, this hike visits the Georgia State Capitol, Underground Atlanta, the Georgia Dome, Philips Arena, CNN Center, Centennial Park, the Georgia Aquarium, and the World of Coca-Cola.

DESCRIPTION

This hike begins in the parking lot opposite **Turner Field,** at the site of the original Atlanta–Fulton County Stadium. From the parking lot, you have a great view of downtown Atlanta and the Olympic flame. Turner Field was built to house the Olympics and then converted to a baseball field to replace the aging Atlanta–Fulton County Stadium. A bronze statue and a plaque commemorate the most historic moment that occurred at the original structure: Henry "Hank" Aaron's 715th home run, which he hit on April 6, 1974, breaking Babe Ruth's long-standing record.

Turn around, cross Georgia Avenue, and enter Turner Field at the black iron gates. Purchase tickets for the stadium tour at **tinyurl .com/bravestours** or at the box office, and view the Braves Museum and Hall of Fame before the tour. In addition to a World Series trophy, the museum has a railroad car that the Braves used in the 1950s and a display on the various fields in which the Braves have played. The tour visits the Braves dugout and bull pen

---

Directions

Take I-75/I-85 South to Exit 246/Fulton Street. At the end of the ramp, turn left on Fulton Street SW. Drive 0.3 mile and turn right on Capitol Avenue SE. Drive 0.4 mile and turn right on Georgia Avenue SE. Enter the Green lot for Turner Field, on the right.

Atlanta Ramble

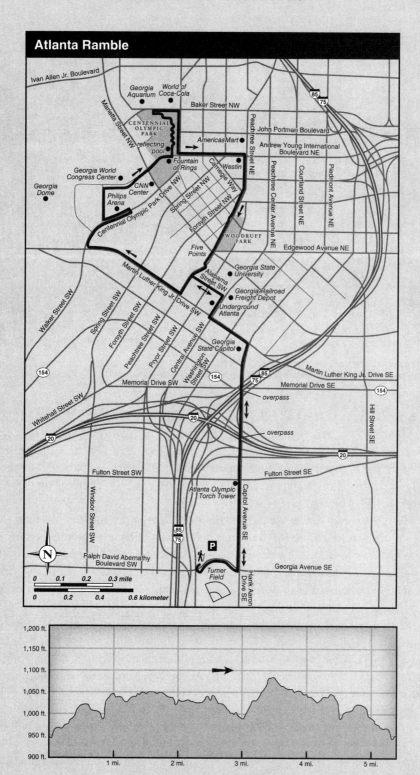

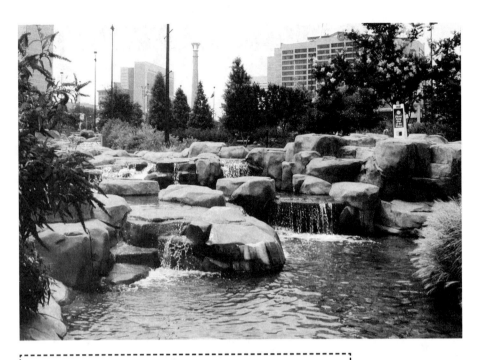

The serene Water Gardens are our favorite part of Centennial Olympic Park.

before taking you to the ball field and then into the locker room. Off-season hours are Monday–Saturday, 10 a.m.–2 p.m. Beginning April 1, tours take place Monday–Saturday, 9 a.m.–3 p.m. and Sunday, 1–3 p.m. Tours are not available on days when the Braves have an afternoon home game. Tours start on the hour, last about an hour, and are not offered on Martin Luther King Jr. Day, Thanksgiving Day, or December 23–January 1.

When exiting Turner Field, turn right on Georgia Avenue SE and then turn left on Hank Aaron Drive SE, crossing under the Olympic rings and passing the flame on your left. At 0.9 mile, the **Georgia State Capitol** (206 Washington St. SW; 404-656-2846; **libs.uga.edu/capitolmuseum**) is on the left. Open Monday–Friday, 8 a.m.–5 p.m. (closed state holidays), the building houses a large number of displays about the cultural and natural history of Georgia, including the state's role in the civil-rights movement. On the grounds are statues of well-known Georgia politicians, including Jimmy Carter, Richard B. Russell, and John B. Gordon, among others. After looping around the grounds, return to Martin Luther King Jr. Drive SW, cross the street, and turn left. At the corner of MLK and Washington Street SW, note the statue honoring the working dogs whose heroism saved many lives during the terrorist attacks on the World Trade Center in New York City. After crossing Central Avenue SW, you'll see the old World of Coca-Cola building on the right, marking the start of Underground Atlanta.

As you leave the area, look across an open area for a mural of whales. Below that is the **1869 Georgia Railroad Freight Depot**, now an upscale event facility. When this depot was completed, it was the tallest building in Atlanta, but a 1935 fire destroyed the second floor. Turn left just before the depot to enter Underground Atlanta.

A potpourri of shops, restaurants, and nightclubs, the three-level **Underground Atlanta** (404-523-2311; **underground-atlanta.com**) is a vast subterranean city within a city. Directly in front of you are an information kiosk and many restaurants. Underground was created at the start of the 20th century, by which time the population of Atlanta had soared to 200,000 people. Crossing the tracks through downtown had become a major traffic snarl, so the government added an iron bridge to speed up traffic. In 1929 the iron bridge was converted to a concrete viaduct, and businesses moved their storefronts to the second story of the buildings.

At the end of the food court, turn left and take the escalator to Kenny's Alley. Turn left again and stroll down Upper Alabama Street SW to Peachtree Street SW, just south of Five Points. Turn left on Peachtree and then right on MLK Drive, and walk 0.4 mile to Centennial Olympic Park Drive NW. Directly in front of you is the white-roofed, red-sided **Georgia Dome,** home of the Atlanta Falcons (1 Georgia Dome Dr. NW; 404-223-9200; **gadome.com**). Turn right on Centennial Olympic Park Drive and continue past the MARTA station until you're standing directly in front of **Philips Arena** (1 Philips Dr.; 404-878-3000; **philipsarena.com**). Home to the NBA Atlanta Hawks and the WNBA Atlanta Dream, Philips is also a popular concert venue. Note the word ATLANTA spelled in white letters in the front of the building. Turn around and walk back to the first road on the right, and turn right.

At the end of this road is one of the three massive buildings that comprise the **Georgia World Congress Center** (285 Andrew Young International Blvd. NW; 404-223-4000; **gwcc.com**). Built on the site of Atlanta's old railroad roundhouse, which was burned during the Civil War, the Congress Center is home to hundreds of industry shows a year. This area was heavily damaged in a 2008 tornado. Turn right and continue down Andrew Young International Boulevard NW, passing **CNN Center** on your right and the **Omni Hotel** and the **Atlanta Chamber of Commerce** on your left.

You're now in the center of Atlanta's **Centennial Olympic Park** (265 Park Ave. West NW; 404-222-7275; **centennialpark.com**). Designed by EDAW and built by Beers Construction and H. J. Russell & Company, the park features the Fountain of Rings, the Great Lawn, Water Gardens, and five unique "quilt plazas" telling the story of the Atlanta Olympics; the Quilt of Remembrance commemorates the 2 people who died and the 118 who were injured when the park was bombed during the 1996 Summer Games. After viewing the Fountain of Rings on the right, turn left and walk to the reflecting pool. With the pool on your immediate left, you'll see a trail almost directly in front of you. This leads to the Water Gardens, our favorite part of the park. Follow the path 0.1 mile to reach the Georgia Agricultural Plaza on Baker Street NW. The **Georgia Aquarium,** the world's largest, opened in November 2005 (225 Baker St. NW; hours and ticket info: 404-581-4000 or geor§iaaquarium.or§). Within the aquarium are nine areas: Cold Water Quest, Georgia Explorer, Ocean Voyager, River Scout, Tropical Diver, Dolphin Tales, Frogs—A Chorus of Colors, the 4D Theater, and Marineland.

The **World of Coca-Cola,** next to the aquarium, is a multimedia presentation designed to both educate and fascinate (121 Baker St. NW; hours and ticket info: 800-676-2653 or 404-676-5151; **worldofcoca-cola.com**). Exhibiting early print ads, modern TV commercials, and everything in between, the displays take you through the development of Coca-Cola's image and products. Turn right on Baker, right again on Centennial Olympic Park Drive, and then left on Andrew Young International Boulevard. On the left is **AmericasMart Atlanta,** one of the largest wholesale markets in the United States (240 Peachtree St. NW; 404-220-3000; **americasmart.com**). On your right, at 210 Peachtree St. NW, is the impressive 73-story **Westin Peachtree Plaza,** a fixture of the Atlanta skyline and home of the most exciting elevator ride in the southeastern United States (404-659-1400; **westinpeachtreeplazaatlanta.com**). The elevator climbs the outside of the building, affording a complete view of the city. At the top, the Sun Dial Restaurant makes a complete revolution every hour.

Turn right (south) on **Peachtree Street,** Atlanta's most famous thoroughfare. When the Fulton County Library comes into view just south of Carnegie Way NE, you'll be entering the oldest part of Atlanta, the **Fairlie-Poplar Historic District.** It was here that the first residential homes were constructed, to be replaced by commercial structures after the Civil War. Today the district is an amalgam of old and new buildings blending together almost seamlessly. Continuing south on Peachtree, you'll see **Woodruff Park** on the left (91 Peachtree St. NE). Watch for the **Coca-Cola Spectacular** sign, atop the Olympia Building (23 Peachtree St. NE), followed by **Five Points,** created by the intersection of Peachtree, Marietta, and Decatur Streets and Edgewood Avenue. (The "fifth point," Whitehall Street, was renamed as an extension of Peachtree.) Continue south on Peachtree two more blocks and turn left into Underground Atlanta. From this point, retrace your steps to Turner Field.

NEARBY ACTIVITIES

Fittingly situated on Auburn Avenue, the center of segregated Atlanta's black business district, the **APEX Museum** (135 Auburn Ave. NE; 404-523-2739; **apex museum.org**) explores the cultural and historical impact of African Americans on Atlanta, the state of Georgia, and the nation. Two blocks past Carnegie Way, turn left on Auburn Avenue NE; the museum is two blocks down, on your right. Open Tuesday–Saturday, 10 a.m.–5 p.m.; $6 adults, $5 students and seniors age 55 and older, free for kids age 3 and younger and museum members.

BIG TREES FOREST PRESERVE TRAIL

IN BRIEF

Big Trees has multiple loops and straight-line trails that can be combined for a wide variety of hikes. A 300-foot climb on the Backcountry Trail is so well done that it seems effortless.

DESCRIPTION

The John Ripley Forbes Big Trees Forest Preserve was created and is managed by the Southeast Land Preservation Trust in partnership with both Fulton County and the state of Georgia, both of which technically own the land. At 30 acres, it is one of the largest undeveloped tracts in the city of Sandy Springs, north of Atlanta. It's named in honor of John Ripley Forbes, a naturalist who worked extensively with local governments nationwide to preserve land. Forbes's legacy in Atlanta includes both the Fernbank Museum of Natural History (see Hike 7, page 45) and the Chattahoochee Nature Center (see Hike 15, page 81).

From the trailhead, the paved path begins an easy descent into the Powers Branch watershed. Immediately visible to the right is the pre-1902 roadbed of Roswell Road, a major Atlanta-area road that permitted area mills access to the railhead in Atlanta and served every town north of the Chattahoochee. The Big Trees Loop splits at a marked intersection

KEY AT-A-GLANCE INFORMATION

LENGTH: 1.2 miles

CONFIGURATION: Loop

DIFFICULTY: Easy

SCENERY: Streamside and watershed views of Powers Branch

EXPOSURE: Mostly shaded

TRAFFIC: Moderate

TRAIL SURFACE: Packed dirt

WHEELCHAIR ACCESS: None

HIKING TIME: 45 minutes

ACCESS: Daily, year-round, sunrise–sunset; free

MAPS: Available at stand at trailhead (look for a stapled multipage handout—the map is on the last page); USGS *Chamblee*

MORE INFO: bigtreesforest.com

FACILITIES: None

SPECIAL COMMENTS: The Big Trees Forest Preserve parking area can be crowded because it also serves as the parking lot for the North Fulton Government Service Center. Dogs must be leashed at all times and cleaned up after—these rules are strictly enforced. The "Nature Trail Guide," available online and at the information box near the entrance, provides a self-guided watershed-education tour describing human impact on water quality and the forest community.

DISTANCE: 5.2 miles from I-285 at GA 400

Directions

Take GA 400/US 19 North (a toll road within the Perimeter) to Exit 5B/Sandy Springs, and merge onto Abernathy Road NW. Drive 1.3 miles and turn right on Roswell Road NE. Drive 2.2 miles and turn right into the North Fulton Government Service Center parking lot. Look for the trailhead at the south end of the parking lot.

GPS INFORMATION

N33° 57.870' W84° 21.780'

7741 Roswell Rd. NE
Sandy Springs, GA 30350

Big Trees Forest Preserve Trail

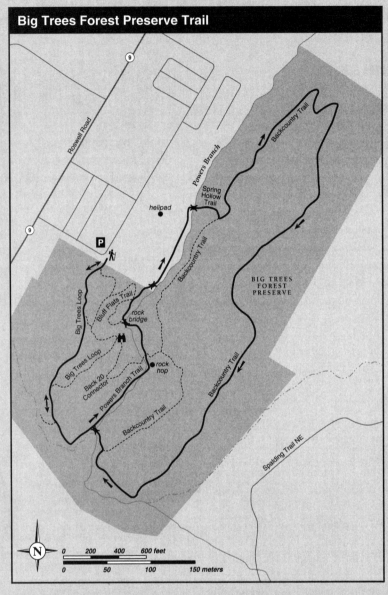

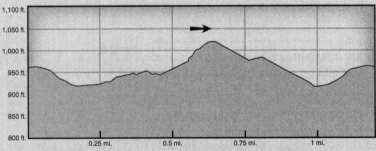

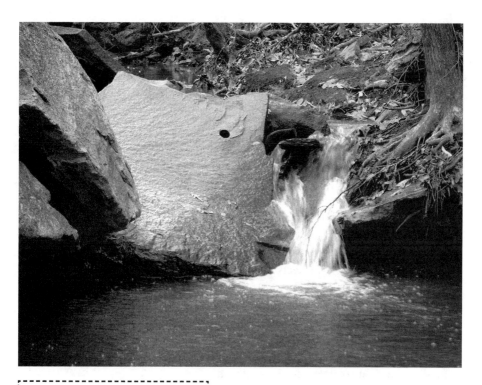

Stones form a cascade on Big Trees Loop.

directly ahead. Continue straight on the chip-covered path lined by a split rail fence as the paved trail bears left. As it descends, Big Trees Loop almost impercep-tibly joins the old roadbed.

Bear right on Powers Branch Trail at 0.1 mile as the Big Trees Loop continues around to the left. As you descend to the creek, Beech Hollow Trail heads right, quickly falling to a loop around a massive American beech. At the bottom is a scenic side view of the creek, near the culvert that carries the stream under present-day Roswell Road. There are tree-stump seats, if you want to spend a few minutes in quiet reflection. As you return to Powers Branch Trail, turn right and descend to a 90-degree left turn as the pathway joins Powers Branch. Continue straight where the Backcountry Connector heads right a few steps after the turn.

Over the next 0.2 mile, the trail climbs about 100 feet on an easy hike into the Powers Branch Watershed. The path twice crosses the stream: once on a wooden bridge, then on an interesting rock-hop—a planned, raised rock path through the water. The stream runs through a concealed culvert beneath a large rock in the center. Kids will love this.

A little more than 0.5 mile into the hike, the boulders get larger, but even an untrained eye can tell that the formation is unnatural. On your left, an old road grade disappears into the modern embankment of the North Fulton Government Service Center. A small cascade in the river makes a pretty photograph, but the telltale drill hole gives away the secret—the falls are artificial. Just past the falls, Powers Branch Trail ends as Spring Hollow Trail turns right, crosses an unrailed bridge over the creek, and rises to the Backcountry Trail. Make a hard left at the end of the brief Spring Hollow Trail.

The Backcountry Trail continues to climb, paralleling the creek. As apartments come into view straight ahead, look down to the left. The creek is now 60 feet below the footpath. A few steps later the trail begins an easy double switch to climb to its highest point, just a few feet after the second switchback. From this point, the treadway begins an easy descent through a second-growth hardwood forest composed of white and post oaks and American beeches, interspersed with native azaleas.

As the hike approaches 1 mile, the footpath begins an easy curve to the right. At the end of the curve, the path runs adjacent to the grade of the Bull Sluice Railroad, built in 1902 to move material to the site of Morgan Falls Dam, one of the earliest hydroelectric projects in Georgia. After work on the dam was completed, the railbed was abandoned. At 1 mile, a path to the left crosses a bridge and makes a switchback ascent to a patio next to a Ford dealership. A small portion of this path runs on the level grade of the old railroad bed.

Just past this bridge, turn left onto the short Backwoods Connector. Cross a wooden bridge, turn to the left on Powers Branch Trail, and follow the path around to the right to return to the trailhead.

NEARBY ACTIVITIES

Heritage Sandy Springs (404-851-9111; **heritagesandysprings.org**), an interpretive farmhouse and museum, is the site of the five freshwater springs for which the city is named. The park, on 6075 Sandy Springs Circle just off Hammond Drive, is open daily, sunrise–sunset.

GRANT PARK LOOP (INCLUDES ZOO ATLANTA)

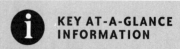

IN BRIEF

Grant Park Loop visits the 1880s-era green space that was the centerpiece of a development of large Victorian homes. The park also houses Zoo Atlanta, whose animals live in near-native habitats.

DESCRIPTION

Each year, more than 2 million people visit Grant Park to see the world-class Zoo Atlanta, view a three-dimensional re-creation of the 1864 Battle of Atlanta, see downtown from a Civil War fort, or just relax in the green space created by Lemuel Grant, for whom the park is named. Grant, who moved to Georgia from Maine in the late 1830s, was one of Atlanta's first residents. He designed a series of defenses around the city that helped the Confederate Army defend the city against a Union onslaught. After the Civil War, Grant played a key role in Atlanta's revitalization. He began work on the park in 1881 and donated it to the city of Atlanta in 1883.

Grant Park (840 Cherokee Ave. SE) has always been open to both black and white visitors, an unusual occurrence in the segregated South. Even the zoo was integrated—sort of (the Atlanta attraction regularly had "black

---

Directions ⟶

Take I-20 East/Ralph David Abernathy Freeway to Exit 59A/Boulevard. At the end of the ramp, turn right on Boulevard SE and drive 0.7 mile to the parking lot, on the right between Confederate and Ormewood Avenues SE. If this parking lot is full, continue south on Boulevard to Atlanta Avenue SE; turn right, right again on Cherokee Avenue SE, and then right a third time, into a second parking lot.

KEY AT-A-GLANCE INFORMATION

LENGTH: 2.4 miles

CONFIGURATION: Loop

DIFFICULTY: Easy

SCENERY: Well-kept historic park with huge trees in a generally upscale downtown area; nationally recognized zoo

EXPOSURE: Partial shade–full sun

TRAFFIC: Heavy, especially in Zoo Atlanta

TRAIL SURFACE: Almost entirely paved

WHEELCHAIR ACCESS: Yes

HIKING TIME: 3.5 hours

ACCESS: Grant Park: daily, year-round, 6 a.m.–11 p.m.; free. See Description for Cyclorama and Zoo Atlanta access.

MAPS: Available at Zoo Atlanta; USGS *Southeast Atlanta*

MORE INFO: Grant Park: 404-546-6813; gpconservancy.org. Atlanta Cyclorama & Civil War Museum: 404-658-7625; atlantacyclorama.org. Zoo Atlanta: 404-624-WILD (9453); zooatlanta.org.

FACILITIES: Restrooms, playgrounds, fast food

SPECIAL COMMENTS: This is an ideal family hike.

DISTANCE: 2.5 miles from the state capitol

GPS INFORMATION

N33° 44.107' W84° 22.170'
Boulevard SE and Ormewood Ave. SE
Atlanta, GA 30308

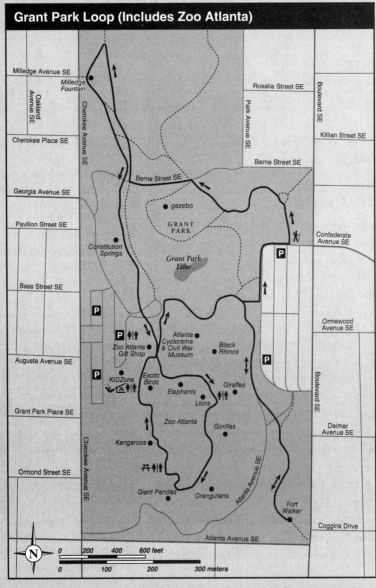

Grant Park Loop (Includes Zoo Atlanta)

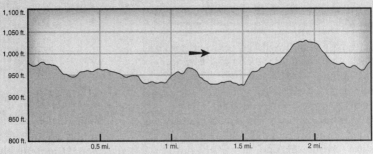

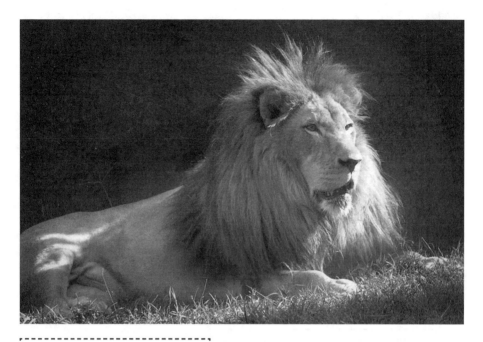

The king of the jungle surveys his domain.

only" days). In 1921 Atlanta added the Cyclorama, a building to house the *Battle of Atlanta* painting. It also moved the Civil War locomotive the *Texas,* which had sat exposed in Grant Park, inside the building.

On a paved road across from the first lane of parking (the lane nearest the entrance), walk through four white posts underneath the spreading crowns of a group of old-growth post oaks. As the paved road begins an easy curve to the left, a side road leaves to the right. The road then curves back to the right as it heads toward a hill with a gazebo on top. Continue to bear right as the road splits in front of the gazebo, and you will reach a five-road intersection. Bear left on a road that descends and then curves right. At 0.3 mile turn right. A few steps down this paved road is a small playground, up on the right. As the road begins to rise, turn right on a paved road; immediately on the left are a massive stone fountain and a park entrance that was added in the early 1900s. Circle the structure, which is being restored by the Grant Park Conservancy, and then make the first left and climb a short way to street level. Two roads enter Grant Park at 45-degree angles from Cherokee Avenue SE, which forms the eastern boundary of the park. This is a popular place to take a picture, but plan to get here later in the day and shoot from the far side of street. Continue circling to the left, descending on the other side of the entrance.

At the end of the road, turn right at the T-intersection and climb to Cherokee Avenue for more views of both Grant Park and the surrounding neighborhood. The area is being rejuvenated thanks to low-interest loans from the city. Turn left and

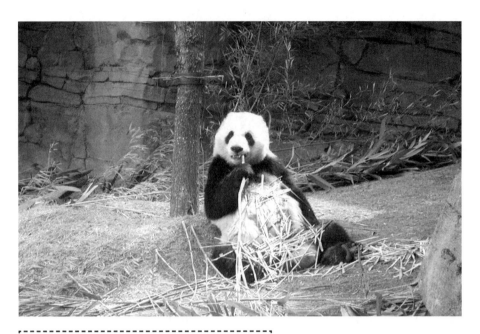

One of Zoo Atlanta's cuddly giant pandas enjoys a snack.

walk on the sidewalk, taking the next left to reenter the park. As this road descends, it curves right, crossing a culvert on a concrete bridge. Just past the bridge is Constitution Spring, which was once one of five mineral springs within the park. A stone bridge sits in a tree-lined open field on the left of the road at 0.8 mile.

The road curves left, coming out at the entrance to **Zoo Atlanta** (800 Cherokee Ave. SE; open daily, 9:30 a.m.–5:30 p.m.; closed Thanksgiving and December 25; $21.99 ages 12–64; $17.99 seniors age 65 and older, military, and college students; $16.99 kids ages 3–11; free for kids age 2 and younger). This nationally recognized zoo allows species to roam freely in specially designed areas intended to mimic the animals' natural habitats. Back in 1984, Atlantans discovered that their Metropolitan Zoo had been named one of the 10 worst in the country. Some spoke of closing it and returning Willie B., a silverback gorilla at the center of the controversy, to his home in Cameroon. Rather than give up, Atlanta hired a new director for the attraction, Terry Maples, who began the arduous task of completely rebuilding the zoo.

Stunning pink flamingos greet visitors just inside the entrance. Close by are elephants, the critically endangered black rhino, and a lion; then it's off to the Ford African Rain Forest. Willie B. died in 2000, but his offspring carry on the strong tradition of the rain forest in Atlanta, where multiple viewing sites allow glimpses into the lives of these stoic creatures. At the end of the rain forest live other animals and reptiles, but follow the path on the left just past a food kiosk to the panda exhibit for a one-of-a-kind treat.

Considered the symbol of peace in its homeland of China, the endangered giant panda was long considered a relative of the raccoon, but DNA testing has proved that it belongs to the bear family. Lun-Lun and Yang-Yang arrived at Zoo Atlanta in November 1999 for a 10-year stay and immediately became stars. The pandas have given birth to three cubs, and their original stay has been extended. A line forms quickly at this exhibit, so plan on a 20- to 30-minute wait.

As you leave, the Panda Veranda is on the left, complete with picnic tables and a McDonald's. If you don't need a break, continue straight ahead to view the zoo's two Sumatran tigers. One of a handful of zoos with a captive-breeding program, Zoo Atlanta is active in the fight to save this nearly extinct species. Fewer than 700 of these big cats are known to exist in the wild or in captivity. As you exit the tiger exhibit, follow the road that bears left toward the Ford Pavilion; then follow the path to the right and make a right into the KIDZone. Immediately after the turn is a marked railroad crossing for a train that young children can ride. Kids can get close to animals in the petting zoo and see kangaroos, but for our favorite exhibit, turn left at Base Camp Discovery and follow the path around to the left. Here, tortoises take their time exploring the habitat created by the zoo. These mammoth prehistoric beasts are fun to watch as they eat, sleep, or walk.

As you leave the KIDZone, turn right; the zoo exit is almost directly in front of you. After you pass through the booths, on your left is the **Atlanta Cyclorama & Civil War Museum** (800 Cherokee Ave. SE). Built in 1921, it houses *The Battle of Atlanta,* a three-dimensional painting in the round, along with a museum featuring the *Texas,* one of the locomotives involved in the Great Locomotive Chase of 1862. Open Tuesday–Saturday, 9:15 a.m.–4:30 p.m.; guided tours every hour on the half hour, except at 12:30 p.m.; $10 ages 13–64, $8 seniors age 65 and older and kids ages 4–12, free for kids age 3 and younger.

After viewing the museum and the painting, exit and turn right. Turn right again on the first concrete path to wind back to the parking lot. Once there, turn right and walk to the southern end of the lot. Follow the road around to the left and then turn right on the paved path at the end of the second lane of parking. This path winds to **Fort Walker,** an earthen outpost along the defenses constructed by Lemuel Grant. This is one of the few remaining intact Civil War sites in the Atlanta metropolitan area. From the top of the hill you'll get a good view of the downtown skyline. Return to the parking lot using the same path you followed to Fort Walker.

4 ISLAND FORD TRAIL

KEY AT-A-GLANCE INFORMATION

LENGTH: 2.9 miles

CONFIGURATION: Loop

DIFFICULTY: Easy, with a couple of moderate climbs into the Chatta-hoochee River watershed

SCENERY: Riverbank views along the Chattahoochee

EXPOSURE: Mostly shaded

TRAFFIC: Moderate

TRAIL SURFACE: Compacted soil

WHEELCHAIR ACCESS: None

HIKING TIME: 1.5 hours

ACCESS: Trail: daily, year-round, sunrise–sunset; headquarters: daily, year-round, 9 a.m.–5 p.m., except December 25; $3 day-use fee

MAPS: Available at visitor center; USGS *Chamblee*

MORE INFO: 678-538-1200; nps.gov/chat

FACILITIES: Restrooms, ball field, some picnic tables, group pavilion

SPECIAL COMMENTS: Headquarters for the Chattahoochee River National Recreation Area are in the former home of Samuel Hewlett, who served on the Supreme Court of Georgia.

DISTANCE: 21.3 miles from the state capitol

GPS INFORMATION

N33° 59.237' W84° 19.552'

1978 Island Ford Pkwy.
Sandy Springs, GA 30350

IN BRIEF

This hike explores the floodplain and water-shed of the Chattahoochee in the vicinity of Island Ford, one of the river's first commonly used fords.

DESCRIPTION

Settlers normally had two options for crossing the Chattahoochee River: they could use one of the many ferries, which cost money, or one of the free fords, where animals, carts, and people made their way across a high, relatively flat area in the river. Fording the river could be a dangerous proposition—high, fast-flowing water could easily drag a cart or person down-stream. Eventually, a ferry did cross the Chat-tahoochee here.

When you visit the river today, it's next to impossible to find the actual location of the ford; the continuous flow requirement of Buford Dam keeps the water high enough to cover most of the rocky ledge that the settlers used. When then-President Jimmy Carter signed the act creating the Chattahoochee River National Recreation Area in 1978, the massive log home of Samuel Hewlett was des-ignated as park headquarters.

Directions ———————————————➤

Take GA 400/US 19 North to Exit 6/Northridge Road. At the end of the ramp, merge onto Northridge Road, cross GA 400, and make an immediate right on Dunwoody Place. Drive 0.6 mile and turn right on Roberts Drive, which crosses back over GA 400. Drive 1.2 miles and turn right at the signed entrance to Island Ford, on Island Ford Parkway. Proceed along the winding drive 1.2 miles to a parking lot at the end of the road.

Island Ford Trail

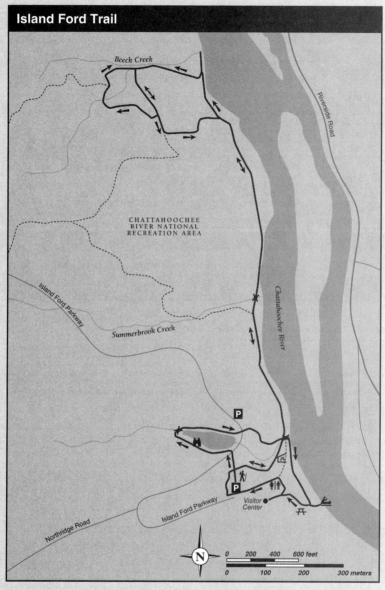

Beech Creek

Riverside Road

CHATTAHOOCHEE
RIVER NATIONAL
RECREATION AREA

Island Ford Parkway

Summerbrook Creek

Chattahoochee River

P

P

Visitor
Center

Island Ford Parkway

Northridge Road

N

| 0 | 200 | 400 | 600 feet |

| 0 | 100 | 200 | 300 meters |

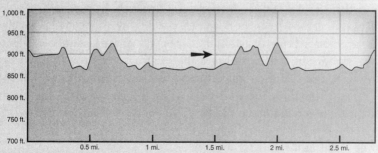

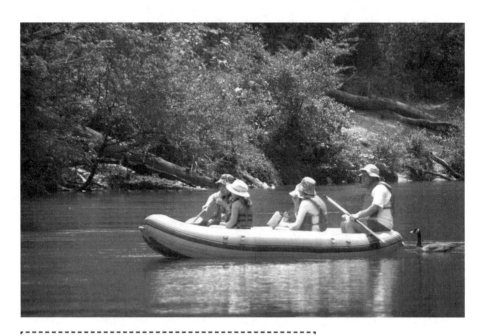

Leisurely float trips are a favorite adventure on the Chattahoochee.

After parking your car, walk to the parking lot on the left as you face Hewlett's home. In the center of the lot, at a brown-roofed information kiosk, is one of the entrances to the Island Ford Trail system. The trail initially falls to a small creek through a mostly pine forest interspersed with oaks. Avoid the side trail that you'll see on the right almost immediately after the start. At 200 feet the trail crosses Island Ford Parkway and then comes to a small pond. Turn left to reach a wooden overlook a few steps away. After enjoying the lakeside view, follow the lakeshore around to the right. Rising to an old dirt road in full sun, the trail reenters the forest at a map stand and easily skirts wetlands at the far end of the pond. Avoid the older trail, which appears to enter the wetland, and take the newer trail that climbs a short hill and then runs level above the pond. Slowly, mature hardwoods replace large pines.

As Island Ford Parkway once again comes into view, watch for a trail on the left before the overlook; this path crosses the paved road. Climb the stairs to a low knoll. This trail quickly leads to the middle parking area, at 0.3 mile. Watch on the right for a red-blazed trail that follows a tributary of the Chattahoochee down to the river's floodplain. About 100 feet after you enter the forest, notice a pretty cascade in the creek on the right. After an easy descent, turn right on the main trail as it meanders along the riverbank. Massive rock outcrops and mature and old-growth trees abound along the banks of the wide, fast-flowing river. When you reach the first outcrop, follow the line into the river; a corresponding shoals churns the water in the Chattahoochee.

The forest opens as you enter a wide expanse of the floodplain that has been converted to Hewlett Field. On the right are picnic tables and a grill. Continue along the river side of the field to a concrete launch and take-out point for kayakers and rafters. Next to the launch is a dock. Turn around and look across Hewlett Field for a sign marking a path to the visitor center. After a thigh-burning climb, follow the trail as it turns left, then right, around the visitor center, returning you to the parking area. Continue past the front of the visitor center, turning right and descending along the same creek as on the descent from the middle parking lot. This time, as you reach the main trunk, turn left and cross a wooden bridge. With the Chattahoochee on your right, the trail follows the river as the hills on either side sometimes narrow the floodplain to a few feet. At 1.2 miles a side trail leaves to the left; soon after, a wooden bridge crosses an active stream. Once you've traversed the bridge, a second trail leaves at a hard left as the main trail bears right. A large rock outcrop lies on the left, with a corresponding shoals in the Chattahoochee on the right. A forest of American beeches and oaks follows as the trail narrows and begins to roll up and down a series of small hills.

As the blue-blazed trail turns inland, a side trail continues along the riverbank down to a deep ravine. Return to the blue trail and turn left. Climbing into the watershed of the Chattahoochee, the trail is easy to moderate. Just before the trail dips to a stream, turn left on a gravel road, which rises to a pathway on the right 0.1 mile later. This trail loops around a forested cove with a stream running through it. At 1.85 miles the trail turns right and descends toward the river. Just before you complete the loop, the trail gets steep for about 25 feet and crosses a creek. Turn right and climb past the trail you just hiked, to a three-way intersection. The red-blazed trail turns right and climbs to Island Ford Parkway. Instead of following that path, bear left on the yellow-blazed trail, which descends into the river valley. Coming out on a low ridge, the trail descends a set of steps back to the river. Turn right to return to your car.

5 JOHNSON FERRY TRAIL

KEY AT-A-GLANCE INFORMATION

LENGTH: 1.9 miles

CONFIGURATION: Balloon

DIFFICULTY: Easy

SCENERY: Long-distance views of the Chattahoochee River and a forested wetland in the river's floodplain

EXPOSURE: Full sun at the start and end of the hike, mostly shaded in between

TRAFFIC: Light

TRAIL SURFACE: Compacted soil

WHEELCHAIR ACCESS: None

HIKING TIME: 1 hour

ACCESS: Trail: daily, year-round, sunrise–sunset; headquarters: daily, year-round, 9 a.m.–5 p.m., except December 25; $3 day-use fee

MAPS: Map stands dot the trail throughout the hike; additional maps available at Island Ford headquarters (see previous hike); USGS *Sandy Springs*

MORE INFO: 678-538-1200; nps.gov/chat

FACILITIES: None

SPECIAL COMMENTS: A National Park Service map indicates—incorrectly—that restrooms are available.

DISTANCE: 19.2 miles from the state capitol

GPS INFORMATION

N33° 56.721' W84° 24.346'

IN BRIEF

This trail explores a floodplain of the Chattahoochee River, including a forested wetland, and then joins the "Hooch" for a hike along its bank.

DESCRIPTION

For more than 20 years, the Chattahoochee Outdoor Center was the summer-fun capital for rafting enthusiasts in Atlanta. Each weekend thousands of people would visit the center, formerly at this hike's trailhead, and take a leisurely float down the Chattahoochee River to one of two take-outs farther south. The center was forced to close in 2002 due to high levels of E. coli (an indication of dangerous pollution) in the river.

From the kiosk at the trailhead, follow the road to descend to a plain that was the parking lot for the outdoor center. The road soon changes from pavement to gravel and continues straight. On your right is the return trail for the loop. Formerly clear of vegetation, the parking lot is in the early stages of natural reclamation. Black-eyed Susans and goldenrods abound in this full-sun portion of the Johnson Ferry Trail. Look for the vestiges

---

Directions ———————————————➤

Take I-285 West to Exit 24/Riverside Drive. At the end of the ramp, turn right. Drive 2.2 miles north on Riverside to Johnson Ferry Road. Turn left at the light and drive 0.2 mile. After you cross the Chattahoochee River, make an immediate right on Columns Drive into the parking lot for the Johnson Ferry North Unit of the CRNRA. Look for a brown kiosk in the center of the north side of the parking lot, opposite the entrance.

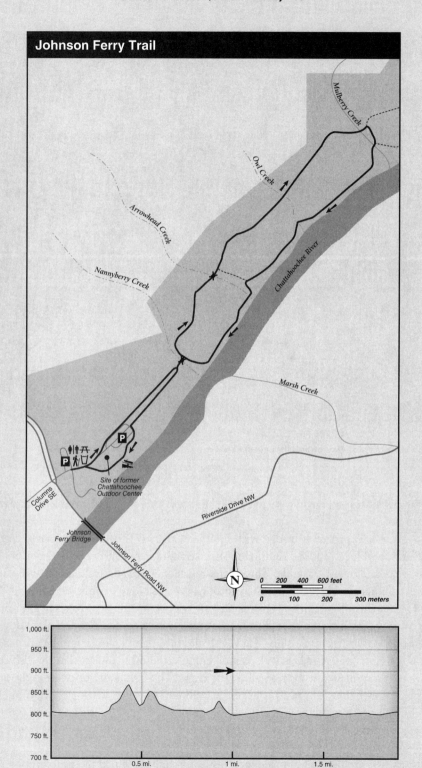

Johnson Ferry Trail

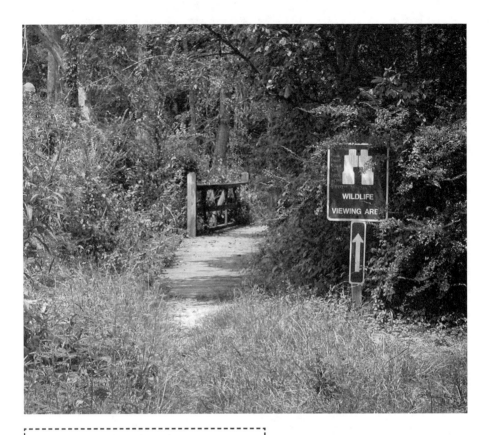

A wildlife-viewing area rewards the patient observer.

of humans—an overgrown picnic table here and there, an old tire, or a decayed exit sign.

As you approach a bridge with a large WILDLIFE VIEWING AREA sign, the parking lot road loops right. Continue straight, crossing the bridge, and make an immediate left at 0.3 mile. Three hundred feet after the turn, a boardwalk first takes you across a stream and then into an up-close view of the wetlands of the Chattahoochee floodplain. Wetlands play an important role in a river's health: during times of high water, they give the river a place to spread out and slow down, reducing downstream erosion. They also provide habitat for a number of small mammals and waterfowl, as well as a breeding ground for insects that the fish eat.

At the end of the boardwalk, turn right. The wetlands, on your right and slightly lower than the trail, continue for about 0.5 mile. They are occasionally visible but are frequently blocked by trees along its edges. On this hike, the forest is made up mostly of white oaks, beeches, and the occasional sycamore tree. The area in and around the wetlands is mostly shaded.

Part of the hike takes place on a historic roadbed, which the trail joins at 0.6 mile, just after you pass two large post oak trees. The wide, nearly level walk is free of traffic noise, and the sounds of nature fill the air: a distant woodpecker tapping a tree in search of food, birds chirping to establish territory, and playful squirrels loudly crunching leaves and sounding like something much bigger.

At 1 mile, the trail turns right. Reaching the bank of the Chattahoochee at 1.2 miles, the pathway makes another hard right, turning to follow the river back to the trailhead. Mostly shaded during this portion of the hike, the Johnson Ferry Trail occasionally breaks into full sun. When the trail runs next to the riverbank, it yields nice long-distance views. You'll also notice a pattern at work: as the trail approaches each of the Chattahoochee's tributaries, it turns right, goes inland about 200 feet to a power-line opening, turns left to cross a bridge, and then turns left again to return to the river. After turning inland the third time, the trail crosses the bridge at the start of the loop, and you are once again in the old Chattahoochee Outdoor Center parking lot.

Continue straight until you see the parking-lot road loop to the left. In the distance, almost straight ahead, is the brown fortlike building that used to house the center. As you approach the building, you'll see a narrow trail to the left at 1.9 miles. This takes you down to a river-access ramp that rafters and kayakers occasionally use. From the ramp, turn around and face the building that formerly housed the outdoor center. Walk up the ramp to the end of the cement, and turn left on a wide trail that swings around to the parking lot. Turn left and climb the paved road to the trailhead kiosk.

6 MIDTOWN ROMP

KEY AT-A-GLANCE INFORMATION

LENGTH: 6.3 miles

CONFIGURATION: Loop

DIFFICULTY: Moderate

SCENERY: Urban landscapes, long-distance views of the city from Piedmont Park and Atlanta Botanical Garden, meadowlike environment in Piedmont Park

EXPOSURE: Full sun

TRAFFIC: Heavy

TRAIL SURFACE: Concrete sidewalks, asphalt pathways, compacted-soil trail in botanical garden

WHEELCHAIR ACCESS: Yes

HIKING TIME: 7 hours

ACCESS: Daily, year-round; see Description for access to specific attractions.

MAPS: USGS *Northeast Atlanta, Northwest Atlanta*

MORE INFO: See Description

FACILITIES: Full facilities at Woodruff Arts Center, High Museum of Art, Margaret Mitchell House, Atlanta Botanical Garden, and Piedmont Park

SPECIAL COMMENTS: Plan this hike around an afternoon show at the Fox Theatre (660 Peachtree St. NE; 404-881-2100; foxtheatre.org), to your left on Peachtree as you return to your car.

DISTANCE: 4 miles from the state capitol

GPS INFORMATION

N33° 47.360' W84° 23.178'

Atlantic Center Plaza: 1215 Spring St. NW
Atlanta, GA 30309

IN BRIEF

This energetic hike takes you through Midtown Atlanta, passing the High Museum of Art, the Woodruff Arts Center, the Atlanta Botanical Garden, Piedmont Park, the Margaret Mitchell House, and Georgia Tech.

DESCRIPTION

The hike begins on Atlanta's first road, **Peachtree Street.** In 1812 Lieutenant George Gilmer left Fort Daniel at Hog Mountain (in present-day Gwinnett County) and began heading south along a low ridge east of the Chattahoochee River, building a road to the site of a Creek village known as Standing Peach Tree. (Some historians believe *peach* is a corruption of *pitch*, as in pine.) When Gilmer arrived, he built Fort Peach Tree, the first building in present-day Atlanta. Over the years, Peachtree Street has been renamed, rerouted, and paved, but it's still very much at the heart of the city.

From the parking area, walk to the corner of Peachtree and 16th Streets NE, and turn right on Peachtree. The **High Museum of Art,** on the right, is one of the best art museums in the southeastern United States (1280 Peachtree St. NE; 404-733-4444; **high.org**). Opened in 1926 in a private home that was donated to the Atlanta Arts Association by

---

Directions ────────────────▶

From I-75 North, take Exit 251A/17th Street. Turn right on 17th Street NW and drive one block to Spring Street NW. Turn left, drive 0.2 mile, and turn left into the Atlantic Center Plaza parking area ($1.25 every 15 minutes, $15 maximum). Walk to 16th and Peachtree Streets NE to begin the hike.

Midtown Romp

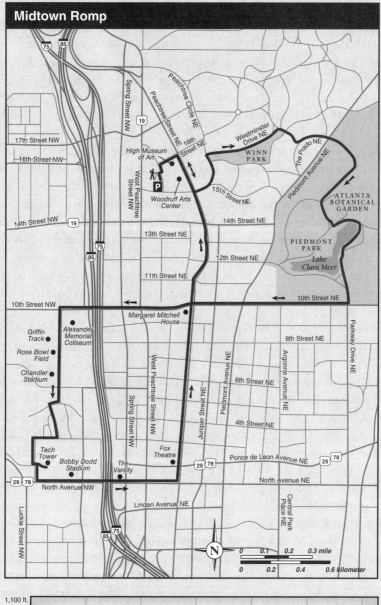

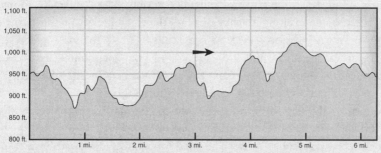

Mrs. Joseph M. High, the museum underwent major expansions in 1955, 1983, and 2005. Today the museum occupies the Meier Building, named for architect Richard Meier, who designed the Atlanta icon; the 2005 expansion, comprising three buildings designed by Renzo Piano, more than doubled its gallery space to nearly 94,000 square feet. The High is open Tuesday, Wednesday, Friday, and Saturday, 10 a.m.–5 p.m.; Thursday, 10 a.m.–8 p.m.; and Sunday, noon–5 p.m.; $19.50 ages 18–64, $18.50 students or seniors age 65 and older, $12 kids ages 6–17, and free for kids age 5 and younger.

Continuing from the High Museum, you'll see Auguste Rodin's sculpture *The Shade* and the impressive **Woodruff Arts Center** (1280 Peachtree St. NE; 404-733-4200; **woodruffcenter.org**). Following a month-long tour of the capital cities of Europe, 122 members of the Atlanta Arts Association were killed when their plane crashed on takeoff from Orly Airport in Paris in 1962. The French government gave the Rodin sculpture to the city of Atlanta in 1968 in memory of those who lost their lives. Today the Woodruff Center houses the Atlanta Symphony Orchestra and the Alliance Theater, respectively, in two buildings: one with a massive metal structure at the entrance and the other, the 14th Street Playhouse, a couple of blocks away.

Cross Peachtree at 15th Street NE to enter the **Ansley Park** neighborhood, developed between 1905 and 1908 by Atlanta businessman Edwin P. Ansley. Turn left on Peachtree Circle NE, walk two short blocks, and turn right on Westminster Drive NE, where you come to the local gem known as **Winn Park** (32 Lafayette Dr. NE). Not even a block wide, it's a focal point of this community. Most days a variety of folks, from young parents to older people, can be found enjoying the park. Playful dogs splash through a small creek, complete with waterfall, that runs lengthwise through the park. Kids will have a blast here, whatever kind of outdoor activity they enjoy. At the end of the park, turn right on The Prado NE, taking the north branch when it splits, and follow it two blocks, crossing Piedmont Avenue NE at a traffic light.

Across Piedmont, at 1.1 miles, is the **Atlanta Botanical Garden** (1345 Piedmont Avenue NE; 404-876-5859; **atlantabotanicalgarden.org**); the road climbs to the entrance. Pay the admission fee and follow the signs to the Dorothy Chapman Fuqua Conservatory and the Fuqua Orchid Center. A variety of exotic plants and animals are housed in the climate-controlled rooms. The Kendeda Canopy Walk takes visitors on an exciting journey through the treetops. Also be sure to visit the Edible Garden. Admission is $18.95 for adults, $12.95 for kids ages 3–12, and free for garden members and kids age 2 and younger. Hours are November–March, Tuesday–Sunday, 9 a.m.–5 p.m.; April–October, Tuesday–Sunday, 9 a.m.–7 p.m. and Thursday, 9 a.m.–10 p.m.; closed major holidays.

Return to the entrance and turn right at the marked entrance to **Piedmont Park** (400 Park Dr. NE; 404-875-7275; **piedmontpark.org**), taking the asphalt path that is closed to vehicular traffic. The road loops around the gardens, coming to the massive stone Millennium Gate on the right, built for the 1895 Piedmont

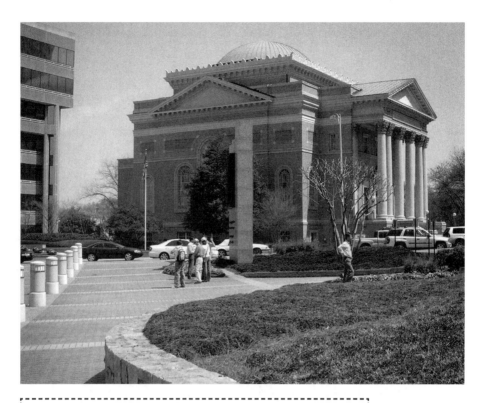

A wide variety of architectural styles are represented in the Arts Center District.

Exhibition, a world's fair–type event. Take the first left, in which direction the path continues as it begins to circle Lake Clara Meer, the park's centerpiece. At 1.7 miles, as the road curves left, look for a small historic grouping of Atlanta's first streetlights (1855) and first street pavement (granite blocks from Stone Mountain). From this triangle, follow the lakeshore as the path curves right, then swings left. As the path bears right at 1.9 miles, a second, straight path branches off, heading straight—follow this to 10th Street NE, and turn right.

Tenth Street begins as a hodgepodge of hotels, businesses, and apartments, but by the time you reach Peachtree Street again, they've been replaced with the massive urban structures typical of cities. After crossing Peachtree at 2.7 miles, you'll see a small, fenced building on the left, looking out of place. This three-story redbrick structure with the white verandas is the apartment building where Margaret Mitchell wrote *Gone with the Wind*. Guided tours take people from the visitor center into the apartment where "Peggy" once sat at a Remington typewriter, weaving many of her personal experiences into a novel about the antebellum South and the changes that the Civil War brought. An informative display on her life and her role in the movement toward integration fill the basement. A museum across the street contains additional information about the book and the movie. The **Margaret Mitchell House** (990 Peachtree St. NE; 404-249-7015;

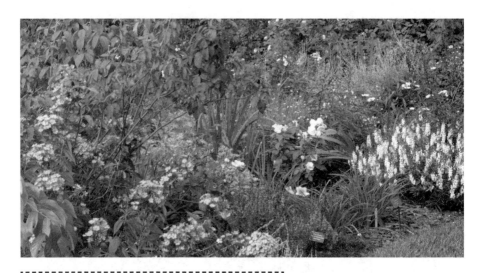

Flowers bloom year-round at the Atlanta Botanical Garden.

margaretmitchellhouse.com) is open daily except January 1, Thanksgiving Day, and December 24 and 25. Tours take place every half hour, 10:30 a.m.–4:30 p.m., 12:30–4:30 p.m. on Sundays; $13 adults, $10 students ages 13–18 and seniors age 65 and older, $8.50 kids ages 4–12.

Continue west on 10th Street NE, crossing I-75/I-85, known locally as the **Downtown Connector.** This high-speed road predates the interstate system—it opened as a limited-access road in 1952, connecting Midtown with the heart of Atlanta. As you leave the bridge, **Alexander Memorial Coliseum** (965 Fowler St. NW), home to **Georgia Tech**'s basketball teams, is on the left. Just past the coliseum, at 3.2 miles, turn left on Fowler Street NW. The Georgia Tech campus is full of life on weekdays but normally calms down on weekends, except when there's a ballgame. Old-growth trees are common, and the campus is an eclectic mix of modern and historic architecture.

Continue south on Fowler to Fourth Street NW, turn right, and then turn left, once again on Fowler Street. At Bobby Dodd Way NW, turn right. Bobby Dodd climbs to Cherry Street NW, where you turn left. Follow Cherry to **Tech Tower,** on the left at the intersection of Cherry Street and Ferst Drive NW. A Georgia Tech landmark, the tower—officially designated as the Lettie Pate Whitehead Evans Administration Building—stands on a portion of the original 4-acre campus. Return to Cherry Street and continue south.

At North Avenue NW, turn left, pass Bobby Dodd Stadium on the left at 4.2 miles, and recross I-75/I-85. On the left, just past the bridge, is an Atlanta dining institution, **The Varsity** (61 North Ave. NE; 404-881-1706; **thevarsity.com**). Known for its unique service ("What'll ya have?") and unique offerings ("Naked Dog Walking"), the restaurant opened its doors in 1928, well before fast food became popular. At Peachtree Street, turn left to return to your car.

MISS DAISY'S ATLANTA 7

IN BRIEF

This hike explores Freedom Park—the largest urban park created in the 20th century—and a series of parks designed by Frederick Law Olmsted for the Druid Hills community in the late 1800s. You'll also visit four major attractions: The King Center, the Fernbank Science Center, the Fernbank Museum of Natural History, and the Jimmy Carter Library and Museum.

DESCRIPTION

Jessica Tandy won the 1989 Best Actress Academy Award for her role as Daisy Werthan, an elderly Druid Hills widow forced to accept an African American (Morgan Freeman) as her chauffeur-helper, in *Driving Miss Daisy*. Based on Alfred Uhry's Pulitzer Prize–winning play, the film depicts the changes that were occurring across Atlanta between 1948 and 1973 as Southern society gradually became integrated. The movie also won the Academy Award for Best Picture of 1989; Freeman was nominated for Best Actor and Dan Aykroyd for Best Supporting Actor.

Begin the hike by crossing the road from the parking lot of **The Carter Presidential Center**—comprising the **Jimmy Carter Library and Museum** and the offices of **The Carter Center**, a

Directions

Take the Downtown Connector (I-75/I-85) to Exit 248C and merge onto Freedom Parkway toward The Carter Presidential Center. Drive 1.3 miles; after you pass under a covered section of the road, Freedom Parkway splits—watch for the brown sign that directs you to bear right for The Carter Presidential Center. Take the first left into The Carter Presidential Center and park in the lot immediately to the right.

KEY AT-A-GLANCE INFORMATION

LENGTH: 9.1 miles round-trip

CONFIGURATION: Double out-and-back

DIFFICULTY: Moderate

SCENERY: Urban parks and skyscrapers; Japanese garden at The Carter Presidential Center

EXPOSURE: Full sun

TRAFFIC: Heavy, except in the Druid Hills portion of the hike

TRAIL SURFACE: Asphalt trail, concrete sidewalk; some compacted dirt in the Druid Hills section of the hike

WHEELCHAIR ACCESS: Yes

HIKING TIME: 7 hours

ACCESS: Daily, year-round; see Description for access to specific attractions.

MAPS: USGS *Northeast Atlanta*

MORE INFO: See Description

FACILITIES: Full facilities at The King Center, the Fernbank Science Center, the Fernbank Museum of Natural History, and the Jimmy Carter Library and Museum

SPECIAL COMMENTS: This hike takes you to the home of the fictional Daisy Werthan, along with the home of playwright-screenwriter Alfred Uhry's real-life grandmother. More important, the hike allows you to reflect on changes that led to integration in the 1960s.

DISTANCE: 2.7 miles from the state capitol

GPS INFORMATION

N33° 45.974' W84° 21.323'

441 Freedom Pkwy.
Atlanta, GA 30307

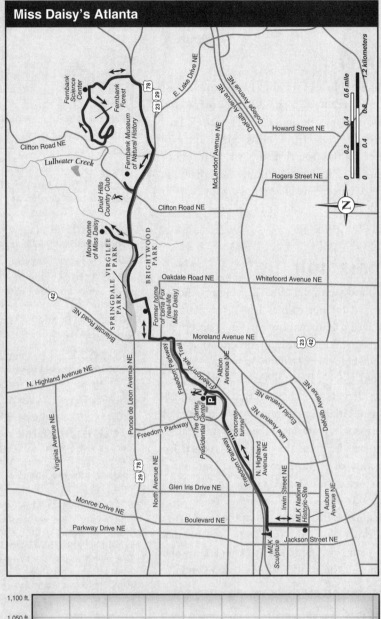

Miss Daisy's Atlanta

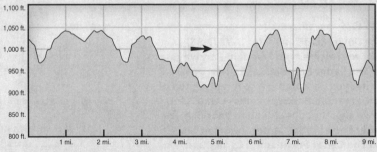

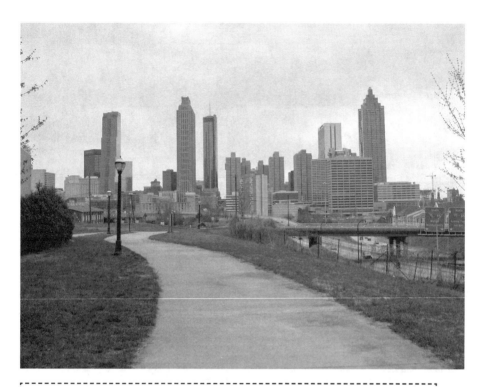

The section of the hike that passes The King Center affords stunning views of the Atlanta skyline.

---

private charitable organization—at the crosswalk to **Freedom Park**. The paved interpretive multiuse trail follows Freedom Parkway and GA 42, which were built on
the right-of-way of a proposed interstate highway that would have connected
downtown Atlanta with Stone Mountain. Despite having purchased the land and
destroying 400 homes, the city, the state, and the federal government were stopped
in their tracks by a group of local residents. The land was subsequently used to
build The Carter Presidential Center, Freedom Parkway, and Freedom Park, a
1.5-mile-long expanse that connects the Carter complex with The King Center and
the Druid Hills neighborhood east of downtown.

Where the Freedom Park Trail crosses Boulevard NE, a black metal sculpture
of the Rev. Dr. Martin Luther King Jr. in silhouette introduces **The King Center**, a
multiblock celebration of the life of the slain civil-rights leader (449 Auburn Ave.
NE; 404-526-8900; **thekingcenter.org**; open daily, 9 a.m.–5 p.m., except major
holidays; free admission). Dr. King was born and grew up in the area known as
Sweet Auburn, the business center of Atlanta's large African American community.
Turn left and walk two blocks south; then turn right on Auburn Avenue NE to
reach the visitor center for the **Martin Luther King, Jr., National Historic Site,** on the
right (404-331-5190; **nps.gov/malu**; hours vary seasonally; free admission). Also in
this multiblock exhibit are Dr. King's grave, his boyhood home, and Ebenezer
Baptist Church. Return to The Carter Presidential Center, but instead of crossing

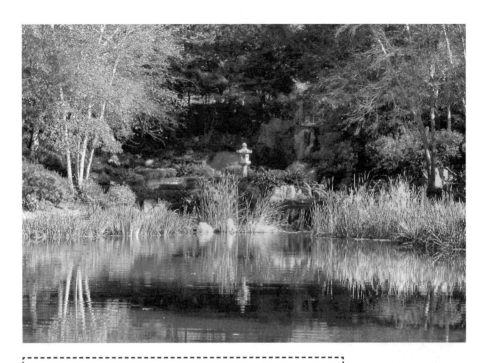

A quiet pond reflects a peaceful garden at The Carter Presidential Center.

back to your car, continue straight to Moreland Avenue NE, where you cross the road at a traffic light and turn left. Walk two blocks, turn right on Fairview Road NE, and watch for **1284 Fairview,** a redbrick Georgian Revival home atop a low ridge on the left. Alfred Uhry based the character of Daisy Werthan on his grandmother, Lena Fox, who once lived at this Druid Hills address.

Continue on to Springdale Road NE and turn left; then make a right at South Ponce de Leon Avenue NE. On your left is **Virgilee Park,** one of five green spaces that Frederick Law Olmsted incorporated into Ponce de Leon, Druid Hills's main thoroughfare (for more information on all five, call 404-377-5361 or visit **atlantaolmsted park.org**). Since the parks' inception, Ponce de Leon has been straightened to improve traffic flow, but the parks are a lasting legacy of Olmsted's vision of picturesque beauty created by combining natural settings with human-made features.

At Oakdale Road NE, Virgilee Park becomes **Brightwood Park,** which ends at Lullwater Road NE. Turn left, cross Ponce de Leon, and turn right, keeping the Druid Hills Country Club on your left. After crossing Clifton Road, you'll see **Deepdene Park** on the left. At the center of the park, a historical marker introduces the only original trolley station remaining in Atlanta, built in 1923.

Take North Ponce de Leon Avenue NE until it dead-ends; turn left and then left again on Artwood Road NE; then turn right on Heaton Park Drive NE. On your left is the **Fernbank Science Center** (156 Heaton Park Dr. NE; 678-874-7102; **fernbank.edu),** which includes Fernbank Forest, a multiacre interpretive Piedmont woodland that gives visitors an idea of what Atlanta was like before it was settled.

Within its gates, an easy 1.1-mile paved loop trail offers a scenic view over the pond. The trail is interpreted, and maps are available at the entrance to the hike. The center's hours vary seasonally; call or check the website for details. Admission is free.

Return to North Ponce de Leon Avenue NE and turn right. Walk to Clifton Road NE and turn right again. On your right is the entrance to the **Fernbank Museum of Natural History** (767 Clifton Rd. NE; hours and admission info: 404-929-6300 or **fernbankmuseum.org**), one of Atlanta's premier family attractions. Inside, dinosaurs greet you in an enormous five-story rotunda. Permanent and special exhibitions adjoin the rotunda on a series of balconies accessed by stairs or an elevator. Among our favorites is "A Walk Through Time in Georgia," which visits each region of the state in five interpretive exhibits and includes a dinosaur gallery of what Georgia might have looked like millions of years ago.

As you leave the Fernbank Museum, turn left, return to Ponce de Leon, and turn right. On your right is the members-only **Druid Hills Golf Club** (740 Clifton Rd. NE). At Lullwater Road, turn right and walk to **822 Lullwater,** a stately brick Tudor that's familiar to movie fans as the *Driving Miss Daisy* house. It's set on a ridge, just as Lena Fox's former home on Fairview is. Turn around and return to Ponce de Leon, crossing at the light, and turn left. Walk two blocks to Moreland Avenue, turn left, and return to The Carter Presidential Center via Freedom Parkway.

Though four presidents—both Roosevelts, Woodrow Wilson, and Jimmy Carter—have close ties to Georgia, only Carter was born here, in the small town of Plains, in the southwestern part of the state. Adjacent to The Carter Center (which is open to the public only by appointment or for special events), the **Jimmy Carter Library and Museum** (441 Freedom Pkwy.; 404-865-7100; **jimmycarterlibrary .gov**) is the first publicly funded presidential library. Inside, a museum follows the life of Carter from his youth to the present day. Open Monday–Saturday, 9 a.m.–4:45 p.m., and Sunday, noon–4:45 p.m.; $8 ages 17–59, $6 students, military, and seniors age 60 and older; free age 16 and younger; closed major holidays.

NEARBY ACTIVITIES

In the warehouse district, near The Carter Presidential Center, **Two Urban Licks** (820 Ralph McGill Blvd. NE; 404-522-4622; **twourbanlicks.com/index-home.htm**) is an upscale Atlanta eatery serving generous portions of "fiery American cooking." Everything we've ever ordered has been exceptional. An important note: They serve dinner only, after 5:30 p.m. From the Carter complex, take the GA 42 West exit. Where Freedom Parkway bears left, continue straight one block and turn right. Follow the signs to the entrance.

8 PALISADES EAST TRAIL

KEY AT-A-GLANCE INFORMATION

LENGTH: 4.75 miles

CONFIGURATION: Loop extended by an out-and-back section along the river north of the Palisades

DIFFICULTY: Moderate

SCENERY: Best long-distance view of the Chattahoochee River in Atlanta

EXPOSURE: Mostly shaded

TRAFFIC: Moderate

TRAIL SURFACE: Compacted soil

WHEELCHAIR ACCESS: None

HIKING TIME: 3 hours

ACCESS: Trail: daily, year-round, sunrise–sunset; headquarters: daily, year-round, 9 a.m.–5 p.m., except December 25; $3 day-use fee

MAPS: At trailhead kiosk and on map stands throughout the park; USGS *Sandy Springs*

MORE INFO: 678-538-1200; nps.gov/chat

FACILITIES: None

SPECIAL COMMENTS: This hike takes in the Fulton County side of Paces Ferry and the remains of an old building at the site of the ferry, along the Chattahoochee River bank.

DISTANCE: 12.9 miles from the state capitol

GPS INFORMATION

N33° 53.274' W84° 26.015'

1425 Indian Trail NW

Sandy Springs, GA 30327

IN BRIEF

This hike follows a ridgetop as it drops to the riverbank at the Whitewater Creek entrance and then easily climbs along the Chattahoochee to East Palisades. The trail leaves the river, climbing to an overlook before returning once again to the riverbank.

DESCRIPTION

From the trailhead kiosk, East Palisades Trail begins an easy descent along a gravel road through a Piedmont hardwood–pine forest. As the ridge ends, the road begins to descend into the river valley. About three-quarters of the way down, the road appears to end—it actually turns right—but our trail continues straight. Watch on the left for Long Island Creek, a large tributary of the Chattahoochee River. As you reach the level floodplain of the Chattahoochee, a side trail on the left that permits river access joins the main trail.

The trail bears right and comes to a second side trail; then you make a wet-footed crossing of a tributary of Long Island Creek. Turn right when the trail reaches an intersection. On the left is the National Park Service bridge to the Whitewater Trail parking area. Spend a few moments looking upstream from the bridge to get a good view of the creek.

Directions ———————————→

Take I-75 North to Exit 256 and turn right on Mt. Paran Road NW. Drive 0.9 mile and turn left on Garmon Road NW. Drive 0.7 mile and, where Garmon Road turns left to become West Garmon Road, continue straight on Northside Drive NW. Drive 0.9 mile and turn left on Indian Trail NW. In 0.4 mile the paved road turns to dirt. Continue another 0.4 mile on the dirt road to the parking area.

Palisades East Trail

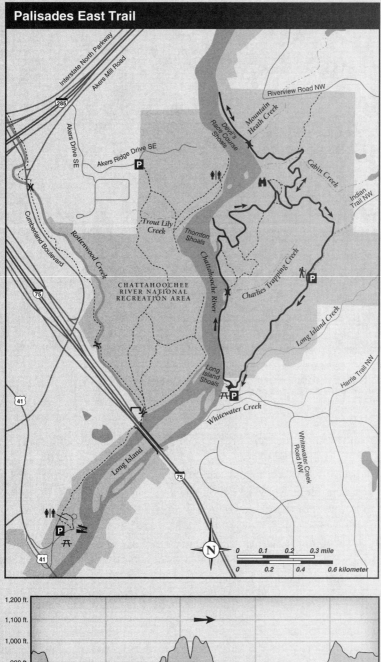

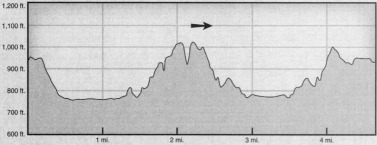

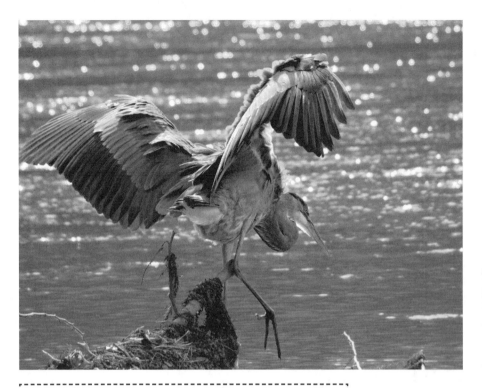

A stately blue heron stalks a meal in the waters of the Chattahoochee River.

As you return to the trail, bear left. The trail curves right and joins the river-bank. Enjoy a good view of the river, including its confluence with Long Island Creek. If you're lucky, you might even glimpse a great blue heron on this section of the trek. Out along Long Island Shoals you may see kayakers in a developed run on this section of the river, and you'll probably see larger waterfowl joining a fisherman or two in a quest for the Chattahoochee's noted marine life.

After Thornton Shoals, at 1 mile into the hike, the footpath turns inland, easily rising to a slightly higher plain before bearing left. At a tributary, the trail bears right and moves inland, coming to a T-intersection at a recently updated map stand. These maps make it possible to vary the hike described here by way of numerous interconnecting short trails. Turn left and continue along the riverbank, approaching the Palisades. Take a few minutes to explore some of the rock grot-toes surrounding the path (the kids will love this) as it ends at 1.3 miles, and then return to the last T-intersection. Turn left and follow the footpath as it begins a moderate-to-difficult climb into the Chattahoochee watershed.

Beginning as a gravel road, the footpath becomes a winding, well-groomed trail as it approaches the top of the ridge. Once at the top, the path curves left, follows the ridgeline out above the Palisades, and then swings back right, ending at a gravel road with a map stand at 1.9 miles. Turn left and follow the road to the second marked intersection; then bear left, descending a set of wooden steps to the East Palisades overlook of Devil's Race Course Shoals. This is the best view of the Chattahoochee River in the Atlanta area. Return to the map stand and turn left.

Watch for a trail almost immediately to the right and turn onto it. It follows the ridge briefly, then turns left at a three-way intersection and begins an extended moderate-to-difficult descent into the river valley. The trail to the right returns you to your car. At 2.4 miles into the hike, the trail curves right and steps over a small rise to a moist, level area replete with ferns and adjacent to a brook. After you step across the brook, the trail again rises, this time to a gravel road. Turning left and recrossing the brook, you'll continue on the roadway to descend to the Chattahoochee. As the road begins to level, it reaches the river's floodplain. On the left, a rock wall encloses a small, square area that once supported a fairly substantial building or bridge.

As you reach the riverbank at 2.7 miles, the trail turns right to follow the river through an area of massive rock outcrops. A few steps later, at a bridge over a small rivulet, is a second cluster of outcrops as massive as the first. This trail continues climbing near the river, past a gravel road on the right and into a bamboo forest. After the trail winds through the large stand, it turns around at 3 miles.

Return to the three-way intersection at the start of the trail's descent into the river valley, but instead of turning, continue straight on the gravel road. This brings you to the gravel road that leads to the parking lot. Turn right and walk 0.3 mile to your car.

NEARBY ACTIVITIES

From the park, take Indian Trail NW back to Northside Drive NW, where you'll turn right. At the intersection with West Garmon Road NW (now on your right), turn left to stay on Northside and follow it 3.1 miles to West Paces Ferry Road NW, where you'll turn left. This takes you through the decidedly wealthy Buckhead neighborhood, which is home to the Georgia governor's mansion. After 1.2 miles, just past Andrews Drive NW, the **Atlanta History Center** is on your right (130 West Paces Ferry Rd. NW; 404-814-4000; **atlantahistorycenter.com**). This museum contains one of the best Civil War exhibits in the nation, along with sections on Atlanta history and golf legend Bobby Jones and a collection of folk art from all over the southeastern United States.

9 PALISADES WEST TRAIL

KEY AT-A-GLANCE INFORMATION

LENGTH: 6.2 miles

CONFIGURATION: Double loop

DIFFICULTY: Moderate

SCENERY: Long-distance winter views, numerous riverside views

EXPOSURE: Full shade on hills, partial shade–full sun along riverbank

TRAFFIC: Heavy along the Chattahoochee, moderate along ridgetop

TRAIL SURFACE: Compacted soil, gravel, short concrete driveway

WHEELCHAIR ACCESS: None

HIKING TIME: 3 hours

ACCESS: Trail: daily, year-round, sunrise–sunset; headquarters: daily, year-round, 9 a.m.–5 p.m., except December 25; $3 day-use fee

MAPS: USGS *Sandy Springs*

MORE INFO: 678-538-1200; nps.gov/chat

FACILITIES: Restrooms at the Paces Mill Entrance and near Akers Mill along the Chattahoochee River

SPECIAL COMMENTS: A helipad was added near the restrooms at the Akers Mill end of the park for medical evacuation. When rafting was more popular on the Chattahoochee, people would often badly injure themselves jumping off nearby Big Rock.

DISTANCE: 12.5 miles from the state capitol

GPS INFORMATION

Akers Drive entrance:
N33° 53.451' W84° 26.901'

Paces Mill entrance:
N33° 52.228' W84° 27.183'

IN BRIEF

The trail follows a high ridge to Rottenwood Creek, where it drops sharply. The footpath explores the riverbank and floodplain of the Chattahoochee near Paces Mill and Akers Mill.

DESCRIPTION

West Palisades connects Akers Mill and Paces Ferry on the west bank of the Chattahoochee River at Devil's Race Course Shoals. Little is known about Akers Mill, but we know quite a bit about John and Hardy Pace. John was a judge, and the first Cobb County election was held in his home. His brother, Hardy, ran the family mill and a nearby ferry. In 1850 the state authorized Hardy to build a dam across the Chattahoochee to impound water to power his mill, and his ferry eventually became both a bridge and a road. Hardy, who died in December 1864, is buried in a private graveyard at the top of Mt. Wilkerson (Vinings Mountain).

Directions ———————————➤

Akers Drive entrance: Take I-75 North to Exit 258/Cumberland Boulevard. Turn right at the end of the ramp, drive 0.5 mile, and turn right on Akers Mill Road. Drive 0.3 mile to Akers Drive SE and turn right at the water mill. Drive 0.2 mile on Akers Drive and turn left at the signed entrance to Palisades West—watch carefully or you'll miss it—and then turn right into the parking lot.

Paces Mill entrance: Turn left on Cumberland Boulevard at the end of the ramp, drive 0.4 mile, and turn left on Cobb Parkway SE. At 0.4 mile turn right at the Chattahoochee/West Palisades/Paces Mill entrance. The road drops below US 41 and curves sharply left at 0.2 mile, passing under Cobb Parkway. You'll reach the parking lot in 0.1 mile.

Palisades West Trail

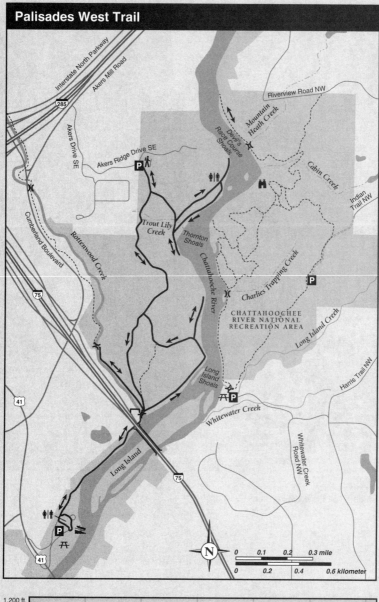

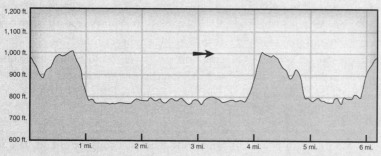

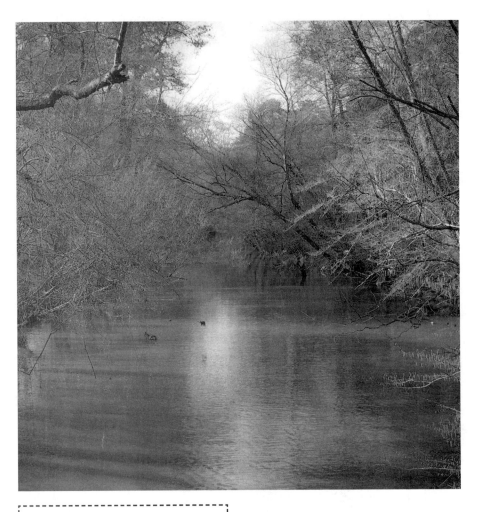

Rottenwood Creek flows calmly along the trail.

As you hike from Akers Mill, the trail enters the forest at the trailhead kiosk and turns right on a gravel road where vehicular traffic is restricted. The road descends, at first gradually, through an upper-Piedmont hardwood forest composed of oaks, American beeches, elms, maples, and pines, mostly shortleaf and loblolly. Underneath the canopy, dogwoods, black cherry trees, and the occasional magnolia tree can be spotted. Continue on the gravel road, which runs along the first ridgetop west of the Chattahoochee. At a three-way intersection less than 0.2 mile into the hike, take a road to the right where you'll see a ROTTENWOOD CREEK sign. Follow this trail as it gradually climbs in full shade. As the trail bears left, a narrow paved path joins it from the right at 0.3 mile.

Soon the footpath bears left, only to sweep back to the right along a mostly level ridgetop. Three roads branch left in quick succession, the last being the road to the confluence of the Chattahoochee River and Rottenwood Creek. At Rottenwood Creek, turn right to explore the level plain of the river on the Bob Callan Multi-Use Trail. Along this level, easy portion of the trail, water forms some cascades and shoals. At the end of the concrete, turn around and head back along the creek side to a right turn on a metal bridge, at 1.8 miles. After you cross, the trail curves left; a bench with an exceptional view of the Chattahoochee River is on the left.

Curving back to the right, the footpath passes under I-75 and follows the bank of the river to an open field at 2.5 miles. Watch on the left for a canoe and kayak take-out, which is the turnaround for this trail. Retrace your steps to the metal bridge, but instead of turning left, continue straight to explore the riverbank. The compacted-soil trail, which is occasionally in full sun, is rooted with repeated rock outcrops that make this section of the hike challenging. You will pass a road on the left at 3.4 miles; the trail ends as you approach the tall palisade of rock 0.2 mile later. Turn around and make a right on the first road. The climb back to the ridgetop is a great 0.4-mile thigh burner. As you reach the top of the ridge, the gravel road bears right.

At 4.5 miles you'll see a ROTTENWOOD CREEK sign on the right. At the next intersection, take the road on the right to explore the Akers Mill portion of the Chattahoochee River National Recreation Area. The trail drops, and the next section of it is concrete. Take a side trail to the right at 4.7 miles; alternatively, continuing straight ahead will also take you to the river. When the trail comes to a T-intersection, turn left. The trail soon curves right to join a gravel road; you'll find restrooms here. Straight ahead, across the surprisingly narrow Chattahoochee, is Big Rock, a massive granite boulder.

Turn left to explore the riverbank, which ends at a sandy spot. Turn around and follow the bank to the Palisades for some excellent river views. As the trail gets rocky and harder to follow, turn around and return to the restrooms. Climb along the gravel road to the ridgetop, and then go straight to return to your car.

NEARBY ACTIVITIES

Six Flags White Water (250 Cobb Pkwy. N, Marietta; 770-424-9283; **sixflags.com /whitewater**) is a great place to cool off after you've hiked West Palisades. As you might have guessed, this is a water-oriented park, featuring the Atlanta Ocean Wave Pool, Captain Kid's Cove, Run-A-Way River, and the Cliffhanger (one of the tallest free-falling waterslides in the world). Return to I-75, drive north to Exit 265, and follow the signs to the park.

10 PAPER MILL TRAIL

KEY AT-A-GLANCE INFORMATION

LENGTH: 3.5 miles; can be extended to almost 12 miles by combining with adjacent Cochran Shoals Park

CONFIGURATION: Loop

DIFFICULTY: Moderate–hard

SCENERY: Views of Sope Creek, which drops to the Chattahoochee River in a long cascade; remnants of the Marietta Paper Mill, on Sope Creek; occasional scenic views throughout the park

EXPOSURE: Mostly shade

TRAFFIC: Light–moderate

TRAIL SURFACE: Many rocky areas, especially near the river and tops of hills; some gravel roads; other portions are hard-packed dirt.

WHEELCHAIR ACCESS: None

HIKING TIME: 2.5 hours

ACCESS: Trail: daily, year-round, sunrise–sunset; headquarters: daily, year-round, 9 a.m.–5 p.m., except December 25; $3 day-use fee

MAPS: Throughout the park and at the Island Ford headquarters building; USGS *Sandy Springs*

MORE INFO: 678-538-1200; nps.gov/chat

FACILITIES: None in the park; however, this hike abuts the CRNRA's Cochran Shoals Unit, which has restrooms.

SPECIAL COMMENTS: Sope (often misspelled as *Soap*) Creek is named for a Cherokee chief who remained in the area after the Trail of Tears.

GPS INFORMATION

N33° 56.270' W84° 26.576'

IN BRIEF

This historic trail offers hikers a variety of options. Only the main path is shared with bicyclists.

DESCRIPTION

From the trailhead, descend a wide gravel road to the first path on the right at 0.1 mile. Watch for a Chattahoochee River National Recreation Area (CRNRA) map and a YOU ARE HERE arrow on a brown post at the intersection. If you haven't hiked Paper Mill recently, please note that there have been extensive changes to the trail system.

As you turn right, the man-made Sibley Pond is on your left, slightly below the trail, which traces the shore to the far end of the lake. Take the trail to your right as you approach a wooden bridge over a small creek to the left, less than 0.1 mile later. The footpath climbs steadily to a ridge where pines have been damaged by borers, but in the new growth lie a wide variety of hardwoods and, for the time being, sun-loving bushes. The treadway begins to drop and turns right at a T-intersection at 0.5 mile. A few feet later, make a right turn as the trail rejoins the main gravel trunk through Sope Creek.

Directions

Take I-75 North to Exit 261, marked as GA 280/ Dobbins AFB/Lockheed, with a separate sign for Delk Road. Turn right on Delk Road SE and drive 1.4 miles. Turn left on Terrell Mill Road SE and drive 1.1 miles; then make a sharp right onto Paper Mill Road SE. Drive 1.1 miles to the signed entrance of the Sope Creek Unit of the CRNRA, and turn right. The trailhead and pay booth are at the far end of the parking lot.

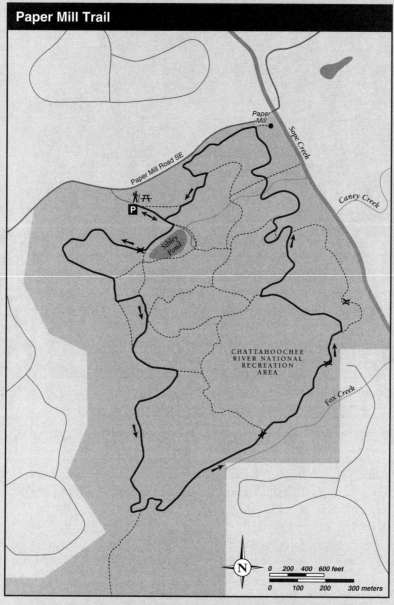

Paper Mill Trail

Paper Mill Road SE

Paper Mill

Sope Creek

Caney Creek

Sibley Pond

CHATTAHOOCHEE RIVER NATIONAL RECREATION AREA

Fox Creek

N

| 0 | 200 | 400 | 600 feet |
| 0 | 100 | 200 | 300 meters |

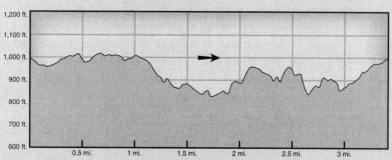

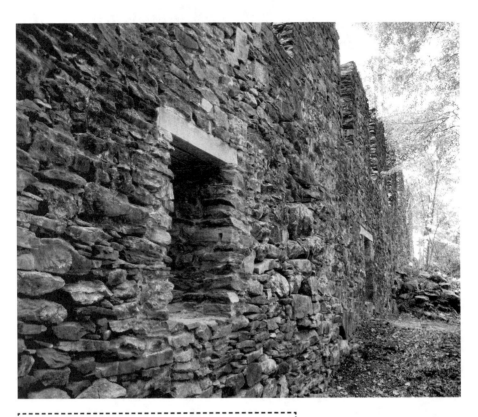

The rocky ruins of the Marietta Paper Mill predate the Civil War.

Over the next 0.5 mile, the gravel road descends steadily, finally curving right at the bottom of the ridge. The main trunk continues straight ahead to Cochran Shoals Trail, but turn right. You will soon see the beginnings of Fox Creek on the right. Over the next 0.7 mile, three trails head to the left and climb toward Sibley Pond—keep straight to follow the creek as it grows. At 1.7 miles the footpath rises and curves left, and a side trail leads off to apartments. The trail joins a wide gravel road 0.1 mile later, making the extended climb out of the river valley. At 2.3 miles turn right and follow this gravel road down to Sope Creek for a photo opportunity. Evidence of Paleo, Archaic, Woodland, Mississippian, Creek, and Cherokee peoples has been found near the creek.

There are two ways to get to the paper mill from here. As you climb up the road that brought you to Sope Creek, a trail heads right. This steep, rocky path is the only difficult section of trail in the park and should be avoided if you have a fear of heights, but it does afford more-scenic views of Sope Creek, especially in winter. If you wish, you can continue up the road to the next trail, which is slightly longer. At the end of this section, at 3 miles, you'll find the Marietta Paper Mill on the right, down a steep embankment. For easier access to the ruins, take the trail to the far side of Paper Mill Road and descend an easier embankment.

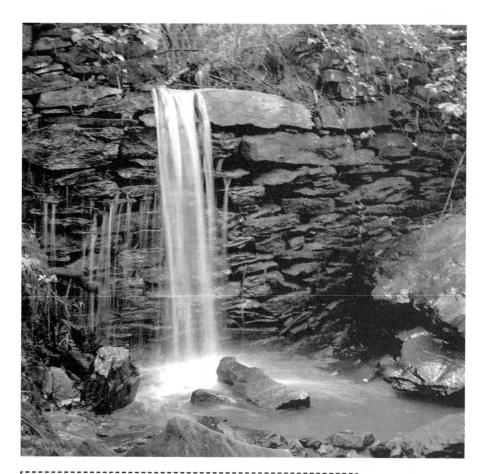

Water seeps through the stones and flows over the top of a historic rock dam.

Built between 1853 and 1855, the paper mill was incorporated as a business in 1859. Because the mill was built from rock, it was sturdier than other mills built in the area, including a gristmill and, later, a sawmill. Their raceways shared water from an upriver dam. Union General Kenner Garrard destroyed the paper mill and gristmill on July 5, 1864, as William Tecumseh Sherman marched toward Atlanta. Rebuilt after the war, the paper mill alternately flourished and struggled with the economy before finally shutting its doors in 1940.

Return to the trail near Paper Mill Road and follow it back to the main trunk. Turn right for a moderate climb to the parking lot.

NEARBY ACTIVITIES

The **Marietta Museum of History** (1 Depot St., Marietta; 770-794-5710; **marietta history.org**) details the rich history of the city and some of the mill owners in the Sope Creek area.

11 POWERS LANDING TRAIL

KEY AT-A-GLANCE INFORMATION

LENGTH: 2.3 miles

CONFIGURATION: Loop

DIFFICULTY: Easy, except on the climb into the watershed, which is moderate

SCENERY: Historical-home site, scenic views of the Chattahoochee River

EXPOSURE: Mostly shaded

TRAFFIC: Moderate

TRAIL SURFACE: Compacted soil, historic roadbed

WHEELCHAIR ACCESS: None

HIKING TIME: 1.5 hours

ACCESS: Trail: daily, year-round, sunrise–sunset; headquarters: daily, year-round, 9 a.m.–5 p.m., except December 25; $3 day-use fee

MAPS: USGS *Sandy Springs*

MORE INFO: 678-538-1200; nps.gov/chat

FACILITIES: Restrooms

SPECIAL COMMENTS: Fishing is popular here, with anglers reporting plentiful brown and rainbow trout and shoal bass.

DISTANCE: 3.3 miles from I-75 North/I-285 Northwest

GPS INFORMATION

N33° 54.217' W84° 26.528'

IN BRIEF

This trail explores Powers Island, in the Chattahoochee River, and then follows the floodplain of the river to a wonderful cove in the watershed. As you return to the trailhead, the path offers scenic views of the river.

DESCRIPTION

In 1819 the Cherokee Nation signed a treaty with the United States that established this section of the Chattahoochee River as its eastern boundary. James Powers established a homestead and a ferry here in 1831. The Cherokees and local settlers gave Powers, who was a gunsmith as well as manager of the ferry and blacksmith shop, a brisk business repairing their weapons. When the Land Lottery of 1832 gave Cherokee territory to settlers from Georgia, Powers moved west across the Chattahoochee in 1833 to Vinings, in newly formed Cobb County. He continued to oversee the ferry's operation. In 1903 the ferry was replaced by a bridge, near where the present-day I-285 bridge crosses the river.

Circle the brown building that formerly housed the Chattahoochee Outdoor Center (closed since 2002) to reach an iron bridge with wooden slats that connects to Powers Island. Kayaks frequently run the course between the

Directions ———————————➤

Take I-75 North to Exit 260/Windy Hill Road, and turn right. Drive 0.6 mile on Windy Hill Road SE and turn right on Powers Ferry Road SE. Drive 1 mile and turn left on Interstate North Parkway. Drive 0.4 mile and turn left on Riveredge Lane NW. Turn left again, at the first driveway past the I-285 bridge over the Chattahoochee River, into the parking lot.

Powers Landing Trail

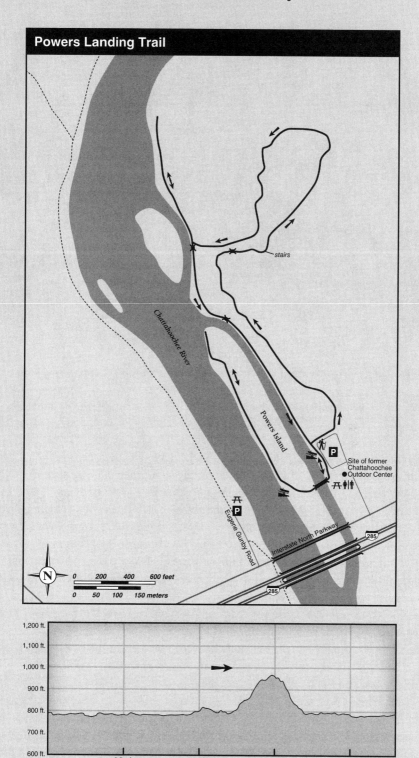

Chattahoochee River

stairs

Powers Island

Site of former
Chattahoochee
● Outdoor Center

Eugene Gunby Road

Interstate North Parkway

285

285

N

| 0 | 200 | 400 | 600 feet |

| 0 | 50 | 100 | 150 meters |

1,200 ft.
1,100 ft.
1,000 ft.
900 ft.
800 ft.
700 ft.
600 ft.

0.5 mi.   1 mi.   1.5 mi.   2 mi.

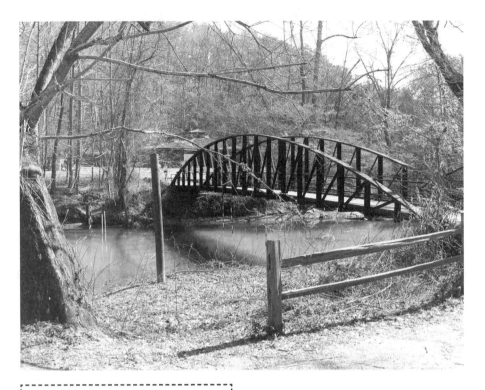

This rustic footbridge leads to Powers Island.

riverbank and the island. After crossing the bridge, join the footpath, which bears right, passing a canoe and kayak launch on the right, then curving back to the left and crossing the narrow island. When you come to a second launch site, on the windward side of the island, views of the river open. Across the Chattahoochee is the popular Cochran Shoals walking trail. Descend the steps for excellent views up and down the river.

Turn around and climb back to the path, heading left at the end of the split rail fence onto a compacted-dirt trail that follows near the riverbank. Passing through a mostly hardwood forest filled with large oak trees, especially close to the shore, the level treadway runs near the riverbank most of the way to the north end of the island. As you near your destination, the footpath heads inland to cross a small creek. Finally coming to a wide channel between two islands, the trail currently ends here. Many years ago this channel did not exist, and it was possible to follow the trail to a deck on the north end of the island.

Return to the start of this trail and turn left. The loop has two entrances—look for the one in the far right corner of the parking lot. Beginning as a wide, level roadway, the pathway approaches an area at 0.9 mile that features an abundance of American beech trees and long poison ivy vines scaling large oak trees. After you cross a creek via a culvert, the footpath reaches a three-way intersection at 1.1 miles. Turn right and begin climbing a narrower trail. On your left is a woodland stream. After you cross a wooden bridge over a tributary, the trail curves right, climbs a set of stairs, and swings left. As you approach a stone wall, ascend to a small, level field that was once a homestead.

On the far side of the former homestead is an old roadbed that was once a driveway. At 1.3 miles the roadbed heads right as the trail continues to climb to a ridgetop. As a second trail heads right, the footpath veers left and begins to climb to an unnamed knoll. From there, the path returns to the woodland stream, now on your left. As the trail descends, the rock outcrops increase, and you can see wildflowers. After a set of wooden steps, the trail returns to the main path in the Chattahoochee floodplain. Turn right, continue to the next map stand, and then turn right again.

Back on a gravel road, watch for a heavily damaged deck on the island, just off the riverbank. The Powers Island portion of the hike once came this far north, but the changing currents of the Chattahoochee have made it impossible to reach the deck. The park ends in an area of large, poison ivy–covered trees. Turn around, return to the map stand, and continue along the riverbank by bearing right.

On the left, at 2.1 miles into the hike, a lone chimney rises, the building that accompanied it long gone. Feel free to explore the area, but watch out for small animals. Return to the path and follow the riverbank back to your car.

NEARBY ACTIVITIES

This is a great hike to take on a Sunday, because afterward you can enjoy brunch at **Ray's on the River** (6700 Powers Ferry Rd., Sandy Springs; 770-955-1187; **rays restaurants.com/raysontheriver**). This upscale Atlanta eatery has been wowing diners for many years, and for good reason: the food is excellent and the prices are reasonable. As you leave the parking lot, turn right on Interstate North Parkway and make a left at the first light, onto Powers Ferry Road. Go under I-285 and turn left at the light to stay on Powers Ferry. After you cross the Chattahoochee River, you'll see Ray's in an industrial park; take the first driveway on the right.

12 REYNOLDS NATURE PRESERVE

 KEY AT-A-GLANCE INFORMATION

LENGTH: 1.8 miles

CONFIGURATION: Loop

DIFFICULTY: Easy

SCENERY: Multiple lakeshore views, forested wetlands, and a 17-foot-circumference white oak that was felled by a storm

EXPOSURE: Mostly shaded, except in the vicinity of the lakes and dam, where it is sometimes fully exposed

TRAFFIC: Light

TRAIL SURFACE: Compacted soil

WHEELCHAIR ACCESS: None on main trail

HIKING TIME: 1 hour

ACCESS: Daily, year-round, 8 a.m.–sunset; interpretive center: Monday–Friday, 8 a.m.–5 p.m. Free admission; donations welcome.

MAPS: Available at trailhead kiosk; USGS *Jonesboro*

MORE INFO: 770-603-4188; reynoldsnaturepreserve.org

FACILITIES: Nature center with native animals; restrooms; picnic areas

SPECIAL COMMENTS: Visitors have many opportunities to see smaller animals, including turtles, tortoises, and a family of beavers, within the park. The preserve offers various programs such as canoeing with Ranger John and building bat houses.

DISTANCE: 7.8 miles from I-75 South/I-285 South

GPS INFORMATION

N33° 36.102' W84° 20.908'

5665 Reynolds Rd.
Morrow, GA 30260

IN BRIEF

Reynolds Nature Preserve, with almost 4 miles of well-made hiking trails, makes for an excellent family hike.

DESCRIPTION

William H. Reynolds Memorial Nature Preserve is built on the estate of William Huie Reynolds, a Clayton County judge who donated 130 acres of land to the county to preserve both forest and wetlands for future generations. The preserve's board of trustees and the county have purchased another 16 acres of adjoining land that was once owned by Judge Reynolds for preservation. Within the boundaries of the park are the Reynolds home, a barn, other outbuildings, numerous ponds and wetlands, a large area of forested hills, and a nature center.

From the trailhead kiosk at the north end of the parking area, follow the paved trail through a mostly pine forest to reach the nature center. Among the pines within the preserve are loblolly, shortleaf, and white. Almost immediately on your right is a trail leading from the Reynolds home; continue straight, toward the nature center. Inside the center are a number of interesting exhibits, including small amphibians and reptiles and an active honeybee hive. As you leave the center, turn right and continue to a paved,

----

Directions ——————————→

Take I-75 South to Exit 233/GA 54/Jonesboro Road. Turn left at the end of the ramp on Jonesboro Road, and drive 0.9 mile to a traffic light. Turn left on Reynolds Road and drive 1.1 miles to the nature-center parking lot. There is an overflow parking area at 0.8 mile.

Reynolds Nature Preserve

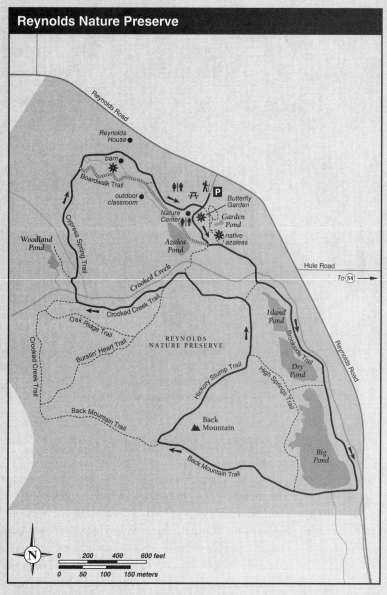

Reynolds Road

Reynolds House

barn

Boardwalk Trail

outdoor classroom

Cypress Spring Trail

Woodland Pond

Nature Center

Butterfly Garden

Garden Pond

native azaleas

Azalea Pond

Crooked Creek

Hule Road

To 54

Crooked Creek Trail

Oak Ridge Trail

Island Pond

Brookside Trail

Crooked Creek Trail

Burstin' Heart Trail

REYNOLDS NATURE PRESERVE

Hickory Stump Trail

High Springs Trail

Dry Pond

Reynolds Road

Back Mountain Trail

Back Mountain

Big Pond

Back Mountain Trail

N

0   200   400   600 feet

0   50   100   150 meters

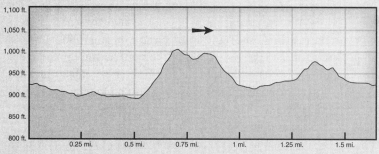

1,100 ft.
1,050 ft.
1,000 ft.
950 ft.
900 ft.
850 ft.
800 ft.

0.25 mi.   0.5 mi.   0.75 mi.   1 mi.   1.25 mi.   1.5 mi.

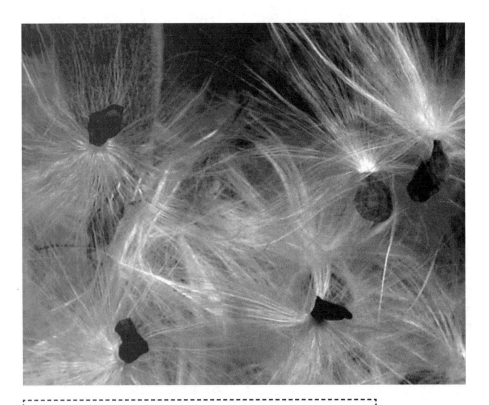

It takes a sharp eye to spot the milkweed bugs hiding among these silky threads.

wheelchair-accessible native-plant garden featuring such plants as American beautyberry, Indian pink, and red buckeye.

Wide, level, and covered in mulch, Brookside Trail—the first named trail in our multitrail loop—begins after the brick-paved native-plant garden, at a marked three-way intersection at 0.1 mile. Three hundred feet past this intersection, Hickory Stump Trail dead-ends into the footpath from the right. Continue straight on Brookside Trail to a series of three man-made ponds: Island, Dry, and Big. Trails cross each pond, forming a dam built by local inmates in the 1930s; then they join Brookside Trail. On Big Pond, a dock allows hikers the chance to view waterfowl, amphibians, and reptiles from the lake. Many turtles, along with geese, ducks, and migratory waterfowl in the spring and fall, call the lake home.

Return to the trail and turn right; walk to the dam and follow Brookside Trail to the right. Views of the lakeshore open to the right as you cross the dam. After the dam, the pathway becomes Back Mountain Trail, and High Springs Trail heads right. Continue on Back Mountain Trail as it begins a moderate-to-difficult climb to a low knob in a Piedmont hardwood forest of oak, hickory, sourwood, sweet gum, black gum, Southern magnolia, and tupelo.

At 0.8 mile, turn right at the signed intersection onto Hickory Stump Trail, a wide, mulch-covered trail, and follow it as it descends the low knob; bear left at the bottom of this easy-to-moderate descent. Turn left onto the marked Crooked Creek Trail at the bottom of the ridge. Where Burstin' Heart Trail heads left, follow Crooked Creek as it bears right and enters an area of larger trees. The path joins the creek that gives the trail its name. Along the creek's bank, the land is heavily eroded from recent storms.

Just past the eroded area, the path climbs to a wide river plain and splits into two trails, with a third trail, Cypress Spring Trail, heading right at an unmarked intersection. Descend Cypress Spring Trail. After passing an unmarked trail on the left that goes to another pond, Cypress Spring Trail splits as it enters a mature-growth forest. Take either footpath—both lead to a boardwalk that crosses a stream in an area of large trees. As the trail curves right at 1.6 miles, the home of William H. Reynolds comes into view on the right; the barn is straight ahead.

Turn left at the end of the house and walk around to the front porch. Originally, this was a four-room, two-story structure with an enclosed staircase; Judge Reynolds added rooms and an attic. Outbuildings include a barn and sheds. As the trail leaves the homestead, it becomes paved. Portable comfort stations and picnic tables sit near the trail in this area. Turn left at the next intersection to return to the parking area.

NEARBY ACTIVITIES

The **Road to Tara Museum** is housed in the Jonesboro Depot Welcome Center (104 N. Main St., Jonesboro; 770-478-4800; **visitscarlett.com/roadtotaramuseum.html**). The original depot figured prominently in the Battle of Jonesboro, a pivotal engagement that marked the end of the Atlanta Campaign. The present stone building, built in 1867, replaced the structure destroyed by Sherman during his March to the Sea. The museum, which displays pieces from the world's largest private collection of *Gone with the Wind* memorabilia, is open Monday–Friday, 8:30 a.m.–5:30 p.m., and Saturday, 10 a.m.–4 p.m.; $7 adults, $6 seniors and children.

13 SILVER COMET TRAIL: MAVELL ROAD TO FLOYD ROAD

KEY AT-A-GLANCE INFORMATION

LENGTH: 8.2 miles round-trip

CONFIGURATION: Point to point or out-and-back

DIFFICULTY: Easy if point to point; moderate if out-and-back

SCENERY: Occasional overlooks into rapidly urbanizing bottomland; pretty view of a creek from a trestle

EXPOSURE: Mostly sunny

TRAFFIC: Heavy; multiuse trail

TRAIL SURFACE: Paved asphalt roadway marked with lanes

WHEELCHAIR ACCESS: Yes

HIKING TIME: 3.25 hours if one-way

ACCESS: Daily, year-round, sunrise–sunset; free

MAPS: Available for purchase at Silver Comet Depot in Mableton (4342 Floyd Rd.; 770-819-3279; silver cometdepot.com) or free at the website below; USGS *Mableton*

MORE INFO: 404-875-PATH (7284); pathfoundation.org/trails/silver -comet

FACILITIES: 3 parking areas with restrooms and phones

SPECIAL COMMENTS: The most popular section of the Silver Comet Trail.

DISTANCE: 6 miles from I-75 North/I-285 Northwest

GPS INFORMATION

Mavell Road: N33° 50.589' W84° 31.002'

Floyd Road: N33° 50.818' W84° 35.200'

Nickajack School: 4555 Mavell Rd. SE Smyrna, GA 30082

Silver Comet Depot: 4342 Floyd Rd. Mableton, GA 30126

IN BRIEF

Hike the level roadbed along the route of the Seaboard Air Line Railroad's *Silver Comet,* one of a family of trains that included the *Orange Blossom Special* of bluegrass-music fame.

DESCRIPTION

The *Silver Comet* was a passenger train that ran on various railroads from Philadelphia to Birmingham, Alabama. The Pennsylvania Railroad and the Richmond, Fredericksburg and Potomac Railroad routed the train in the Northeast and Mid-Atlantic, while the Seaboard Air Line Railroad routed the train in the Deep South. Shortly after service was inaugurated in 1947, the *Silver Comet* gained national

----

Directions ———————————→

Mavell Road trailhead: Take I-285 South to Exit 16 and turn right on South Atlanta Road. Drive 0.4 mile and turn left on Cumberland Parkway. Drive 0.6 mile to South Cobb Drive and turn right. Drive 0.4 mile and turn left on Cooper Lake Road SE. Cooper Lake Road winds 0.7 mile to Mavell Road SE, on the left—watch for a sign on the right for Nickajack Elementary School. Turn on Mavell Road and drive 0.3 mile. Turn left into the Silver Comet Trail parking lot, past the Nickajack Elementary School parking lot on the left, just before the Creekside at Vinings condominiums.

Floyd Road trailhead: Take I-285 South to Exit 16 and turn right on South Atlanta Road. Drive 0.4 mile and turn left on Cumberland Parkway, which becomes the East–West Connector after 0.6 mile. Drive a total of 6.3 miles on Cumberland/East–West, then turn left on Floyd Road. Drive 0.7 mile, turn right on Floyd Road, and make an immediate right into the Silver Comet parking lot, just past the Silver Comet Depot bike shop.

Silver Comet Trail: Mavell Road to Floyd Road

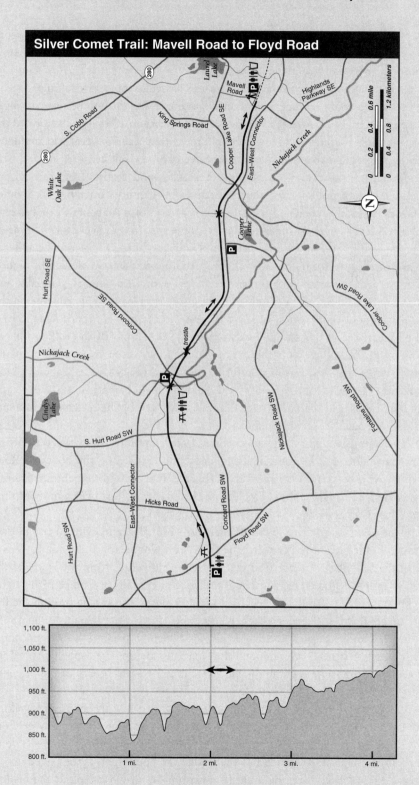

attention when segregationist "Dixiecrats" left the 1948 Democratic National Convention in Philadelphia and rode the train to Birmingham, where they nominated Strom Thurmond for president.

As competition from airlines and cars sent passenger-rail service into decline in the 1960s, the route became a combined passenger–freight line before passenger service ended in 1969. After CSX ended freight service in 1988 and abandoned the track, it lay idle until the state of Georgia, three counties, and several state and local interest groups came together to build the Silver Comet Trail in 1998.

Today the trail draws hikers, joggers, skaters, and cyclists from throughout the Atlanta metropolitan area to southern Cobb County. Traveling 61.5 miles from Mavell Road to the Georgia state line, where it joins Alabama's Chief Ladiga Trail, the Silver Comet traverses a railroad grade that never exceeds 4%. Some of the grade is uphill for an extended stretch if you start at the Floyd Road trailhead, but as you depart from the Mavell Road trailhead, the trail descends slightly through a predominately pine forest intermixed with tulip poplars, pin oaks, and invasive mimosa trees. Almost immediately, a side trail leads to apartments on the left. Throughout this portion of the trail you can see homes, apartments, farms, and businesses. The railroad bed was originally carved out of the rolling hills of the Georgia Piedmont, with the debris from the cut used to span bottomland farms. The Atlanta and Birmingham Air Line, a subsidiary of the Seaboard, built the section of track from Howell's Yard (Atlanta) to Rockmart in 1904. An early example of these cuts can be seen at 0.3 mile, followed by the raised embankment of a railroad bed across bottomland.

There are a number of improved trail-access points along the way, many from apartments and housing developments, but at 0.7 mile the Fontaine Road Parking Area Access Trail comes in from the left. Just beyond that entrance, a rest area allows you to take a quiet break from the busy trail. Just over a mile into the hike, Silver Comet Trail crosses a bridge over a creek.

A short distance past the 2-mile mark, the asphalt trail begins to rise noticeably, curving left and then crossing the East–West Connector at 2.4 miles. This is one of the few places on the trail where the path diverges from the route of the original railroad grade. As you leave the trestle, the Silver Comet turns right, quickly regaining the railroad bed. Shortly after the trestle, a side trail on the left takes hikers down to Heritage Park, where they can visit the remains of an 1840s woolen mill and explore additional trails. On the climb back to the Silver Comet, watch on the left for a well-defined dirt road just before the asphalt path. Turn left on this dirt road and climb the hill, watching for paths to explore on the left, near the hilltop.

Once you've returned to the Silver Comet, turn left and continue walking west on the asphalt path. In less than 0.1 mile you come to a trestle over Concord Road. In winter and early spring, the Concord Covered Bridge is visible to your left on the trail. At the end of the bridge, on your right, is the paved access to the Concord Road parking area. If you want an up-close look at the bridge,

> This stretch of the Silver Comet is the busiest, so be prepared to share the trail.

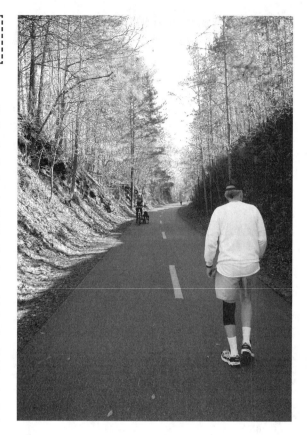

climb to the parking area and bear right to reach the public road; then turn right. Carefully follow the road 0.2 mile downhill to the bridge, built in 1872. Turn around and climb the hill to the parking area and turn left. When you reach the Silver Comet Trail, turn right.

Now the Silver Comet Trail begins to curve slowly left, coming to a trestle over Nickajack Creek. Note that the old railroad ties of the trestle have been covered with wooden slats and paved. Following this trestle, the pathway begins an extended climb over the next 1.2 miles to the Floyd Road Parking Area. Passing a deep valley on the right at 3 miles, the trail passes under Hurt Road 0.1 mile later, then enters a deep cut carved out of stone. This formation—rock overlain with a few inches of Georgia clay—is typical of the geology throughout the Piedmont and southern Blue Ridge Mountains.

Exiting the cut, you'll find a park bench at 3.3 miles. The trees, mostly older oaks, are bigger here, although the forest is second-growth. Walking along a ridge created by the roadbed, you come to a traffic light–controlled intersection with Hicks Road at 3.8 miles. A small sitting area with a picnic table and park bench are on the right at 4.2 miles, just before the trail intersects Floyd Road, which is also controlled by a traffic signal. If you're hiking out-and-back, the picnic area is your turnaround point. If you've done the hike as a one-way with a shuttle, enter the Floyd Road Parking Area through a small sitting area next to the Silver Comet Depot bike shop, across Floyd Road on the left, or continue 0.1 mile west on the Silver Comet to reach another entrance to the Floyd Road parking area.

NEARBY ACTIVITIES

More hiking trails traverse **Heritage Park** (see Hike 17, page 90).

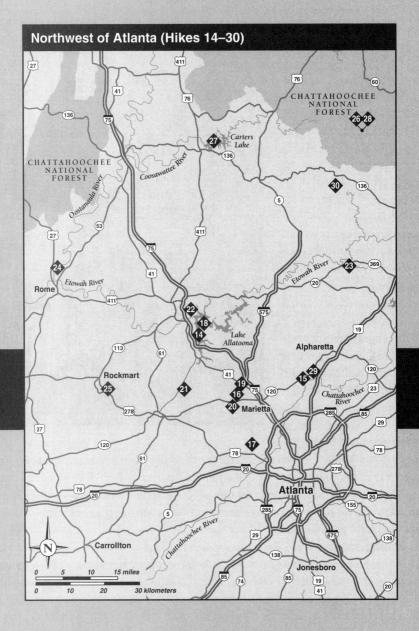

Northwest of Atlanta (Hikes 14–30)

NORTHWEST OF
ATLANTA

14 ALLATOONA PASS TRAIL

KEY AT-A-GLANCE INFORMATION

LENGTH: 3 miles round-trip

CONFIGURATION: Out-and-back with 2 smaller loops

DIFFICULTY: Moderate

SCENERY: Allatoona lakeshore, with excellent long-distance views; deep railroad cut

EXPOSURE: Full sun–partial shade at the lakeshore, shady near the cut

TRAFFIC: Moderate

TRAIL SURFACE: Gravel, hard-packed dirt

WHEELCHAIR ACCESS: None

HIKING TIME: 2 hours

ACCESS: Daily, year-round, sunrise–sunset; free

MAPS: USGS *Acworth*

FACILITIES: Nearest are at Red Top Mountain State Park, 1 exit north on I-75

MORE INFO: 770-975-0055; georgiatrails.com/gt/allatoona_pass

SPECIAL COMMENTS: Nearby Cartersville affords a number of additional hiking opportunities. Contact the Bartow County Convention and Visitors Bureau (800-733-2280; visitcartersvillega.org/na/hiking _and_geocacheing).

DISTANCE: 26.1 miles from I-75 North/I-285 Northwest

GPS INFORMATION

N34° 6.835' W84° 42.903'

Lake Allatoona Inn:
632 Old Allatoona Rd. SE
Cartersville, GA 30121

IN BRIEF

Climb to the tops of two mountains separated by a railroad pass to view the site of the last Civil War battle in the Atlanta area. This trek includes a long, scenic lakeshore walk.

DESCRIPTION

Deep Cut, the local name for Allatoona Pass, was built by slaves during the construction of the Western and Atlantic Railroad. Union General William Tecumseh Sherman, who first rode his horse through the cut while working as a surveyor in 1844, recognized during the Atlanta Campaign that a well-entrenched force could hold the narrow pass against the attacks of a much larger army, choking off supply lines in the process. Sherman avoided a direct attack during the Atlanta Campaign, marching on Kennesaw Mountain from the west. He then directed his engineering chief, Captain Orlando Poe, to fortify the ridge above the pass after taking it in June 1864. On October 5, 1864, Confederate General Samuel French

- -

Directions ———————————————→

Take I-75 North to Exit 283/Allatoona Road/ Emerson. Turn right at the end of the ramp. At 0.5 mile the road veers left, crosses railroad tracks, and then curves right—*don't* take the road to the right just before the railroad tracks. At 0.8 mile the modern railroad tracks run to the right, down a steep embankment. At 1.4 miles the road curves sharply right and enters a small community. The parking lot for Allatoona Pass is on the left, 0.1 mile after the curve, across the road from the Lake Allatoona Inn. Go to the second driveway and enter. From your car, walk to the brown gate at the northwest end of the parking lot. A small path lies on the left side of the gate.

Allatoona Pass Trail

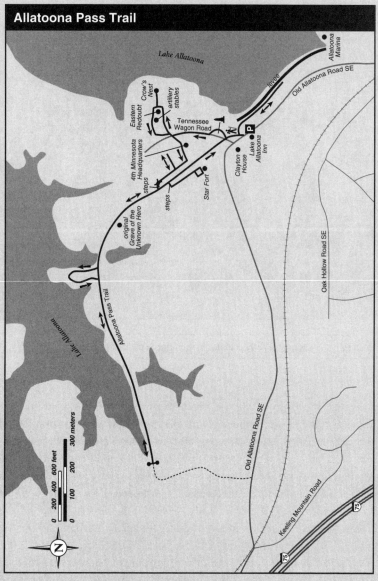

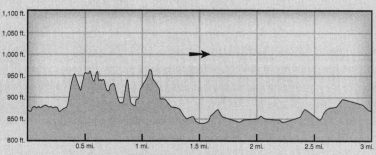

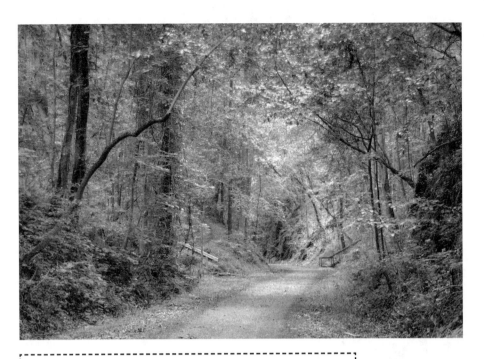

The tranquil trail through Allatoona Pass belies its tumultuous Civil War past.

tried to capture the Union star fort above Allatoona Pass, along with the stores and munitions that were so desperately needed by fellow general John Bell Hood's troops. French returned empty-handed, and his group suffered 799 casualties.

At the start of this exciting interpretive trail is a map of the area on which the trail has been superimposed. Directly behind you is the Clayton House, a two-story home with a wide porch that served as a hospital for both the Union and Confederate armies. As you continue, the paved path turns to gravel as you walk toward Deep Cut, and you encounter an immense curtain of bamboo on your left. On your right, additional interpretive signs describe the battle.

From these signs, turn around and walk out onto a substantial 15-foot levee built to impound the waters of Lake Allatoona. A chain across the entrance prevents vehicular traffic. As you walk the levee, the lake comes into view past Allatoona Marina, which is on your right. Return to the trail and turn right. Almost immediately, the pathway turns right again, descending to a small area dedicated to monuments from the states whose men fought this battle. Alabama, North Carolina, Mississippi, Texas, Missouri, Illinois, and Iowa mark the site— no Georgia troops fought in this battle.

Return to the trail and turn right to immediately begin climbing a gravel road to the top of the mountain. The Tennessee Wagon Road connected the Chatta-hoochee River to Chattanooga. Allatoona, the small community at the southern terminus of the road, was a thriving railroad town at the start of the Civil War.

Much of the town was destroyed when the US Army Corps of Engineers built Lake Allatoona.

As the road climbs and curves left, you can see the Eastern Redoubt across a deep gully to the right. This is the fort commissioned by Captain Poe to extend the defensive line for the Allatoona depot. Used to store Union rations, the depot and warehouses held enough livestock and flour to feed 100,000 men for 10 days.

Atop the hill is a four-way intersection. Turn right and climb a flight of railroad-tie stairs. A few steps down, the trail splits into a loop—take the trail to the right. This wide, shady, well-defined interpretive treadway gives visitors a glimpse into the logistics behind a battle. The trail splits two more times. Each time, take the trail to the right, signed as the trail to the Crow's Nest.

Soldiers used a complex treetop flag system to communicate to Sherman's stronghold at Kennesaw Mountain. Flag systems were maintained for secret communications and in case a telegraph line was cut. During the battle, Sherman ordered the transmission of an uncoded message—TELL ALLATOONA HOLD ON. GENERAL SHERMAN SAYS HE IS WORKING HARD FOR YOU— well aware that French would intercept the communication and be concerned about the presence of Yankees to his rear. Sherman, afraid the attack was a ruse to draw him out of Kennesaw, never left his stronghold.

Follow the signs to the Eastern Redoubt, where a wooden bridge crosses the entrenchments used to create the fort. A short wooden fence atop the earthen mound provided additional protection for soldiers. Turn right and follow the marked trail to the artillery stables. Turn around and return to the pathway. Turn left on the trail, returning to the Tennessee Wagon Road. Cross the road and continue to the headquarters of the 4th Minnesota Regiment. Lieutenant Colonel John Tourtellotte was in charge of troops stationed at Allatoona before Union General John Corse arrived, just before the battle.

Walk 100 feet for your first view of Deep Cut. Notice the two levels of the pass. Railroad workers removed the soft top layer, and then slaves from local plantations removed the solid rock. As the trail turns right and descends to the cut, a side path leads off to the right. Two hundred feet from the main trail, the path overlooks a steep valley and begins circling to the right. Notice entrenchments on your left, used by Union forces during the battle. Confederates from the valley charged this Union line, failed to breach it, and retreated. Union gunfire from here killed many Confederate soldiers in the assault on the star fort.

Return to the main trail, turn right, and continue descending into the cut. Approaching the bottom, the trail turns and dips rather dramatically, crossing a small drainage ditch on a stone-and-dirt bridge. Turn right and follow the level, shaded railroad bed 0.1 mile to the Grave of the Unknown Hero, on the left. This was the original site of the grave of a soldier who died in battle. It was moved when Allatoona Dam was constructed, but for many years engineers on the Western and Atlantic maintained the grave. Return to the railroad bed and then turn left.

At 1.2 miles most of the path is fully exposed to sun as it begins to skirt Allatoona's lakeshore. A few steps ahead, turn right on a side trail to explore a peninsula of the lake. At the peninsula's point, you'll notice a pole with an extended flat top where an eagle has built an aerie. Scan the lake to see similar poles and nests. Return to the railroad bed and turn right. At 1.8 miles a gate across the road, marking the end of the Allatoona Pass Trail, is your sign to turn around and return to Deep Cut.

Back in the cut, wooden stairs on the right at 2.6 miles begin a moderate-to-steep ascent that takes you to a star fort. A wooden walkway bridges entrenchments surrounding the fort's sally port (entrance). The Confederate attack came along a low ridge that is to your right as you step off the bridge. At the height of the battle, men from smaller surrounding redoubts retreated to the fort as the Confederates overran those positions. Imagine 700 men huddled within these confines, surrounded by the enemy, under fire, and running low on ammunition.

Take the wooden walkway to exit the fort, and then follow the trail back to the steps. At the bottom of the steps, turn right. Continue straight ahead to return to your car.

NEARBY ACTIVITIES

The **Etowah Indian Mounds Historic Site,** featuring six earthen mounds and a museum with a film, is nearby in Cartersville (813 Indian Mounds Rd. SW; 770-387-3747; **gastateparks.org/etowahmounds**; open Wednesday–Saturday, 9 a.m.–5 p.m., closed January 1, Thanksgiving, and December 25; admission $3.50–$5.50). To get there, take I-75 North to Exit 288 and follow the brown signs.

CHATTAHOOCHEE NATURE CENTER TRAIL

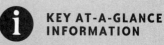

IN BRIEF

This hike explores the Chattahoochee River above Bull Sluice before climbing into the watershed. The hike ends at the Discovery Center, where visitors can learn about the natural world.

DESCRIPTION

We're frequently asked about good hikes for beginners. The Chattahoochee Nature Center has just such a hike. Offering a deep-woods experience in an in-town setting, the nature center also has a number of natural-history and animal exhibits designed to keep the kids engaged, and many of the trees and plants have signs identifying them. We usually hike these trails two or three times a year.

Enter the Chattahoochee Nature Center from the Discovery Center, at the right rear of the parking lot. This "green" area is a wonderful introduction to the story of the Chattahoochee River and the work of the center.

If you arrive early, large waterfowl can often be spotted from a wetlands boardwalk. Turn right as you leave the center, and follow the concrete–asphalt road to a gated chain-link fence near a traffic light–controlled

---

Directions

Take GA 400/US 19 North to Exit 6/Northridge Road. Turn right on Northridge, cross back over GA 400, and then take the first right on Dunwoody Place. Drive 1.2 miles and turn right on Roswell Road, which crosses a bridge over the Chattahoochee River at 0.5 mile. At the end of the bridge, turn left on Azalea Drive. Drive 1.7 miles to a traffic light and turn left on Willeo Road. Drive 0.6 mile, then turn right into the Chattahoochee Nature Center; follow the road around to the parking lot.

KEY AT-A-GLANCE INFORMATION

LENGTH: 2.5 miles

CONFIGURATION: Loop

DIFFICULTY: Easy

SCENERY: Excellent views of Bull Sluice; lake and river views

EXPOSURE: Full sun in developed areas, mostly shaded elsewhere

TRAFFIC: Moderate

TRAIL SURFACE: Compacted soil, pavement in developed areas

WHEELCHAIR ACCESS: Discovery Center and garden trails only

HIKING TIME: 1.5 hours

ACCESS: Monday–Saturday, 10 a.m.–5 p.m.; Sunday, noon–5 p.m.; closed Thanksgiving and December 24–25. Admission: $8 adults, $6 seniors, $5 children ages 3–12, free for children age 2 and younger and CNC members. No pets.

MAPS: Free with nature-center admission fee

MORE INFO: 770-992-2055; chattnaturecenter.org

FACILITIES: Restrooms, picnic tables, Discovery Center

SPECIAL COMMENTS: On summer weekdays kids can have a blast at Camp Kingfisher, offering nature hikes, swimming, canoeing, and science-education activities.

DISTANCE: 9.6 miles from GA 400 North/I-285 North

GPS INFORMATION

N34° 0.239' W84° 22.949'

9135 Willeo Rd.
Roswell, GA 30075

Chattahoochee Nature Center Trail

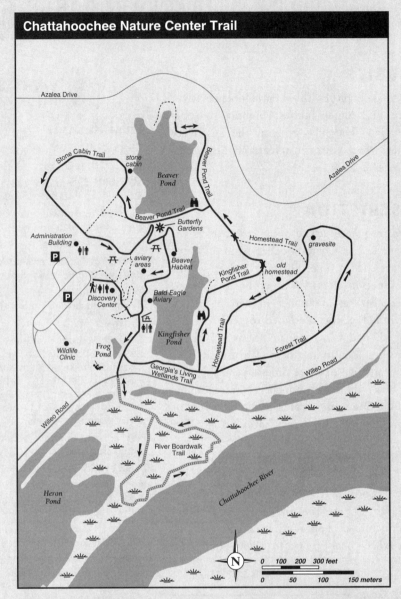

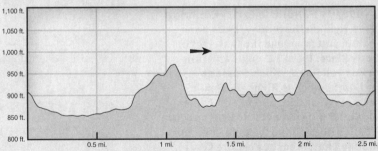

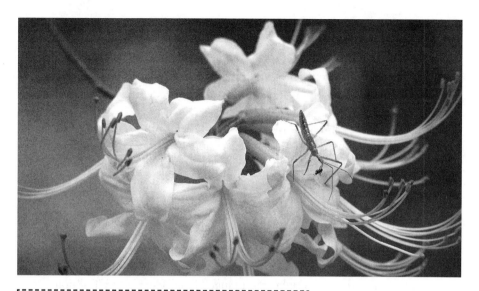

A pink azalea provides a perch for a walking stick feasting on a fly.

intersection, at 0.2 mile. Cross with the light to a second unlocked chain-link gate on a boardwalk.

Jutting into the Chattahoochee and frequently in full sun, the boardwalk is a great place to study the area's unique wetland plant life. Turn right at the first intersection and follow the boardwalk as it wraps around to the left. Bull Sluice Lake, on the river, opens on the right at 0.4 mile, affording hikers prime opportunities to view wildlife. On one crisp morning, we spotted a pair of ospreys, a great blue heron, and numerous smaller birds. Named for a waterfall that was completely covered when the lake was formed, Bull Sluice was created by Atlanta's first hydroelectric project, Morgan Falls Dam.

As you continue around the boardwalk loop, head down a short side trail on the right to an A-frame-roofed area with seats. Here you can enjoy long-distance views of the Chattahoochee before the boardwalk curves left again to explore an inland estuary. After returning to the starting point and crossing the road, pass through the chain-link gate and turn right almost immediately, following a concrete path down to an overlook on Kingfisher Pond.

As the path continues through "Georgia's Living Wetlands," interpretive displays discuss the importance of protecting the fragile riverine wetlands, or riparian zones. Water-loving trees, including river birches, black walnuts, and water oaks, have been planted to show visitors what a healthy riverine wetland looks like.

After a second overlook, which houses a re-creation of southeast Georgia's Okefenokee Swamp (complete with bald cypress trees), the trail splits—take the red-blazed trail on the right. Called the Forest Trail, this pathway immediately begins to climb into the watershed of the Chattahoochee River through a fully shaded pine–hardwood forest. Watch for American beeches and loblolly pines, which form a canopy over Southern magnolias and dogwoods. A dirt road cross-cuts the path where it jogs slightly to the right. A white-blazed crossover trail heads left at 0.9 mile, but continue straight ahead to a Civil War–era grave at 1.1 miles. At the grave, the trail circles left, climbing to its highest point, where an orange-blazed trail intersects it. Bear left on the orange trail, which immediately begins a gradual descent.

After passing a white crossover trail on the left, you'll notice an old home-stead on the right, apparent by the home's chimney. After you pass another white crossover trail that heads right, the orange- and red-blazed trails end. Turn right on the blue-blazed Kingfisher Pond Trail, climbing to an interpretive area at 1.4 miles. A cutaway into the mountain, along with an interpretive sign, displays the layers of soil typical in the Piedmont section of Georgia.

Bearing left at a side trail down to an amphitheater, the footpath once again begins an easy climb to a wooden bridge over a gully. Just before the bridge, a white crossover trail joins the path from the right, and the bridge makes a 90-degree left turn. As the pathway swings right, the orange-blazed Homestead Trail joins from the right just before you cross another wooden bridge. Kingfisher Pond Trail ends at Beaver Pond. Bear right on the green-blazed Beaver Pond Trail, which follows the pond's shore as it easily climbs to a bridge at 1.6 miles. Just past the bridge, you'll see houses on the right; the trail quickly ends. Turn around and return to the three-way intersection with the blue-blazed trail; turn right to continue on the green-blazed trail, crossing an earthen dam in full sun. On the far side of the dam, a concrete walkway joins the trail on the left, but continue straight to the end of the lake and bear right on the yellow-blazed Stone Cabin Trail at 1.9 miles.

The trail bears left at an open field through a forest that includes sweet gums and tulip poplars, and then it descends gradually to the entrance, where the path is paved with concrete. Turn left and follow the walkway around to the right to reach the Bonnie Baker Butterfly Gardens. Plants in this area have been specially chosen for their ability to attract butterflies. Among the flora are blazing stars, Carolina silver bells, yarrows, purple coneflowers, and the aptly named butterfly bushes. Briefly returning to the green trail, the concrete walkway then takes a hard right to continue to a side trail on the right, which leads down to a beaver habitat. After visiting the beavers, turn around and return to the main trail, where you'll turn left. The path leads through a raptor sanctuary—a permanent home for owls and hawks unable to return to the wild after having been injured—and then ends at a massive habitat for a pair of American bald eagles. Follow the trail back to the Discovery Center.

NEARBY ACTIVITIES

The **Roswell RiverWalk** (770-641-3705) is a linear park with many access points that follow the Chattahoochee. It is currently 3 miles long but is being extended.

CHEATHAM HILL TRAIL 16

IN BRIEF

The trail follows a gravel road from Burnt Hickory to Dallas Highway and then parallels a low ridge to Cheatham Hill. After taking you to explore Civil War entrenchments, the trail descends to Kolb's Farm Trail, returning to Dallas Highway along a paved road. On the return to the trailhead, the hike leaves the main trunk and explores the watershed of Noses Creek.

DESCRIPTION

Union General William Tecumseh Sherman's Atlanta Campaign had stalled at the western side of Kennesaw Mountain. To the south, Confederate General John Bell Hood had prevented Sherman's favorite move: an end run around the Confederate line at Kolb's Farm. Now Sherman's massive army was sitting beneath the bastion of the mountain. Feeding the men was a logistical nightmare: deep in enemy territory, some of the troops were stationed up to 8 miles from the railhead. Sherman decided to launch an assault against a broad front stretching from the base of Big Kennesaw Mountain down to Cheatham Hill. He hoped to find a hole in the Confederate line—an improbable situation, given that his adversary was General Joseph Johnston, an expert at defense.

As dawn broke on June 27, 1864, the Union Army began a coordinated attack against

i KEY AT-A-GLANCE INFORMATION

LENGTH: 5.6 miles

CONFIGURATION: Balloon

DIFFICULTY: Easy

SCENERY: Civil War battlefield, with the massive Illinois Monument at the site of the heaviest fighting; entrenchments; John Ward Creek

EXPOSURE: Full sun–full shade

TRAFFIC: Moderate

TRAIL SURFACE: Gravel, compacted soil, pavement

WHEELCHAIR ACCESS: None

HIKING TIME: 3 hours

ACCESS: Trails: daily, year-round, sunrise–sunset; hours for visitor center and battlefield grounds vary depending on season (see nps .gov/kemo/planyourvisit/hours.htm for details); free

MAPS: At visitor center; USGS *Marietta*

FACILITIES: None

MORE INFO: 770-427-4686; nps.gov/kemo

SPECIAL COMMENTS: Throughout the hike you'll find interpretive markers with extensive information on the Battle of Kennesaw Mountain. The paved portion of the hike has both markers and monuments and runs just east of the actual battle line.

DISTANCE: 10.9 mile from I-75 North/I-285 Northwest

Directions ———————————————→

Take I-75 North to Exit 265/North Marietta Parkway, and turn left. Drive 2.1 miles and turn right on Polk Street. Drive 1.6 miles and turn right on Burnt Hickory Road NW. In 1 mile enter the parking lot, on the left.

GPS INFORMATION

N33° 57.800' W84° 35.623'
Burnt Hickory Rd. NW and
Old Mountain Rd. NW
Marietta, GA 30064

Cheatham Hill Trail

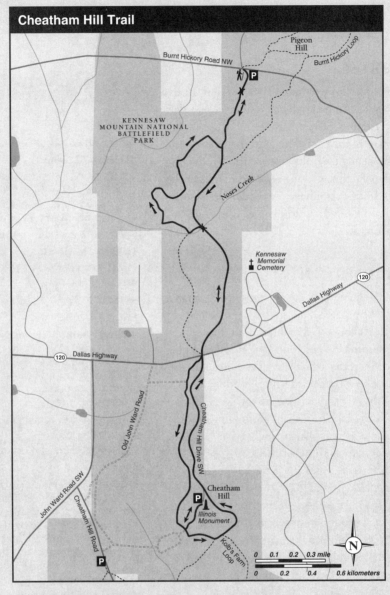

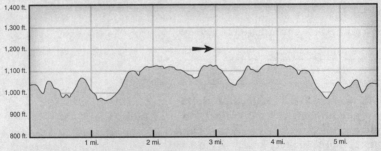

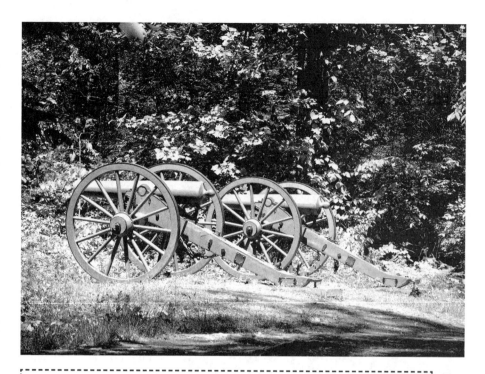

These cannons fired on Union troops as they advanced on Confederate forces at Cheatham Hill.

Confederate entrenchments, starting at Big Kennesaw and quickly moving south to Cheatham Hill. Our trail roughly follows just west of the main Confederate line from south of Pigeon Hill to Cheatham Hill. At the start of the hike, a field on the left just past a split rail fence is where Union soldiers attacked a Confederate skirmish line manned by the recently transferred Georgia 63rd Regiment. The skirmish line was designed to warn troops of the approaching enemy. However, the men of the 63rd stood their ground against an overwhelming force. As the Confederate line evaporated, other members of the regiment charged, only adding to the carnage. Still, as the Union line neared the Confederates, it slowed, eventually withdrawing because the position became unsustainable.

On the left, an interpretive marker bears additional information on the battle. After passing the first field, Cheatham Hill Trail begins climbing along a gravel road, with alternating cleared fields that tend to attract a wide variety of birds. The trail descends, quickly entering a pine forest (mostly shortleaf and loblolly) mixed with white oaks and American beeches—a typical second-growth forest of the Georgia Piedmont. At the start of the hike are some large post oaks; hickory joins the mix later on. At the bottom of the first hill, the road crosses a stone bridge and then climbs as it curves right, then left. At 0.3 mile the return footpath heads right, promptly followed by another side trail on the left after the last field. From this point to Dallas Highway, the wide road runs through the forest but is only occasionally shaded.

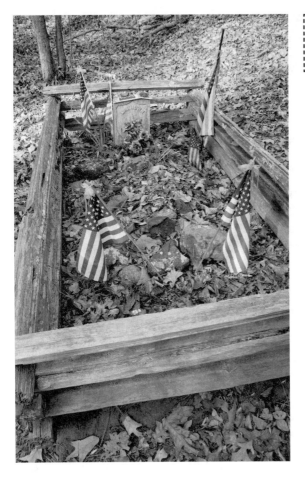

> No longer unknown: In 2009 the identity of the Union soldier buried here was confirmed.

At Noses Creek (named for a Cherokee chief who lived nearby), the roadway crosses the clear stream on a wooden bridge with no rail. Notice the stonework supports under the bridge, which obviously predate the current structure. Following the creek, the gravel road begins an extended moderate climb in full sun to Dallas Highway. Be careful when you cross the highway: the intersection has no traffic light, and drivers tend to speed.

After it crosses the road, the trail passes through a split rail fence, and immediately on your right a sign indicates that Cheatham Hill and Kolb's Farm are straight ahead. After a short stretch through a mostly pine forest, the trail breaks into the full sun of an open field, 50–100 feet west of the paved-road entrance to Cheatham Hill. On the morning of June 27, 1864, there was fighting along a line between where the path and the road now run.

The trail dips to adjoin the paved road at an artillery battery at 2 miles, separated from traffic by a brown gate to prevent vehicular access. To the left is the Cheatham Hill parking lot—the path continues straight, and you soon reach an open field. At a four-way intersection in the middle of the field, turn left and climb to the Illinois Monument, a large, bold memorial to Union General George Thomas's men, who were ordered to charge Cheatham Hill. After climbing the steps and viewing the monument, circle to the left. Below the monument runs an improved tunnel, dug by Union soldiers who were trying to blow a hole in the Confederate line.

As you circle left of the monument, the path climbs to a series of Confederate entrenchments known as the Dead Angle. Hundreds of Union dead who had charged the Confederates lay strewn in front of the entrenchments, but the

Confederate line held, handing the Union Army its worst defeat of the Atlanta Campaign. At the top of the hill, turn left to follow the path along the entrenchments until you come to Mebane's Battery, an artillery position that anchored the right end of Confederate Corps Commander Benjamin Franklin Cheatham's line. The hill was named in his honor following the success of the Confederate Army.

Turn around, keeping the Illinois Monument to your right as you follow the footpath left along the ridge. At the end of the ridge, the trail begins an extended moderate descent, passing a Union soldier's grave that was discovered in 1938 by Civilian Conservation Corps workers who were improving the area. The headstone has long read UNKNOWN, but in 2009, after five years of researching burial records in Georgia, Illinois, and Washington, D.C., an amateur historian and park volunteer named Brad Quinlin identified the soldier as Private Mark Carr.

At 2.8 miles Cheatham Hill Trail turns left, briefly joining Kolb's Farm Loop (see page 103) for 0.1 mile as it continues to descend. At the second intersection, Kolb's Farm Trail turns right and Cheatham Hill goes straight, quickly curving left and beginning a moderate climb to a parking lot at 3.1 miles. From here, follow the paved road, which bears right, and walk past a series of interpretive markers and monuments before you cross Dallas Highway.

After crossing the bridge over Noses Creek, turn left on a compacted-dirt path, which enters the full shade of a diverse hardwood forest that runs between the creek on the left and a forested wetlands on the right. At 4.6 miles the trail turns right and begins to climb into the watershed of Noses Creek on a good thigh burner to the top of a knoll. From here the trail begins a series of easy ups and downs; turn left on the main trunk at 5.3 miles to return to the trailhead.

17 HERITAGE PARK TRAIL

KEY AT-A-GLANCE INFORMATION

LENGTH: 3.5 miles round-trip

CONFIGURATION: Out-and-back

DIFFICULTY: Easy

SCENERY: This trail affords great riverside views most of the way, rising near the end to a beautiful "above it all" vista. Historical buildings stand near the trail.

EXPOSURE: Shaded except for the initial 0.3 mile, which is fully exposed

TRAFFIC: Moderate

TRAIL SURFACE: Gravel turning to packed dirt at the end; boardwalk over wetlands

WHEELCHAIR ACCESS: None

HIKING TIME: 2.5 hours

ACCESS: Daily, year-round, sunrise–sunset; free

MAPS: USGS *Mableton*

MORE INFO: 770-528-8810; prca .cobbcountyga.gov/parksh-m.htm

FACILITIES: Restrooms at visitor center; picnic tables along the hike

SPECIAL COMMENTS: This area developed into an industrial center because of water power and the nearby Western and Atlantic Railroad. The Heritage Park Trail connects to the Silver Comet Trail at the Concord Woolen Mill ruins.

DISTANCE: 8 miles from I-75 North/I-285 Northwest

GPS INFORMATION

N33° 50.338' W84° 32.5438'

60 Fontaine Rd. SE
Mableton, GA 30126

IN BRIEF

This historic road explores a portion of Confederate General Joseph Johnston's Smyrna Line and the remains of an old woolen mill. Hikers can view Ruff's Mill and continue on to see Concord Covered Bridge.

DESCRIPTION

From the parking lot, walk toward the stone-and-wood interpretive center. Here you'll find detailed information on the historic sites along the trail, along with a viewing platform that overlooks the wetland marsh formed by Nickajack Creek. From the building, walk to the northwest corner of the parking area, where the trail enters the woods and gradually descends a compacted-soil path. After an S-curve at the start of the treadway, two immense beech trees on either side of the trail shade the area.

The path gradually drops to a marsh traversed by a wooden boardwalk. It's easy to spot various small wetland birds here. About 200 feet farther along, a more substantial iron bridge with wooden planking carries you across Nickajack Creek. Look left as you cross, and you'll see water cascading over shoals. Immediately after you cross this bridge, turn left at an unmarked intersection of four trails.

Directions ⟶

Take I-285 South to Exit 16/South Atlanta Road, and turn right. Drive 0.4 mile and turn left on Cumberland Parkway, which becomes the East–West Connector after 0.6 mile. Drive a total of 3 miles on Cumberland/East–West and turn left on Fontaine Road SE. Drive 0.5 mile and make a right into the parking lot. Follow the parking lot around to the far side of the visitor center.

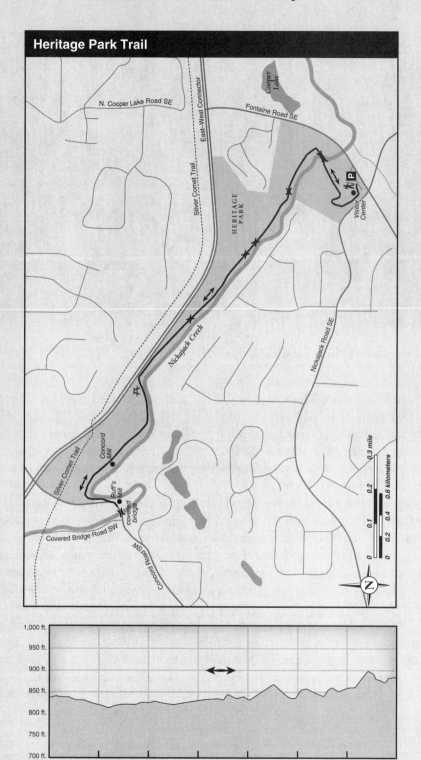

Heritage Park Trail

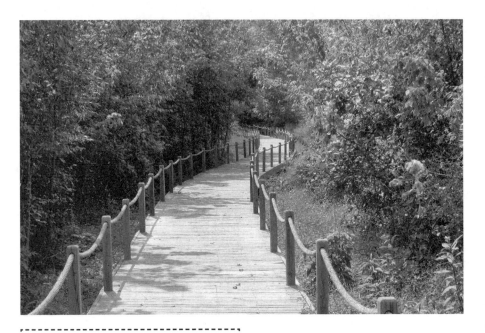

Boardwalks abound on the trail in Heritage Park.

Now a gravel road, the trail begins to parallel Nickajack Creek, on your left. Following the Battle of Kennesaw Mountain, Confederate General Joseph Johnston pulled back to a secondary defensive position known as the Smyrna Line, the southern end of which was formed by Nickajack Creek. Soldiers stationed on this part of the trail on July 3, 1864, came under artillery fire in the morning. This was the only fighting in this vicinity.

The first in a series of scenic creekside vistas comes into view at 0.4 mile. Photographers will want to get here before noon for the best pictures. Shortly past the scenic view, houses are visible across the creek and up a hill. At 0.5 mile the trail crosses the first of a string of small wooden bridges across tributaries of Nickajack Creek. Immediately after the first bridge, a side trail leads right. The bridge at 1.1 miles is longer than the others, spanning a creek, a wetland area, and another creek. On an early-fall morning, you may see a number of large waterfowl in this area.

About 0.2 mile after the wetlands, the pathway turns sharply left and the traffic noise grows very loud. At this point, the East–West Connector, a major Cobb County thoroughfare, is up the embankment to the right. A few steps past the turn is a picnic table, and just beyond that is an excellent view of the creek. The far riverbank is a wall of river-worn granite, common in the Georgia Piedmont. As you continue down the treadway, the traffic noise subsides. At 1.6 miles the historic woolen mill comes into view.

Water from Nickajack Creek powered the Concord Woolen Mill, a three-story building made of fieldstone and cement. Today only part of the structure remains. Built before the Civil War by Robert Daniel and Martin Ruff, the mill produced wool for the Confederacy and was among Sherman's targets during the Atlanta Campaign. Union soldiers destroyed it in 1864 shortly after they captured it. Following the war, the mill was rebuilt. In 1872 industrialist Seaborn Love and others purchased the mill and a portion of the surrounding land, which included housing for mill workers.

By 1916 the property had been sold to Annie Johnson, a Rome, Georgia, social activist who wanted to revitalize the mill by bringing in Russian Jewish immigrants who needed work. Unfortunately, her plan failed; the mill was abandoned and fell into disrepair. When the East–West Connector and the nearby Silver Comet Trail were built, metal supports were added to what remained of the building to ensure that blasting would not further damage the walls. Take time to explore the mill and a nearby outbuilding.

Returning to the path, you'll find two unmarked paved trails heading right as you pass the mill. These connect Heritage Park to the paved, mixed-use Silver Comet Trail. As you continue, the path rises slowly and steadily; a number of side trails lead both left and right. At 1.7 miles there is a long-distance view from the trail, now 100 feet above Nickajack Creek. Five hundred feet farther on, the trail makes a hard left turn and begins an easy descent to Ruff's Mill and Concord Bridge.

Known as Daniel and Ruff Mill when it was built before the Civil War, the mill was known simply as Ruff's Mill by the time Sherman's troops arrived in 1864. Unlike the Concord Woolen Mill, Ruff's gristmill survived the Yankee invasion and prospered after the war, eventually being sold and run as Martin's Feed and Grain. When owner Asbury Martin left, he moved lock, stock, and millworks to another site—all that's left are the mill building and the miller's house, both of which are privately owned.

At the roadway, turn left and walk down about 100 feet to the Concord Covered Bridge. One of the shorter remaining covered bridges in Georgia, this one spans 130 feet between two stone abutments. Two modern concrete piers give the heavily used bridge additional support in the center. Built in 1872, the structure features queen post trusses and was completely renovated in 1983.

An earlier bridge spanned Nickajack Creek in this spot as early as 1848. On July 3, 1864, Confederate soldiers stationed on high ground just south of the bridge came under Union attack. They were driven from the ridge, crossed Concord Bridge, and re-formed a line on the north side of Nickajack Creek. The following day, the Battle of Ruff's Mill was fought about 1.5 miles from the gristmill.

Turn around and retrace your steps to your car.

NEARBY ACTIVITIES

The paved multiuse **Silver Comet Trail** (see Hike 13, page 70, and Hike 25, page 124), which connects to Heritage Park at Concord Woolen Mill, is open daily, sunrise–sunset.

18 IRON HILL LOOP

**KEY AT-A-GLANCE
INFORMATION**

LENGTH: 3.8 miles

CONFIGURATION: Loop

DIFFICULTY: Easy

SCENERY: Lakeshore, historic
open-pit iron mines

EXPOSURE: Partial shade, some
full sun

TRAFFIC: Light

TRAIL SURFACE: Gravel

HIKING TIME: 2 hours

ACCESS: Daily, year-round, 7 a.m.–
sunset; $5 state-park fee

MAPS: Red Top Mountain State Park,
USGS *Allatoona Dam*

MORE INFO: 770-975-0055;
gastateparks.org/redtopmountain

FACILITIES: Limited on trail; park has
restrooms, picnic tables, and
camping.

SPECIAL COMMENTS: Although this is
listed as a multiuse trail, a majority of
the users are hikers.

DISTANCE: 24.5 miles from I-75
North/I-285 Northwest

GPS INFORMATION

N34° 8.384' W84° 42.034'

IN BRIEF

Enjoy a great family hike on a wide, lightly used trail with little elevation change. Two open-pit iron mines lie along the route.

DESCRIPTION

Metals were an early driving force in the settling of Georgia. Among the more important native metals are iron, gold, and bauxite (aluminum ore). The state's iron heritage is celebrated at Red Top Mountain State Park with the Iron Hill Loop, a multiuse gravel trail that explores two open-pit iron mines, one dating from the 1830s and another that operated at the turn of the 20th century. The name of the park refers to the color of the earth in these mountains—a dark red that indicates the presence of iron.

From the trailhead at the far end of the parking lot, the trail drops a few steps to the loop. You may hike the loop in either direction, but this description assumes that you're walking the trail clockwise. Turn left to follow the pathway as it drops almost imperceptibly through a mixed forest of pines and hardwoods including oaks, maples, hickory trees, and sweet gums.

At 0.1 mile a tributary begins to form on your right, and as the trail drops slowly, the tributary drops quickly until a large valley has formed. The trail leaves the valley and comes into full sun at 0.2 mile, cutting across Iron Hill Cove Road at an angle. The easy descent

----

Directions ————————————————————→

Take I-75 North to Exit 285/Red Top Mountain Road. Turn right at the end of the ramp and drive 2.9 miles to the marked entrance to the Iron Hill parking area.

Iron Hill Loop

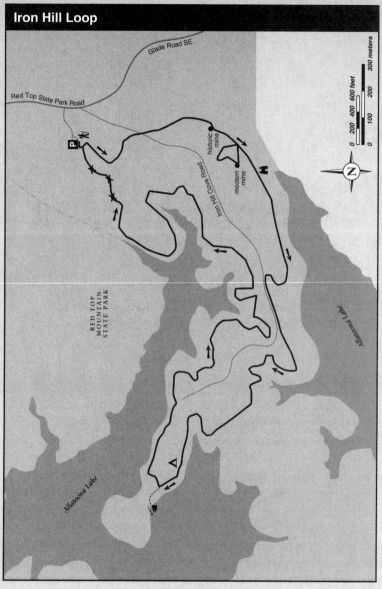

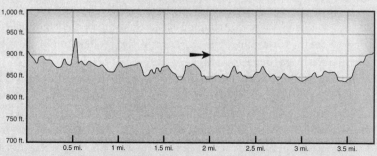

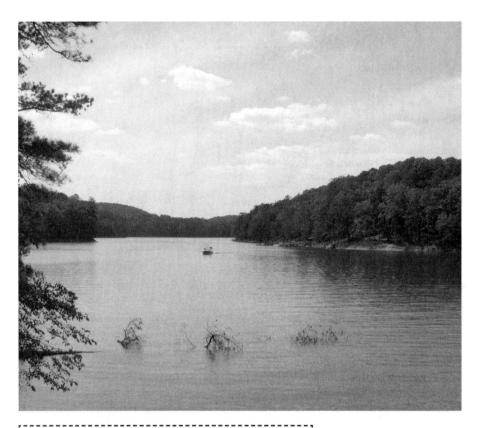

Much of the Iron Hill Loop runs alongside beautiful Lake Allatoona.

continues across the road. About 0.2 mile later, the older, historic iron mine is on the right, appearing to be an overgrown road leading into a large bowl. Note that the road in the mine is level and free of rocks and roots, thus making it easy to cart large amounts of dirt from the open pit to a furnace (such as nearby Cooper's Furnace), where it could easily be converted into pig iron for shipping. Pig iron would then be further processed to remove impurities at one of the foundries that used iron from Cass County (now Bartow County).

You come to a second mine, commonly called the modern mine because it operated into the early 1900s, through a large clearing on the right at 0.7 mile. Unlike that of the historic mine, the iron ore in the modern mine is visible and easily identifiable by its deep-red color.

A tributary of the Etowah River forms Lake Allatoona, on the left side of the trail as it descends gradually from the site of the modern mine. As the path bears right, it winds through an old campground complete with an unused boat ramp. Proposed in the 1930s, the construction of Lake Allatoona began in 1941, only to be delayed by World War II. Built as a watershed lake, Allatoona was designed to hold back the waters of the Etowah, which had regularly flooded the

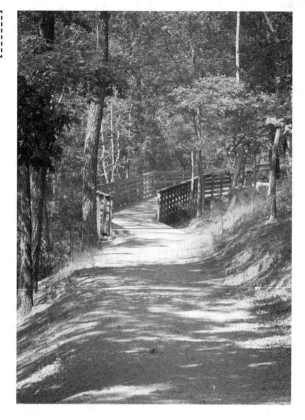

One of the trail's three bridges, which serve to protect sensitive wetlands

city of Rome. During the fall and winter, when rainfall is at its lowest, the lake is partially drained. Spring rains fill the lake instead of inundating the relatively flat land of the river valley. In 1947, only months before the dam was complete, the Etowah flooded for the last time.

Over the next 2 miles the pathway follows the lakeshore, leaving it only occasionally. At 1.3 miles the trail turns left and crosses a peninsula, rejoining the lakeshore 0.4 mile later. Around the 2-mile mark, the trail crosses a much smaller peninsula, quickly rejoining the lakeshore for another 1.6 miles. Now in a quiet cove, the pathway leaves the lake for the last time at 3.6 miles, beginning an easy extended climb. Three bridges carry hikers across sensitive wetland areas at 3.7 miles before returning to the trailhead.

NEARBY ACTIVITIES

Mark Anthony Cooper, an early supporter of railroads, built an iron furnace near the Lake Allatoona Dam. To get there, take Red Top Mountain Road out of the park and past I-75 to US 41. Turn right on US 41 and drive 2.1 miles to Old River Road; then turn right and drive 0.3 mile to the **Cooper's Furnace Day Use Area** (free admission; closed December 1–March 1).

The Iron Hill Loop makes up only a fraction of the 16-plus miles of hiking trails in Red Top Mountain State Park. The **Homestead Trail** starts at the visitor center and explores 5.7 miles of lake coves and mountaintops (see the second edition of this book for a full profile). The **Lakeside Trail** explores an arm of the lake and visits a homestead (the Vaughn Cabin).

19 KENNESAW MOUNTAIN: BURNT HICKORY LOOP

KEY AT-A-GLANCE INFORMATION

LENGTH: 5.9 miles

CONFIGURATION: Loop

DIFFICULTY: Hard

SCENERY: 360-degree views, including Atlanta and Stone Mountain to the east; Pine Mountain, Lost Mountain, and the mountains of Georgia's Valley and Ridge section to the west and northwest; and the Allatoona Mountains to the north

EXPOSURE: Mostly shaded, except on peaks, where the trail gets full sun

TRAFFIC: Heavy

TRAIL SURFACE: Rocky soil on the mountains, gravel and compacted soil on the return trip

WHEELCHAIR ACCESS: None

HIKING TIME: 2.5 hours

ACCESS: See page 85 for details.

MAPS: Available at visitor center and Marietta Welcome Center (770-429-1115); USGS *Marietta*

MORE INFO: 770-427-4686; nps.gov/kemo

FACILITIES: Visitor center–museum with restrooms and water. A kind resident regularly leaves a bucket of water for dogs along the trail on the return trip to the visitor center.

SPECIAL COMMENTS: This was Georgia's first Important Birding Area.

DISTANCE: 11.4 miles from I-75 North/I-285 Northwest

GPS INFORMATION

N33° 58.970' W84° 34.6957'

900 Kennesaw Mountain Dr.
Kennesaw, GA 30152

IN BRIEF

The Burnt Hickory Loop is the most challenging trail in this book, and one of the most rewarding in the Atlanta area.

DESCRIPTION

On July 27, 1864, Union General William Tecumseh Sherman engaged Confederate forces under the command of General Joseph Johnston along a 5-mile front on the west side of Kennesaw Mountain, Little Kennesaw Mountain, Pigeon Hill, and Cheatham Hill. This battle marked the worst defeat of the Union Army during the Atlanta Campaign. Kennesaw Mountain National Battlefield Park commemorates the fight.

The first mile of the Burnt Hickory Loop, known as Kennesaw Mountain Trail, climbs 600 feet to the top of Big Kennesaw (the mountain's local name), following a combination of gravel roads and compacted-dirt paths. Keen eyes will spot Civil War–era entrenchments over the first 0.5 mile of the footpath. A historic road crosscuts a modern gravel road at 0.3 mile. Confederate forces used this road to drag artillery to the mountaintop. For a scenic view at 0.6 mile, take a brief walk down an

----

Directions ⟶

Take I-75 North to Exit 267B/US 41/Cobb Parkway. At the end of the circle, merge onto the Canton Road Connector. Drive 1.1 miles and turn right on the Church Street Extension. Drive 0.6 mile and turn left on Old US 41. Drive 1.2 miles and, at the traffic light, turn left on Stilesboro Road NW. Make an immediate left into the Kennesaw Mountain National Battlefield Park parking lot. Walk toward a brown kiosk between the visitor center and Kennesaw Mountain Drive.

Kennesaw Mountain: Burnt Hickory Loop

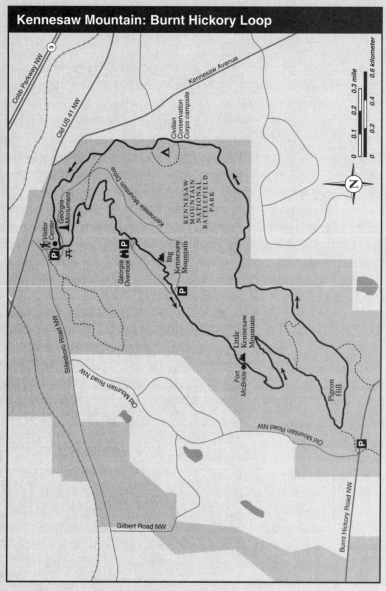

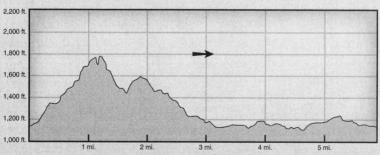

unmarked path on the left. On clear days, the Georgia Dome and the "King and Queen" towers of the Concourse Corporate Center in Sandy Springs are visible from this vantage point.

The trail climbs a set of iron-railed concrete steps and turns left on a sidewalk. As you follow the sidewalk to the right, the view to your left opens for an expansive long-distance vista of Atlanta. (On one memorable day while we were admiring the view, an American bald eagle skirted the mountain 40 feet below.) It was from this site that Sherman first observed Atlanta, then home to a mere 10,000 residents. It had taken him less than two months to move 60 miles from Ringgold to Marietta, but it would him take more than two months to move the 12 miles from Marietta to Atlanta.

As you continue on the sidewalk, steps leave to the left; climb them to the massive Georgia Overlook. Dedicated on the 100th anniversary of the Battle of Kennesaw Mountain, the structure honors all Georgia-born generals who fought in that conflict. Continue straight ahead to reach the top of Kennesaw Mountain. Although this trail sees heavy use, you won't encounter as many hikers past the Georgia Monument as you will earlier in the hike.

From the memorial, the footpath, which is initially paved, quickly reverts to a rocky, root-strewn dirt trail as it passes Civil War–era cannon along the ridgelike mountaintop. The men stationed here saw the 100,000-man Union Army fill the valley beneath them as Sherman moved into position for battle. At 0.9 mile the path breaks into full sun as it reaches the crest of Kennesaw Mountain and then begins a moderate-to-difficult descent to Kennesaw Mountain Drive. Almost immediately, a side trail leads left. Continue straight along the scenic ridge of Big Kennesaw. At 1.4 miles, the trail descends stairs to Kennesaw Mountain Drive, which you can follow back to the visitor center for a total hike of 2.4 miles.

Across the road are a small parking lot and an interpretive sign telling the story of Little Kennesaw Mountain, which looms before and below the scenic overlook. The footpath descends a flight of concrete steps, joining a rocky dirt trail at the bottom. The rocky soil here stunts tree growth, so you'll see massive post oaks and shortleaf pines that are only 30 feet tall. At 1.6 miles the trail reaches the gap between Big and Little Kennesaw and begins a moderate-to-difficult climb to the top of Little Kennesaw, alternating between sections of partial shade and full sun.

Four cannons that occupy the top of Little Kennesaw (1.9 miles) at Civil War–era Fort McBride mark the start of the most difficult portion of the trail. The National Park Service has repeatedly reworked the steep-sided and rock-strewn trail in this area to make it easier to navigate, albeit with limited success. In 2005 the trail was completely reblazed and marked, with only a few switchbacks. A pine blowdown that is slowly being overgrown at 2.7 miles marks the gap between Little Kennesaw and Pigeon Hill.

Massive boulders atop extended sheets of granite form the top of Pigeon Hill, the only area on Burnt Hickory Loop that saw extensive fighting during the Battle of Kennesaw Mountain. Union troops were repulsed before reaching the

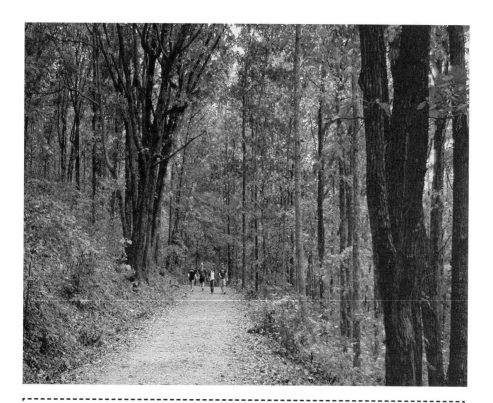

This switchback provides a level respite from the steep climb up Kennesaw Mountain. Sweeping views from the mountaintop await those who complete the trek.

top of the mountain. The hill drew its name from the passenger pigeon, a now-extinct bird that once nested here, blackening the skies during migrations. At 3 miles, turn left at a brown sign that reads simply EAST. This marks the return trail to the visitor center.

Descending gently over the next 0.3 mile, the trail swings left and joins a gravel road at a signed intersection. Turn left to follow the relatively level gravel road through a second-growth hardwood forest punctuated with loblolly pines and native magnolias (Southern grandiflora). At 4.2 miles you'll see houses to the right; a few steps farther, a wooden fence prevents you from accidentally walking into somebody's backyard. Along this fence, a caring soul leaves a plastic bucket with water for thirsty dogs.

After the fence ends at 4.8 miles, the gravel road continues to the marked Kennesaw Mountain Civilian Conservation Corps (CCC) campsite to the left, just past a gravel road that also heads left. The men who lived at this camp made many of the initial improvements to the park and discovered the grave of a Union soldier at Cheatham Hill (see Hike 16, page 85). A few steps past the level campsite are the remains of the headquarters building. Almost nothing remains of the CCC camp, whose modular buildings were transported to house workers elsewhere.

Leaving the gravel road at 5.1 miles, the trail bears left, then right at a map stand 0.1 mile ahead, continuing past a blowdown courtesy of the southern pine beetle. As traffic noise increases, the trail bears left, entering full sun in an open field at 5.7 miles. The traffic light at the park entrance is off to the right, and the visitor center comes into view shortly as the trail slowly curves left alongside an open field. Just before the visitor center, you'll see the Georgia Monument on the left, across the paved Kennesaw Mountain Drive.

NEARBY ACTIVITIES

Marietta offers some of the best antiques shopping in the state, around the antebellum square 1 mile east of the visitor center. Near the historic depot downtown are the **Marietta Museum of History** (1 Depot St.; 770-794-5710; **mariettahistory.org**) and the **Marietta Gone with the Wind Museum: Scarlett on the Square** (18 Whitlock Ave.; 770-794-5576; **gwtwmarietta.com**).

KOLB'S FARM LOOP

IN BRIEF

The trail explores the north end of a Civil War battlefield. It's also designed to attract birds, from the common yellow finch to the stunning scarlet tanager.

DESCRIPTION

Kennesaw Mountain National Battlefield Park was the first site in Georgia to be designated as an Important Bird Area. Migratory birds use the park extensively during the fall and spring, as do year-round species. Among the birds you may spot along the trail are warblers, thrushes, and tanagers. Larger birds include orioles, rails, and hawks.

Turn right on a gravel road, passing around a brown gate that excludes vehicular traffic, and immediately begin a short, moderate climb to the trail's high point, a ridge some 30 feet above and 600 feet behind the parking lot. On the east side of this ridge, on July 27, 1864, about 8,000 Union troops under the command of General George Thomas began to assemble for a frontal assault on a heavily fortified Confederate line at Cheatham Hill (see Hike 16, page 85), about 0.4 mile due

- -

Directions ──────────→

Take I-75 North to Exit 265/North Marietta Parkway, and turn left. Drive 2.1 miles and turn right on Polk Street. Drive 1.9 miles and turn right on Whitlock Avenue/Dallas Highway. Drive 1.3 miles and turn left on John Ward Road SW. Drive 0.6 mile and turn left on Cheatham Hill Road. Drive 0.4 mile to the parking lot, on the right. After you park, walk to the south end of the lot on a compacted-soil trail to reach a large rock in a gravel road: this marks the start and end of Kolb's Farm Loop.

KEY AT-A-GLANCE INFORMATION

LENGTH: 5.5 miles

CONFIGURATION: Loop

DIFFICULTY: Moderate

SCENERY: Portions of a Civil War battlefield, prime creek views

EXPOSURE: Alternating full sun and full shade on the west side, mostly full shade on the east side

TRAFFIC: Heavy; horses allowed on portions of the trail

TRAIL SURFACE: Compacted soil, some gravel

WHEELCHAIR ACCESS: None

HIKING TIME: 3 hours

ACCESS: Trails: daily, year-round, sunrise–sunset; hours for visitor center and battlefield grounds vary depending on season (see nps.gov/ kemo/planyourvisit/hours.htm for details); free

MAPS: Available at visitor center; USGS *Marietta*

MORE INFO: 770-427-4686; nps.gov/kemo

FACILITIES: Water on trail near Kolb's Farm

SPECIAL COMMENTS: Kennesaw Mountain National Battlefield Park was Georgia's first Important Birding Area. The park maintains 18 miles of interpretive trails.

DISTANCE: 12.5 miles from I-75 North/I-285 Northwest

GPS INFORMATION

N33° 55.948' W84° 36.269'

Kolb's Farm Loop

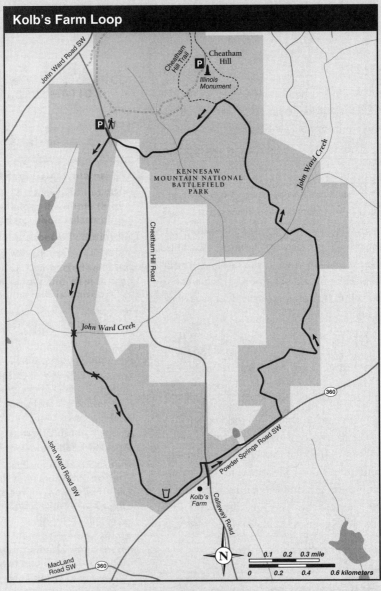

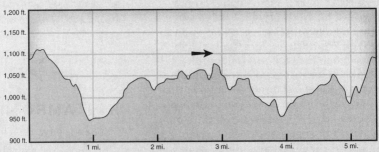

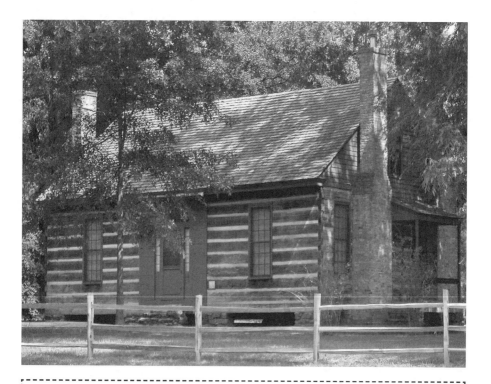

Built in 1836, historic Kolb's Farm was used by the Union Army as a headquarters during the Civil War. As many as 20 buildings, including this dogtrot cabin, stood within the current park boundary.

east of this spot. The ensuing battle was the Union Army's worst defeat during the Atlanta Campaign.

The trail levels and begins to descend through a second-growth forest composed mostly of red maples and several varieties of pines, with native dogwoods especially visible alongside the road. At 0.8 mile the trail begins a moderate-to-difficult descent to John Ward Creek as the forest becomes mostly pine, including a number of tall, ramrod-straight loblollies. About halfway down the hill is the first cleared field, designed to attract birds. It's not unusual to see at least a couple of birders on the west side of the loop trail.

As it approaches the creek, Kolb's Farm Loop begins to level and a gravel road heads right at just under 1 mile. This road is a walk-around for horses, which would destroy the wooden-planked boardwalk ahead. About 0.1 mile later, the pathway becomes a boardwalk a few inches above a marshy area surrounding John Ward Creek. After crossing the creek and more marshland, the boardwalk ends and the gravel horse path returns. The smell of honeysuckle wafts through the air, and you can see homes off to the right.

Approaching 1.2 miles, the trail in this area has been reworked, so mind the markings and continue on the newer trail, straight ahead, skirting the end of a field. As the trail curves right, a large stand of bamboo grows on the right. Returning to the forest at 1.5 miles, the loop begins a 0.3-mile climb. At the peak of this hill,

Kolb's Farm Trail curves slowly right, and the sound of traffic noise grows louder, continuing for the next mile as the pathway parallels Powder Springs Road.

Undergrowth increases and Virginia creeper and wild grape abound. A working water fountain on the right, at 2.4 miles, is ready to quench the thirst of hikers and dogs. Immediately after passing the water fountain, you can see the road and a subdivision across the street. These homes were built on the site of major fighting in the Battle of Kolb's Farm. A few steps farther on is the first view of the farm itself.

Peter Valentine Kolb came to Cobb County in the 1830s. He built a dogtrot cabin, composed of an open center hall with four rooms, two on either side. Kolb was wealthy compared to others in the area—he had enough money to build four fireplaces. Sometime after 1845 he enclosed the dogtrot, now an open center hall. In the early 1960s, the National Park Service restored the cabin to its appearance at the time of the Battle of Kennesaw Mountain. At this point the loop trail begins to skirt the northern edge of the battlefield.

After a gravel road heads right, the pathway reaches Cheatham Hill Road. Turn right at the paved road and cross Powder Springs Road at the traffic light. Continue to a small parking lot just east of Kolb's Farm. Historical markers describe the battle and the house that stands here, in addition to a small family cemetery. Do not approach the house, which is a private residence.

Return to the light, cross Callaway Road, and then turn left. Cross Powder Springs Road, continue north from the road, and turn right onto a stone-walled walkway that leads to an open field. The path roughly parallels an entrenchment held by Union troops during the battle. These men fired on Confederate General John Bell Hood's right flank as he attacked the Union's Army of the Ohio, under the command of General John Schofield, on June 22, 1864. Historical markers on the right side of the trail use maps to tell the story of the battle in depth.

Turning left at 2.7 miles, the trail becomes forested and reenters heavy shade. Signs indicate that the trail goes to the visitor center and Cheatham Hill, guiding hikers to make the turn. After reaching a ridgetop at 2.9 miles, the trail begins an extended moderate descent to John Ward Creek. You'll see houses on the left 0.2 mile later; then you'll enter a steep-sided ravine with large trees.

After the loop trail narrows and rounds a large granite boulder, it becomes heavily rooted and rocky. To cross a ravine, Kolb's Farm Loop makes a short, steep descent to a stone-and-dirt bridge, then quickly ascends before continuing to John Ward Creek.

The pathway turns to gravel roadbed at 3.5 miles, and you'll occasionally see houses on the right. The final descent to John Ward Creek traverses a valley. At 3.9 miles the trail splits. On the left the footpath climbs a low ridge and parallels the second trail, which runs adjacent to the river. If the river is running high, the trail to the right will be blocked. After 0.2 mile the trails rejoin on the ridge. If you took the trail to the right, turn right at the three-way intersection.

At John Ward Creek, two bridges stand about 100 feet apart to take you across. After the second bridge, a trail enters from the right. Over the next 0.5 mile, you'll encounter four Y-intersections—always take the trail to the left as you follow a wide, roadlike path. At 4.8 miles, cross an earthwork that was held by Maney's Brigade during the Battle of Kennesaw Mountain. Turn left when the trail reaches a T-intersection 0.2 mile later. From this point on, several side trails on the right lead to Cheatham Hill. After crossing a stone bridge at 5.1 miles, the trail begins climbing to the Kolb's Farm Loop parking area, curving left and then bearing right as it leaves the roadbed 500 feet after the bridge. The final moderate ascent brings you to Cheatham Hill Road. Cross the street and turn right to return to your car.

NEARBY ACTIVITIES

Kennesaw Mountain National Battlefield Park has a museum discussing the battles fought in or near what is now the park, in addition to describing the entire Atlanta Campaign. In the visitor center, the museum is open daily, 8:30 a.m.–5 p.m., except January 1, Thanksgiving, and December 25.

21   PICKETT'S MILL TRAIL

KEY AT-A-GLANCE INFORMATION

LENGTH: 3.1 miles

CONFIGURATION: Loop

DIFFICULTY: Moderate

SCENERY: Multiple creekside settings with cascades

EXPOSURE: Full shade for most of the trail

TRAFFIC: Moderate

TRAIL SURFACE: Compacted soil, gravel, historic roads

WHEELCHAIR ACCESS: None

HIKING TIME: 2 hours

ACCESS: Thursday–Saturday, 9 a.m.–5 p.m.; closed January 1, Thanksgiving, and December 25; $3–$5 entrance fee

MAPS: Map with marker descriptions and troop movements available for purchase at visitor center; USGS *Dallas*

MORE INFO: 770-443-7850; gastate parks.org/pickettsmillbattlefield

FACILITIES: Visitor center with restrooms and a small museum; picnic tables

SPECIAL COMMENTS: This 765-acre park features Civil War earthworks and 4 miles of hiking trails. The visitor center shows an excellent video presentation on the Battle of Pickett's Mill.

DISTANCE: 31.5 miles from I-75 North/I-285 Northwest

GPS INFORMATION

N33° 58.429' W84° 45.551'
4432 Mt. Tabor Church Rd.
Dallas, GA 30157

IN BRIEF

This trail explores the site of a decisive Confederate victory during the Atlanta Campaign, then takes hikers down the path Union soldiers trod as they advanced down a valley toward the Confederate Army's right flank. Most of the entrenchments were built after the battle.

DESCRIPTION

The Battle of Pickett's Mill was a mistake. General William Tecumseh Sherman had hit on a successful plan—engage the enemy while outflanking them—and tried to duplicate it here in the rolling hills south of Kingston, Georgia. Union troops had engaged the Confederates at New Hope Church, west of Pickett's Mill. Sherman ordered General George Thomas to find the left end of the Confederate line and outflank Confederate General Joseph Johnston once again. Thomas and a subordinate, General O. O. Howard, mistook a salient in the Confederate line for

Directions ———————————→

Take I-75 North to Exit 277/GA 92 (Acworth). At the end of the ramp, turn left and immediately move to the right lane. Drive 0.3 mile to the traffic light; then turn right on Lake Acworth Drive and follow it 3.8 miles to Cobb Parkway. Turn right and move into the left lane. Continue 1.5 miles and then turn left on Dallas–Acworth Highway. Drive 6.3 miles and turn left on Mt. Tabor Church Road. Drive 0.5 mile and turn left at the marked entrance to Pickett's Mill Battlefield Historic Site. The visitor center is 0.6 mile down the road, on the left. Park and then walk to the entrance of the blue wood-and-stone visitor center. After paying the $3–$5 entrance fee, exit the other side of the building and follow a concrete path to the trailhead, a wooden-deck overlook.

Pickett's Mill Trail

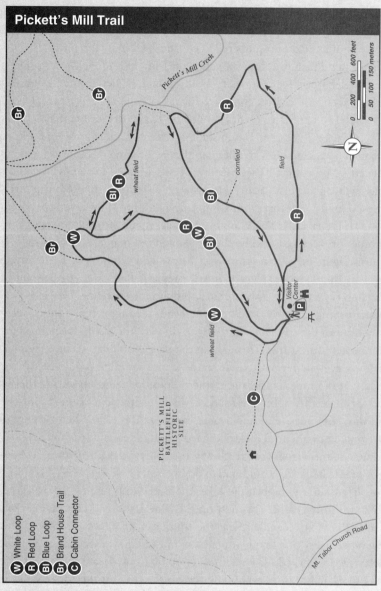

Pickett's Mill Creek

cornfield

field

wheat field

wheat field

Visitor Center

PICKETT'S MILL
BATTLEFIELD
HISTORIC
SITE

Mt. Tabor Church Road

0   200   400   600 feet
0   50   100   150 meters

W White Loop
R Red Loop
Bl Blue Loop
Br Brand House Trail
C Cabin Connector

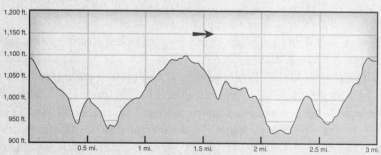

the end of the line and ordered an attack—against the best tactical commander in the Western Theater, Patrick Cleburne. Cleburne once defeated Sherman himself, although Sherman had outnumbered Cleburne 10 to 1 at the time.

Advancing under fire down a valley on May 27, 1864, Union soldiers were trapped by Cleburne's men. Some Yankees did take higher ground, eventually continuing the advance, but they too were forced back. A second wave of Union soldiers, intended to reinforce the first, ended up to the east of the main attack. After withstanding heavy losses, the Union soldiers retreated under cover of darkness. The loss was such a stinging blow to Sherman that he omitted it from his memoirs.

Pickett's Mill contains three separate trails—blazed in red, white, and blue—covering each of the historically important sites within the 765-acre park. This narrative combines the three trails into one hike. From the overlook, follow the Red Loop to the right. Quickly joining a gravel road, the trail descends through a mostly pine forest punctuated by the occasional red maple. After 0.1 mile the Red Loop turns right. Before the turn, just below you to the left, is the area where fighting was the heaviest. Here Confederates repelled three Yankee attacks, but there was no time for the Confederates to build a trench line.

After turning right, the Red Loop descends through a pine forest. Burn marks on the bottom of the trees have nothing to do with the Civil War but tell the story of a more recent forest fire. Throughout the park, you can see entrenchments near each of the developed trails. The first one is on the right, at 0.2 mile. A cornfield on the left, at 0.3 mile, marks the farthest Union penetration during the Battle of Pickett's Mill. At this point the road curves left into the cornfield and ends, but the pathway continues, entering a pine forest on the right side of the road. Less than 0.1 mile later, the trail makes a sharp left and descends to a bridge over a dry creek; then it turns rocky as it climbs to a low ridge through a forest of red maples, American beeches, and native dogwoods.

Just less than 1 mile into the hike, the Blue Loop rejoins the Red Loop, and the latter trail turns right. Turn left on the Blue Loop and continue an extended climb over the next 0.6 mile. Near the trail, at 1 mile, are the rifle pits that the Confederate cavalry quickly dug in an attempt to delay a secondary Union attack. The delay tactic worked—a combined force of Confederate infantry and cavalry had time to establish a line some 500 feet to the rear. As the trail climbs, it again passes through territory that Union soldiers held for some of the battle, then rejoins the Red Loop and continues past the overlook at the trailhead.

Now on the White Loop, the path curves right just past the visitor center. A few feet after the center and to the right, in a mostly pine forest, is a historic road. Off to the left are additional entrenchments. The gravel road continues downhill but gradually levels, coming to a side trail at 1.7 miles that rejoins the main trail 0.2 mile later. When you reach a Y-intersection at 2 miles, take the path to the left. Less than 100 feet on, the path makes a sharp right, entering the forest and leaving the gravel road at an AREA CLOSED sign. The path briefly descends to the site of a federal artillery emplacement.

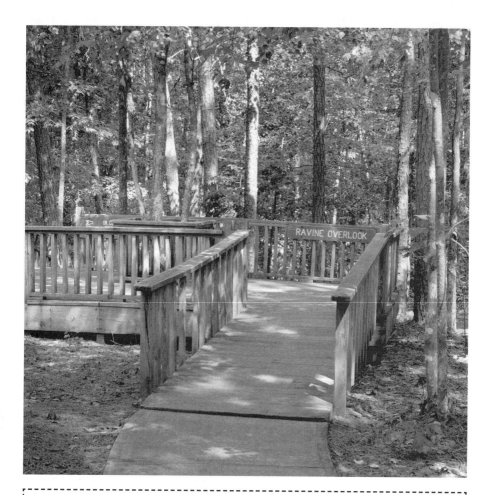

A peaceful overlook at Pickett's Mill confutes this Civil War battlefield's sobriquet, "Hell Hole." More than 2,000 men lost their lives here.

Turn around and retrace your steps to the Y. Turn left and follow the mostly level path 0.1 mile, where the White Loop heads right. Continue straight, descending easily to a road on the left—turn left even though that road continues straight. Now descending much more steeply, the trail enters Little Pumpkinvine Creek Valley, so called because the winding river resembles a pumpkin vine when viewed from above. The Georgia legislature officially renamed the stream Pickett's Mill Creek in the 1990s.

In this area, the Union assault formed late in the afternoon on May 27, 1864. Take a few minutes to enjoy the now-serene surroundings. Retrace your steps to the top of the hill and turn left on the combined red, white, and blue trails, where the trail enters the ravine. The next 0.5 mile takes hikers along the path that Union soldiers used to advance on Confederate positions in the vicinity of the visitor center. A relatively small number of Confederates, entrenched at the tops of the hills on either side, poured deadly fire on the advancing Yankees. Union

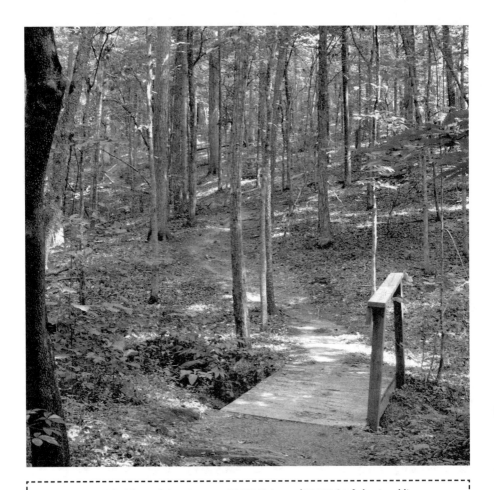

As you cross a creek at the park, imagine some 14,000 Union and 10,000 Confederate soldiers converging in this area for a night of battle. An eventual Confederate victory bought a costly one-week reprieve from the Union's advance on Atlanta.

commanders, who had charged the Confederate line three times, decided to dig in and hold their positions. Supporting drives did not weaken the Confederate line, and under cover of darkness the Yankees retreated.

As you leave the valley, the trailhead is directly in front of you.

NEARBY ACTIVITIES

The **Silver Comet Trail** (see Hike 13, page 70, and Hike 25, page 124) is 9 miles south of Pickett's Mill on GA 92. From the park, turn left on Mt. Tabor Church Road; then turn left on Due West Road, turn right on GA 92, and drive 7 miles.

PINE MOUNTAIN TRAIL: EAST LOOP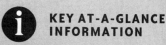

IN BRIEF

This loop trail offers additional hiking to Cooper's Furnace, Lake Allatoona Dam, and a US Army Corps of Engineers museum. The hike ascends from 800 feet of elevation at the trailhead to 1,562 feet of elevation at the David G. Archer Overlook.

DESCRIPTION

Not to be confused with the Pine Mountain Trail in F. D. Roosevelt State Park, south of Atlanta (see Hike 56, page 268), this Pine Mountain Trail is adjacent to Lake Allatoona, near Cartersville. From a map kiosk in the parking lot, the East Loop climbs to the intersection of the 0.6-mile Cooper's Furnace connector less than 0.1 mile into the hike. Head right and continue climbing to a marked three-way intersection. Bear right to hike the trail counterclockwise.

During the first 0.3 mile, the trail parallels GA 20 Spur but does not run close to it. As the path turns left and away from the road, it climbs to Whiskey Point, which according to local legend was the site of a moonshine operation in the 1950s. The return trail can be seen across the valley, especially if other hikers are on the trail.

Just a few steps before Whiskey Point, the trail begins to descend. The path then crosses a stream on a bridge, turns left, and crosses the same stream on a second bridge. Known as

---

Directions ⟶

Take I-75 North to Exit 290/GA 20. At the end of the ramp, turn right on GA 20. Take the first right onto GA 20 Spur and travel 3.2 miles to the parking area, just past Bartow Beach Road SE on the right.

KEY AT-A-GLANCE INFORMATION

LENGTH: 3 miles

CONFIGURATION: Loop

DIFFICULTY: Hard

SCENERY: Great views of the Etowah River Valley from the top of Pine Mountain

EXPOSURE: Partial shade–full sun

TRAFFIC: Light

TRAIL SURFACE: Gravel and compacted soil

HIKING TIME: 1.5 hours

ACCESS: Daily, year-round, sunrise–sunset; free

MAPS: USGS *Allatoona Dam*

MORE INFO: 770-387-5626; visitcartersvillega.org/na/hiking _and_geocacheing

FACILITIES: None

SPECIAL COMMENTS: This hike offers one of the best workouts in the Atlanta area.

DISTANCE: 37.6 miles from I-75 North/I-285 Northwest

GPS INFORMATION

N34° 10.617' W84° 44.228'

GA 20 Spur and Bartow Beach Rd. SE
Cartersville, GA 30121

Pine Mountain Trail: East Loop

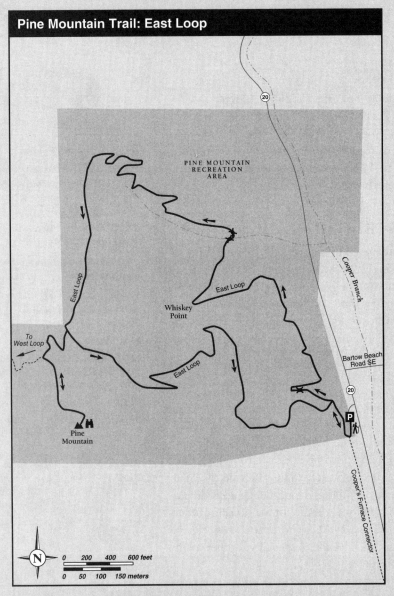

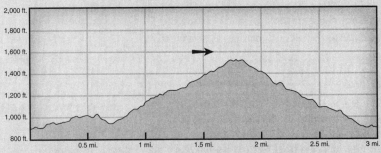

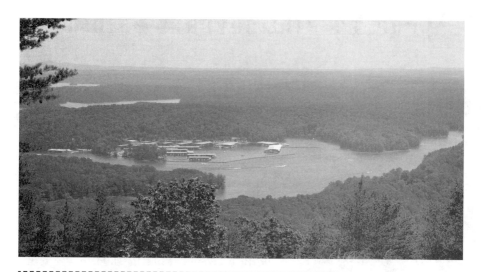

A scenic overlook bestows views of multiple arms of Lake Allatoona from the top of Pine Mountain.

Double Bridges, this area is a pleasant place to enjoy the surrounding hardwood forest. From here the trail rises easily until it curves right and then quickly jogs left near a low point, leaving the hardwoods (and the stream) at 0.7 mile. The forest quickly becomes only partially shaded by pine trees, and rock outcrops become more common. At 0.8 mile you reach the first in a series of switchbacks. These switchbacks carry hikers to the ridgeline at 1.1 miles.

As the final switchback turns left, the pathway climbs steadily as it runs below the ridge of Pine Mountain to a Y-intersection at 1.5 miles. Bear right at the Y and continue climbing 0.3 mile on this trail until it enters full sun at the David G. Archer Overlook atop Pine Mountain. Archer, who serves as Cartersville's city attorney, was instrumental in getting the trail built. From the overlook, hikers enjoy a stunning view of the Etowah River Valley and a small area that is worth exploring for a couple of additional views. Return to the Y and make a sharp right to return to the loop trail. On the downhill section, from the top of Pine Mountain to the trailhead, the elevation drops some 700 feet in about a mile. The trail winds a bit but is easy to follow. As you near the trailhead, the forest returns to Piedmont hardwoods.

NEARBY ACTIVITIES

Cartersville is home to the world-class **Booth Western Art Museum**, comprising a fine collection of Western and Civil War art (501 Museum Dr.; hours and admission info: 770-387-1300 or **boothmuseum.org**). The museum's Millar Presidential Gallery features a brief biography of each president, along with a photograph or painting and a handwriting sample. Take I-75 North to Exit 288/Main Street; then turn left and drive 2.3 miles. Turn left at Wall Street and follow the signs two blocks to the parking area.

23 POOLE'S MILL COVERED BRIDGE

KEY AT-A-GLANCE INFORMATION

LENGTH: 1.1 miles round-trip

CONFIGURATION: Out-and-back

DIFFICULTY: Easy

SCENERY: Covered bridge; falls and cascades along Settingdown Creek

EXPOSURE: Full sun

TRAFFIC: Moderate

TRAIL SURFACE: Compacted soil, pavement

WHEELCHAIR ACCESS: Limited

HIKING TIME: 1 hour

ACCESS: Daily, sunrise–sunset; closed late November–spring; free

MAPS: USGS *Matt*

MORE INFO: 770-781-2215; tinyurl.com/poolesmillpark

FACILITIES: Restrooms, picnic tables with grills, pavilion rental, playground

SPECIAL COMMENTS: Poole's Mill is 1 of 12 covered bridges in Georgia.

DISTANCE: 31 miles from GA 400 North/I-285 North

GPS INFORMATION

N34° 17.350 ' W84° 14.521'

7725 Poole's Mill Rd.
Ballground, GA 30107

IN BRIEF

This trail meanders down a ridge to Poole's Mill Covered Bridge and explores Settingdown Creek, the waterway that the bridge spans. The cascading falls after the bridge on the left are a great place to enjoy the creek.

DESCRIPTION

A Cherokee trading path ran about 1 mile north of Poole's Mill. In 1804, under terms laid out in the Treaty of Tellico, this path became the federal highway that connected Savannah to Nashville. By the time Cherokee chief George Welch established the first mill on the site in 1820, traffic was steadily increasing on the road. Welch sided with the Treaty Party, advocating removal of the Cherokee people, which the party felt was inevitable, and hoping to secure better terms. He left Georgia soon after signing the supplement to the Treaty of New Echota on March 1, 1836. According to the Historical Society of Forsyth County, the federal government reimbursed Welch $719.50 for the gristmill.

Directions ⟶

Take GA 400/US 19 North to Exit 12B/ McFarland Parkway West, and circle around to merge on McFarland. Travel 1.3 miles and turn right on Union Hill Road. In 0.3 mile turn left on Mullinax Road, which becomes Post Road after 2.1 miles and then becomes Tribble Road after 8.1 miles. Drive a total of 9.1 miles on Mullinax/Post/Tribble; then turn left on Watson Road. Drive 0.3 mile and turn right on Heardsville Road. At 2.1 miles Heardsville Road becomes Heardsville Circle; continue straight on Heardsville Circle another 0.7 mile and turn right on Poole's Mill Road; then make an immediate left into the parking lot.

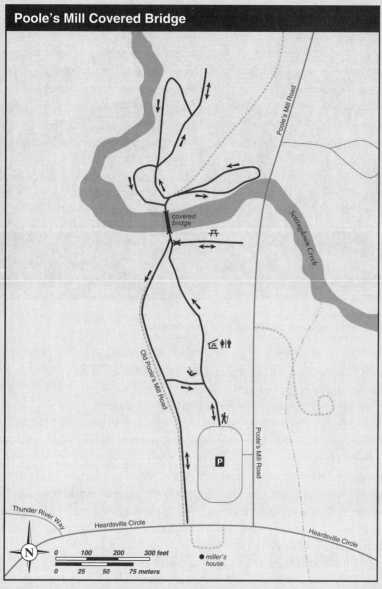

Poole's Mill Covered Bridge

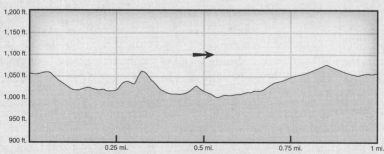

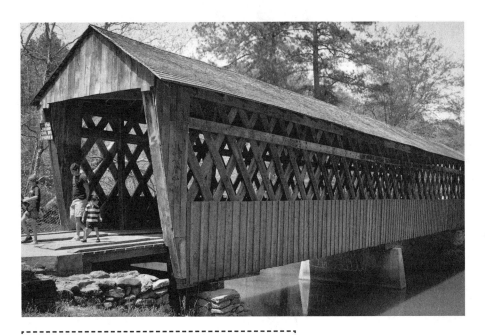

The historic covered bridge at Poole's Mill is 1 of 12 in Georgia.

Jacob Scudder was an entrepreneur with a number of businesses in a town known as Scudders near the intersection of Matt Highway and Old Federal Road, north of Poole's Mill. Today little remains of the small town, but it was Scudder, a white man, who took over Chief Welch's mill. Scudder, who married Welch's sister-in-law, purchased the land from the man who won it during the Sixth Georgia Land Lottery. He added a sawmill to the existing gristmill and, shortly before he died, transferred the title to his sons, who then sold it to a Dr. D. L. Pool (nobody really knows why landmarks bearing the doctor's name are spelled with an *e*). By the time the mill ceased operations in 1947, electricity had replaced water as the power source of choice, and chickens had replaced grain and cotton. The mill was burned down by vandals in 1959.

Since the Old Federal Highway was north of the mill, Poole's Mill Bridge began as a simple wooden structure to span Settingdown Creek between the mill and the main road. In 1899 the bridge was washed away, and the county contracted a millwright to build a new bridge. He quit before completing the project, and Bud Gentry was hired. Gentry is generally credited with building the bridge.

From the trailhead kiosk at the north end of the parking lot, the compacted-dirt trail meanders through a children's playground with swings and slides. At the top of the knoll, a "trail tree" marked the way to the bridge before the county opened the park in 1997. A pavilion to the right of the trail contains the park's restrooms.

From the knoll, the trail splits—one side goes directly to the bridge, while the other leads to a small garden area maintained by the county. Just before the bridge, the trails rejoin and asphalt-paved roads enter from the left and right. Turn right and walk along Settingdown Creek to reach the modern bridge over the creek. Photographers will find good places to take pictures of the covered bridge from along the bank, especially as sunset approaches. Picnic tables line the creek.

Return to the bridge at 0.3 mile and cross it; then turn right and follow the road on the other side, as far as the modern bridge. From this side you can exit the park and carefully walk to the center of the modern bridge for an excellent view of the covered bridge. Be extremely careful with young children, though, because drivers frequently speed here. Return to the covered bridge, and turn right on the original roadway connecting Poole's Mill to Old Federal Highway. To get an idea of what roads were like before modern paved roads became popular in the 1920s, follow this rough path down to the chain-link fence that marks private property at 0.6 mile.

Turn around and watch for a well-worn path heading right, about halfway back to the bridge. Turn right and follow it over two sets of rock outcrops, down to the bottom of a set of cascading falls typical of North Georgia. A chain-link fence prevents visitors from following the riverbank to the right, so turn left and begin climbing a series of rocks as the water shoots through, around, and over the rocks in the river. Just below the top of the rock, watch for metal spikes driven into the granite, as if to anchor a structure.

Return to the bridge and cross it, but instead of following the trail back, continue straight on the paved road as it rises to the modern street. Across the street on the left is the house where the miller lived. Mills in North Georgia were often operated by a man other than the owner, and part of the miller's compensation was a home. This house is privately owned—do not approach it. Return down the path to a crossover trail on the left, just before the playground, and take it to return to your car.

NEARBY ACTIVITIES

The **Cumming Fairgrounds** (770-781-3491; **cummingfair.net**) hosts many events throughout the year, including a rodeo and a steam, antique-tractor, and gas-engine exposition. The **Cumming Country Fair and Festival**, held at the fairgrounds in early October, offers a look back at Cherokee history. Exhibits include a seven-sided Cherokee council house and Blackburn's Tavern, one of the town's few remaining original buildings, which was restored and moved to the fairgrounds; a covered bridge permits access to this area. Additional displays include an extensive collection of pre-1930 steam-powered building equipment, two working mills, a blacksmith shop, and a 1940s-era cotton gin. We particularly enjoy the working sawmill, which demonstrates how the one at Poole's Mill would have worked. Be sure to spend a few minutes at the quilting bee.

24 ROME HERITAGE TRAIL

KEY AT-A-GLANCE INFORMATION

LENGTH: 8.6 miles round-trip

CONFIGURATION: Out-and-back

DIFFICULTY: Moderate

SCENERY: River views

EXPOSURE: Full sun most of the way

TRAFFIC: Light–medium

TRAIL SURFACE: 12-foot-wide poured concrete throughout

HIKING TIME: 3.5 hours

ACCESS: Daily, year-round, sunrise–sunset; free

MAPS: USGS *Rome North*

MORE INFO: 706-291-0766; rfpra .com/trails.htm; georgiatrails.com/gt /heritage_trail_system

FACILITIES: Restrooms in Ridge Ferry Park

SPECIAL COMMENTS: Restaurants and Starbucks Coffee nearby

DISTANCE: 60 miles from I-75 North/I-285 Northwest

GPS INFORMATION

N34° 17.098' W85° 9.957'

755 Braves Blvd. NE
Rome, GA 30161

IN BRIEF

Part of a much longer trail, the Rome Heritage Trail traverses the downtown area of Rome, Georgia.

DESCRIPTION

Like its Italian namesake, Rome, Georgia, is built on seven hills. The city center, however, lies at the confluence of three rivers, where the Etowah and Oostanaula form the Coosa. This hike takes place entirely along the Oostanaula River, although the other two rivers are visible from the Robert Redden Footbridge.

The Rome Heritage Trail is part of the much longer Heritage Trail System, which began in 1976 as a 1-mile hike in Heritage Park—the first Rails-to-Trails project in Georgia. In 1992 Rome moved to create a citywide trail network encompassing the Heritage Trail downtown and the Pinhoti Trail west and north of the city. The first new section was

----

Directions ⟶

Take I-75 North to Exit 290/GA 20. Turn left at the end of the ramp and follow GA 20 for 2.3 miles to North Tennessee Street. Turn left and then immediately right onto the ramp for US 41/US 411/GA 20. (*Warning:* Merging at the end of this ramp can be difficult.) Once you're on the road, follow US 411 for 18.9 miles. In Rome, take the Second Avenue exit, which merges into Turner McCall Boulevard in 0.8 mile. Follow Turner McCall Boulevard 1.4 miles to Broad Street. Turn left on Broad and move to the right lane. In 0.2 mile, turn right on Riverside Parkway and follow it to State Mutual Stadium, 2 miles ahead on the left. Park anywhere and find the trail on the northwest side of the stadium.

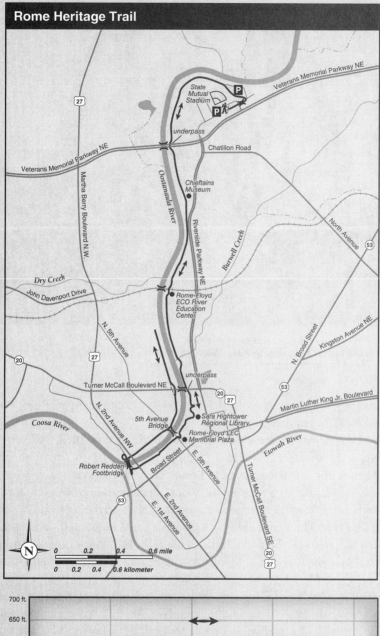

Rome Heritage Trail

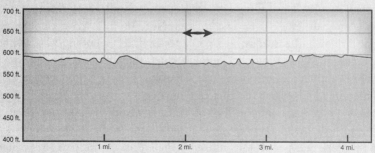

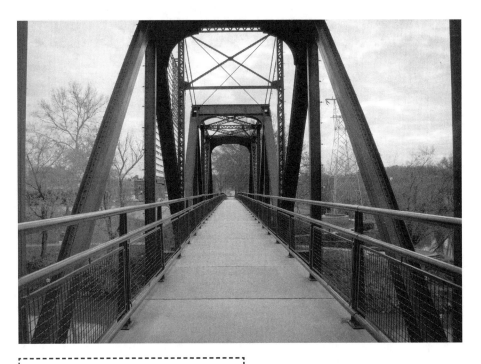

Rome's Robert Redden Footbridge beckons hikers.

completed in 1998, and today the 4.3-mile trail connects many of Rome's attractions and most downtown government buildings.

The hike begins at **State Mutual Stadium** (755 Braves Blvd. NE; 706-368-9388; **tinyurl.com/statemutualstadium**), completed in 2003 to attract the minor-league Macon Braves baseball team to Rome. From the parking lot in front of the stadium, a bridge crosses a deep ravine to additional parking. Turn left at the end of the bridge and, keeping the ravine to your left, walk to the park entrance by the Oostanaula River. The ravine feeds a low, marshy area on the left, while breaks in the trees yield views of the river. Trails to the right lead to the river for fishing.

At 0.9 mile the trail curves right and passes under Veterans Memorial Parkway NE. Before the bridge, a paved trail heads left, returning to the stadium. After passing through a fairly dense forest, the trail opens 1.3 miles into the hike; **Chieftains Museum** is on your left (501 Riverside Pkwy. NE; 706-291-9494; **chieftainsmuseum .org;** open Friday and Saturday, 1–5 p.m.; $5 adults, $3 seniors, $2 students). The former home of Major Ridge, a Cherokee chief, the museum tells the story of the Ridge family and its role in evicting the Cherokee Nation from Georgia in 1838—part of the forced relocation of American Indian tribes from the South to Oklahoma throughout the 1830s along the Trail of Tears. A wealthy landowner, Ridge owned a ferry near his home, only a few steps ahead on the trail in **Ridge Ferry Park.**

In this park many trails join and leave the Heritage Trail, either leading to the river or to parking lots. After passing a paved road to Riverside Parkway, the trail passes under a low railroad bridge before reaching the **Rome-Floyd ECO [Etowah-Coosa-Oostanaula] River Education Center,** at 1.9 miles (393 Riverside Pkwy. NE; 706-622-6432; **romeecocenter.com;** open Monday–Friday, 1–5 p.m., other days and times by appointment; free). Kids will enjoy taking a break at the nearby "tree house," a few steps farther on the trail.

Just before the US 27 bridge, at the 2.4-mile mark, a cluster of restaurants on the left is a good place to break for lunch. Return to the trail and continue under the US 27 bridge to downtown Rome. The first major building on the left is the **Sara Hightower Regional Library** (205 Riverside Pkwy. NE), at 2.7 miles. The Heritage Trail rises to join the parking lot, which it skirts to the right before briefly joining a road. From this point on, the trail is mostly in full sun.

On the left, just before the Fifth Avenue Bridge at 2.9 miles, the **Rome–Floyd County Law Enforcement Center Memorial Plaza** honors local police officers and firefighters who lost their lives in the line of duty. When you're done looking at this moving collection of monuments, turn around and cross at the traffic light directly in front of you (crossing near the Fifth Avenue Bridge is much less safe). The trail passes the historic city hall, courthouse, and civic center before passing a cement structure on which the flood levels of 1932 and 1946 are marked; the level of the historic flood of 1886 was too high for this structure and is marked on a building. The newest addition to the trail is a display about the three rivers of Rome; the display is located just before the Second Avenue Bridge, under which the trail passes.

At 3.2 miles the trail turns left and then makes a U-turn onto the **Robert Redden Footbridge.** Originally a swing trestle for the Central of Georgia Railway, the bridge was paved in place in 1976 (see **railga.com/oddend/romebridge.html** for more information). The original swing mechanism is visible under the center pier.

Once over the bridge, the trail circles left, dropping to the bottom of a massive berm built to protect the city from floodwaters. Today the rivers are controlled to prevent flooding by upstream dams forming Carters Lake (Oostanaula) and Lake Allatoona (Etowah). The trail swings left, passes under the Redden Footbridge, and then splits into two trails. Choose the path closest to the river—it affords excellent long-distance river views and passes under two bridges before rejoining the other path. The trail passes under the US 27 Bridge and continues along the top of a berm until it reaches a water station at 4.3 miles. At this point, retrace your steps to your car.

NEARBY ACTIVITIES

Our favorite section of the **Pinhoti Trail** runs north from James H. "Sloppy" Floyd State Park, south of Summerville (2800 Sloppy Floyd Lake Rd.; 706-857-0826; **gastateparks.org/jameshfloyd;** $5 state-park fee). From Rome, take US 27 North 18.7 miles to Sloppy Floyd Lake Road, turn left, and drive 3.2 miles to the park. Access is at the end of the Marble Mine Trail.

25 SILVER COMET TRAIL: ROCKMART

 KEY AT-A-GLANCE INFORMATION

LENGTH: 9.5 miles round-trip

CONFIGURATION: Out-and-back

DIFFICULTY: Moderate

SCENERY: 2 large creeks in the city of Rockmart, railroads, slate quarry

EXPOSURE: Full sun

TRAFFIC: Light; multiuse trail

TRAIL SURFACE: Concrete

WHEELCHAIR ACCESS: Yes

HIKING TIME: 4 hours

ACCESS: Daily, year-round, sunrise–sunset; free

MAPS: Available for purchase at the Silver Comet Depot bike shop in Mableton (4342 Floyd Rd.; 770-819-3279; silvercometdepot.com) or free at the website below; USGS *Rockmart North, Rockmart South*

MORE INFO: 404-875-PATH (7284); pathfoundation.org/trails /silver-comet

FACILITIES: Portable toilet at parking lot, restrooms in Rockmart City Hall

SPECIAL COMMENTS: Few hikers outside of Cobb County use the Silver Comet Trail. Rockmart has lots for kids to see and do, making this a great family hike.

DISTANCE: 38.2 miles from I-75 North/I-285 Northwest

GPS INFORMATION

N33° 58.616' W85° 0.267'

IN BRIEF

The Silver Comet Trail in Rockmart follows the old Seaboard Air Line Railroad tracks—now a concrete hiking and biking trail—to the old slate quarry and into downtown Rockmart. More than 100 years old, the city offers a delightful break, whether you stop for lunch or just to window-shop.

DESCRIPTION

Unlike the section of the Silver Comet Trail between Mavell Road and Floyd Road (see Hike 13, page 70), the trail in the vicinity of Rockmart is only lightly used. The railroad bed in Rockmart is significantly older than that near Mavell Road. Seaboard needed a railroad from Atlanta to Alabama, but rather than build the route themselves, they purchased an existing line from Alabama to Cartersville, Georgia, and built the additional track from Rockmart to Atlanta in 1904. Coot's Lake Beach, for which the trailhead is named, is a pay-per-use facility adjacent to the trailhead.

Walk to the front of the parking lot and turn right. A short access trail makes a short

----

Directions ⟶

Take I-75 to Exit 265/Marietta Parkway/GA 120 West, and turn left. Drive 2.3 miles and turn right on Whitlock Avenue/GA 120 West, which becomes Dallas Highway and then Charles Hardy Parkway. Drive a total of 14.4 miles on this combined road and then turn right on GA 120 West, which becomes US 278/GA 6 and is signed east–west as Jimmy Lee Smith Parkway, Jimmy Campbell Parkway, and Rockmart Highway. Drive 15.3 miles on this combined road and turn right on Coot's Lake Road. Drive 0.1 mile to the trailhead parking lot, on the right just behind Coot's Lake Beach.

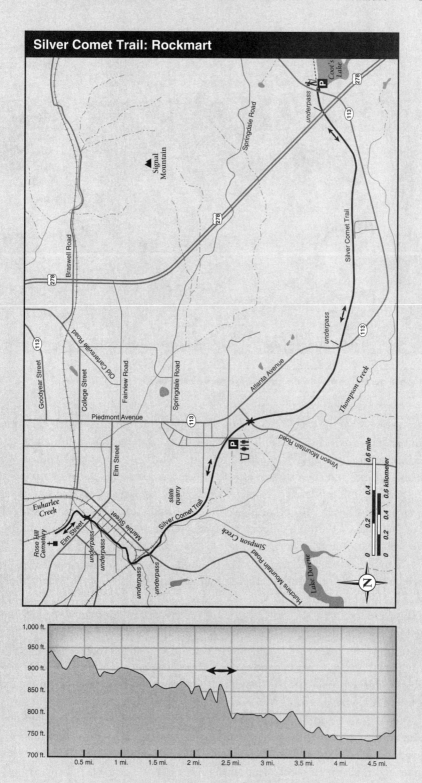

Silver Comet Trail: Rockmart

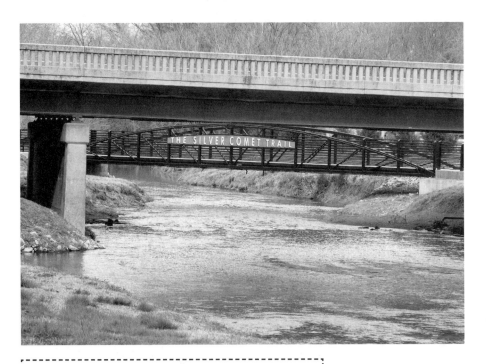

The trail crosses Euharlee Creek on a stylishly signed wooden bridge.

drop to the Silver Comet. Turn left on the wide, concrete-paved path and almost immediately cross Coot's Lake Road at an intersection with no traffic light. After the intersection, the Silver Comet curves right, leaving the original roadbed of the Seaboard Line, and then curves back to the left as it begins a fairly sharp descent to a narrow, unlit underpass. As the trail exits the underpass, it begins an equally steep rise and returns to the original roadbed. You'll notice various mature pines near the trail as the path imperceptibly descends almost the entire distance to downtown Rockmart.

Watch down the hill on the left for an old shed at 0.3 mile. Sheds like these were common throughout North Georgia and the Blue Ridge Mountains before the 20th century. The shed is a good example of form following geography: because mountain fields were frequently far apart, farmers would build a small shed for each field rather than storing all their equipment in a single barn. On the right, past the shed, sharp cliffs expose the red Georgia clay in a man-made cut. At mile marker 34, the trail gently curves right. The Silver Comet's raised roadbed after the curve is made of the debris that was removed to create the railroad cut. At 0.9 mile the trail crosses McDowell Road, a two-lane dirt road.

At 1.5 miles another cut begins, where the roadbed has been dug out of the mountain. At 1.8 miles the trail passes under the Atlanta Avenue; after this, you'll see additional cliffs that were created when the railroad was built. The trail slowly curves right, passing a small, clear pond on the left and crossing Vinson Mountain

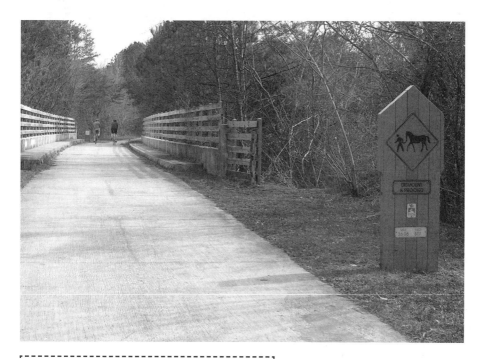

The Silver Comet is the very definition of a multiuse trail.

Road on a trestle. In the middle of the trestle, look left to see the entrance to the Van Wert parking lot.

Van Wert, originally the seat of Paulding County, is pretty much a forgotten town. When Polk County split off in 1851, Dallas became Paulding's county seat and Cedartown became Polk's county seat, leaving Van Wert to struggle without the additional revenue generated by being a government center. In 1872 Seaborn Jones sealed the fate of struggling Van Wert when he donated land to form the village of Rockmart. The railroad built a depot in Rockmart and bypassed Van Wert.

Just past the trestle, the Van Wert parking-area-access trail heads right, quickly descending to the parking lot. The Silver Comet begins a long, gradual curve left as the area known as White Bottom opens on the left; a sign on the trail identifies the area as Ma White's Bottomland. The Whites owned most of the land, and when her husband died, Ma White continued to run the farm.

The Silver Comet begins a sweeping curve to the right as it joins Thompson Creek at 3.5 miles. From this point on through the city of Rockmart, the trail runs near this creek or the larger Euharlee Creek. Notice that the creek runs through a gorge carved from slate on your left. Rockmart Slate Quarry, complete with a railroad siding, is ahead on the right. One of the reasons the railroad ran to Rockmart was that it could generate income hauling slate from this quarry. Formed some 600 million years ago, a vast ancient sea deposited layers of sediments that over time became slate. A popular roofing material until the 1920s, slate was replaced by asbestos shingles. By that time a new use had been developed for the rock—it was used as an aggregate to strengthen cement.

At 3.8 miles the trail appears to rise to a road. But just before you begin the climb, a second paved trail heads left. Take this second trail and travel under Hutchins Mountain Road. After the underpass, which the Silver Comet shares with nearby Simpson Creek, the landscape opens into a wide, level plain populated by massive oak trees. Continuing on the left, Simpson Creek runs alongside the trail to its confluence with the lyrically named Euharlee Creek. Shortly after the confluence, Silver Comet Trail curves abruptly to the right, passing under other tracks also owned by CSX. On the right, after an easy climb, you'll see a cotton gin at Beauregard Street, where the trail becomes the Rockmart Riverwalk, lined with black lampposts.

Passing under Church Street, the Silver Comet enters downtown Rockmart. In recent years this town has undergone a remarkable transformation, in part thanks to the increasing use of Silver Comet Trail. Upscale shopping and new restaurants join a century-old church and a police station. A wooden bridge crosses Euharlee Creek, giving hikers access to Seaborn Jones Park. Dedicated in 2002, the park is a great addition to Silver Comet Trail, with picnic tables and large open areas. Turn right and continue to the bridge over Euharlee Creek to take the Silver Comet north out of the city. As the trail curves left, Rose Hill Cemetery lies up a hill on the left. At this point, turn around to head back to your car.

NEARBY ACTIVITIES

Take a few minutes while in downtown Rockmart to pay your respects to the residents of the town who fought and died in American wars, including both World Wars, the Korean War, and the Vietnam War. The moving **Veterans' Memorial,** on Church Street, is only a few steps from the Rockmart trailhead.

SPRINGER MOUNTAIN LOOP 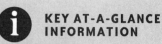 26

IN BRIEF

This trail combines the start of the Appalachian Trail and the Benton MacKaye Trail to form a loop that begins and ends at the popular FS 42 parking lot.

DESCRIPTION

The Appalachian Trail (AT) is a 2,000-plus-mile hiking adventure from Maine to Georgia that many people start but few finish. Benton MacKaye conceived the idea of a trail along the eastern ridge of the Appalachian Mountains in 1921 after hiking Vermont's Long Trail. MacKaye, a Harvard-educated forester, left the Appalachian Trail Conference in the 1930s and formed the Wilderness Society with a group of fellow conservationists.

When the Georgia portion of the hike was originally laid out, it extended to Mt. Oglethorpe, near Jasper. There were many problems with the final 15 miles of the original

- -

Directions

Take I-75 North to Exit 260 and merge onto I-575. At the northern border of Cherokee County (30.7 miles), limited-access I-575 becomes full-access GA 515. Drive a total of 55.7 miles on I-575/GA 515 to First Avenue, and turn left. Drive 0.1 mile and turn right on GA 52 East. Drive 3.7 miles and turn left on Big Creek Road, which becomes Doublehead Gap Road at 8.5 miles. Drive a total of 15.3 miles on Big Creek/Doublehead Gap and then turn right on FS 42, a gravel road; watch for Pleasant Hill Baptist Church on the left and the signed entrance to Blue Ridge Wildlife Management Area on the right. Drive 6.5 miles on FS 42 to the day-use parking area for the Appalachian Trail/Springer Mountain, on the left. To reach the trailhead, walk to the brown-roofed building in the northwest corner of the parking lot.

KEY AT-A-GLANCE INFORMATION

LENGTH: 4.4 miles

CONFIGURATION: Loop

DIFFICULTY: Moderate, mostly because of the rocky uphill climb to Springer Mountain

SCENERY: Long-distance views into the Amicalola River watershed from Springer Mountain and into the Etowah River watershed from Ball Mountain

EXPOSURE: Mostly shaded

TRAFFIC: Heavy from the parking area to Springer Mountain; the Benton MacKaye portion of the trail is lightly used.

TRAIL SURFACE: Compacted dirt

WHEELCHAIR ACCESS: None

HIKING TIME: 3 hours

ACCESS: Daily, year-round, sunrise–sunset; free

MAPS: Fannin County Chamber of Commerce (800-899-6867); USGS *Amicalola, Noontootla*

MORE INFO: 770-297-3000; tinyurl.com/springermtn

FACILITIES: Primitive outhouse at Springer Mountain Shelter

SPECIAL COMMENTS: Hiking opportunities abound in this area, home to the Appalachian and Benton MacKaye Trails. In April you may run into AT thru-hikers. You'll need to wear hunter's orange during deer season (September–November).

DISTANCE: 91 miles from I-75 North/I-285 Northwest

GPS INFORMATION

N34° 38.255' W84° 11.711'

Springer Mountain Loop

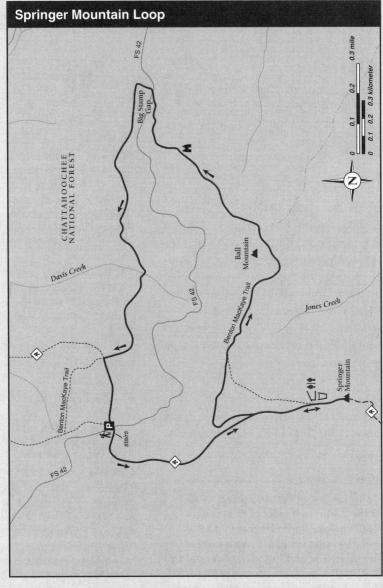

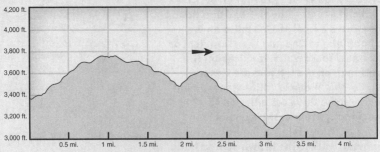

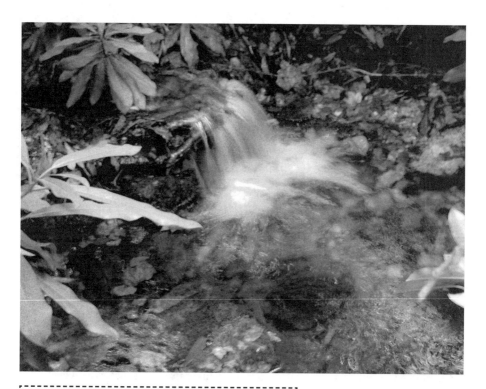

A small cascade on Davis Creek, near the Benton MacKaye Trail

hike, so the end of the trail was rerouted to Springer Mountain, in Chattahoochee National Forest. Additionally, as a result of this rerouting, Amicalola Falls could serve as the access point for long-distance hikers.

Originally known as Penitentiary Mountain, Springer Mountain probably gets its name from one of two sources: John Springer, the first Presbyterian to be ordained minister in Georgia (in 1790), or William G. Springer, an early settler of Carroll County, Georgia. Whichever man was so honored, the name began to appear near the start of the 20th century. In 1959 the Georgia Appalachian Trail Club rerouted the end of the Appalachian Trail to Springer Mountain.

Twenty years later, the Benton MacKaye Trail Association was formed to create a trail along the western ridge of the Appalachians, also beginning at Springer Mountain and running through Georgia and Tennessee. Today the trail is 288 miles long; two additional intersections with the AT occur in Great Smoky Mountains National Park, on both the North Carolina and Tennessee sides of the park.

From the brown trailhead kiosk in the FS 42 parking lot, walk left—crossing the lot—descend a set of wooden steps, and cross FS 42. As the pathway reenters the woods, the forest is predominantly oak, tulip poplar, and American beech trees; watch for holly and hemlocks as well. Almost immediately, the Appalachian Trail begins a moderate climb along a ridge to the peak of Springer Mountain. The familiar white rectangular blaze is used throughout to mark the Appalachian Trail. On the right is the first of a number of good views into the Amicalola–Coosa River watershed.

An 8-foot rock wall at 0.2 mile is adjacent to Springer Mountain Loop. Just past the wall is a tree that animals hollowed out and occasionally populate. Continuing on the AT, you'll get additional long-distance views that are perhaps best in the winter and early spring. In this area, rock-lined culverts have been carefully crafted to move water away from the rocky, rooted trail. At the marked intersection with the Benton MacKaye Trail, on the left, continue straight ahead toward Springer Mountain.

A second trail, also on the left, takes overnight hikers to the Springer Mountain Shelter. Continue straight ahead to the top of the mountain. The trail winds through a boulder-strewn area before coming out on solid rock with an unimpeded long-distance view to the southwest, making it an excellent place to watch the sunset. Two markers indicate the start of the AT: one features a 1930s-style hiker, courtesy of the Georgia Appalachian Trail Club, and another shows a map of the trail, courtesy of the US Forest Service.

After spending a few minutes enjoying the view, return to the white diamond–blazed Benton MacKaye Trail, turn right, and begin an easy descent as the trail follows the curve of the mountain. In less than 0.1 mile, embedded in a rock on your right, a memorial plaque tells hikers about MacKaye's legacy. An easy-to-moderate ascent marks the start of Ball Mountain, which the Benton MacKaye skirts just beneath the peak. As the trail begins its descent to Big Stamp Gap, winter views through a deciduous forest off to the right, at 2 miles, foreshadow the scenic highlight of the trail at 2.4 miles. About 200 feet down a marked side trail is an excellent view of the northeast Georgia mountains.

Crossing FS 42 at 2.8 miles into the hike, the trail continues downhill, making a sweeping turn to the left and running parallel to but beneath the US Forest Service road. The trail repeatedly runs through rhododendron thickets so full that they actually form a canopy over the trail, protecting it from the summer sun. The first canopy, at 3.1 miles, indicates that a stream parallels the trail on the left. The trail makes a wet-footed crossing of the stream at 3.3 miles. Over the next 0.3 mile, the path crosses streams twice, and you'll get a couple of low-light opportunities to photograph cascades near the trail. At 4 miles, turn left on the AT at the signed intersection to return to the parking lot on FS 42.

NEARBY ACTIVITIES

Ellijay is home to the **Georgia Apple Festival**, held the second and third full weekends in October. You can buy anything made from an apple at the festival, or you can simply browse the shops on Winesap Way or Granny Smith Street. For more information, contact the Gilmer County Chamber of Commerce (706-635-7400; **gilmerchamber.com/apple**).

TALKING ROCK NATURE TRAIL

IN BRIEF

One of four developed trails in the Carters Lake area, this footpath takes hikers to a stunning overlook of the lake's reregulation pool and Georgia's Valley and Ridge section.

DESCRIPTION

The Talking Rock Nature Trail begins as a short, moderate downhill hike through two brown posts placed to exclude vehicles. The trail moderates as it bears left, making a U-turn deep into a forested cove. On the left, after the turn, an area has been cleared and replanted with trees and shrubs designed to attract wildlife, including deer, squirrels, turkeys, and songbirds. The trail is interpreted, with signs pointing out some of the improvements.

Past the feeding area, the trail bears right, following a small creek on the right down to a three-trail intersection. Straight ahead, a park

----

Directions

Take I-75 North to Exit 260 and merge onto I-575. At the northern border of Cherokee County (30.7 miles), limited-access I-575 becomes full-access GA 515. Drive a total of 43 miles on I-575/GA 515 to GA 136; then turn left and immediately move to the right lane. At 0.2 mile turn right on GA 136. Move to the left lane, drive 0.2 mile, and bear left. At 2.1 miles turn right on GA 136, at Bart's Bait and Tackle. Drive 10 miles, turning right at the visitor-center sign. Bear left at 1.9 miles; the road to the right leads to the visitor center. The guard shack is directly in front of you. Pay a $4 entrance fee, which gives you access to the Northbank Recreation Area, including this trail, the dam overlook, and a picnic area. Trail parking is 0.2 mile ahead, on the left. Look for an overhead TALKING ROCK NATURE TRAIL sign 20 feet down the hill.

KEY AT-A-GLANCE INFORMATION

LENGTH: 2.4 miles

CONFIGURATION: Balloon

DIFFICULTY: Moderate

SCENERY: Beautiful long-distance views into Georgia's Valley and Ridge section, and of the reregulation pool for Carters Lake

EXPOSURE: Mostly shaded except toward the overlook, where the trail enters full sun

TRAFFIC: Moderate

TRAIL SURFACE: Compacted soil

WHEELCHAIR ACCESS: None

HIKING TIME: 1.25 hours

ACCESS: Daily, year-round, sunrise–sunset; $4 day-use fee

MAPS: Available at the visitor center (down the road to the right before the trailhead); USGS *Oakman*

MORE INFO: 706-334-2248; tinyurl.com/acecarterslake

FACILITIES: None on trail; restrooms at visitor center

SPECIAL COMMENTS: Other trails at Carters Lake include the Hidden Pond Songbird Trail (0.6 mile), Tumbling Waters Nature Trail (1.7 miles), Oak Ridge Nature Trail (1.2 miles), Ridgeway Mountain Bike Trail (6 miles), and Amadahy Trail (3.5 miles). You'll need to wear hunter's orange during deer season (September–November).

DISTANCE: 66.3 miles from I-75 North/I-285 Northwest

GPS INFORMATION

N34° 36.548' W84° 39.889'

Talking Rock Nature Trail

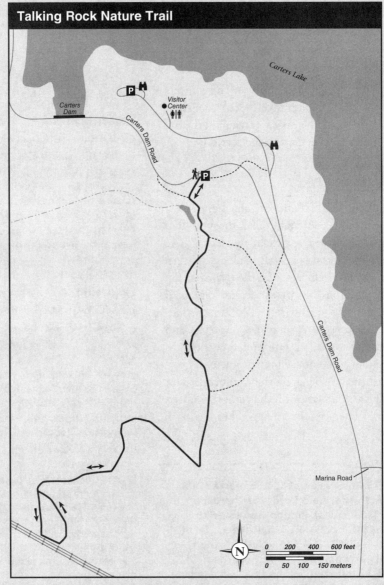

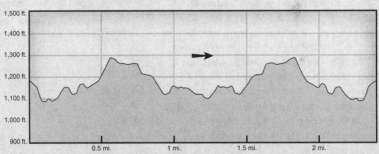

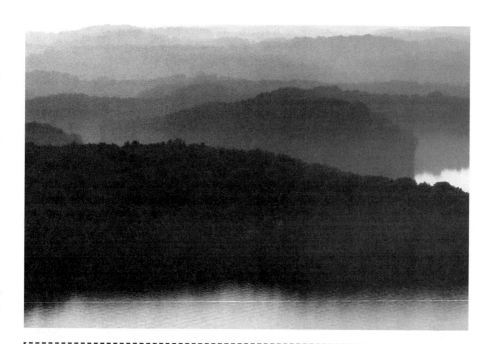

In the valley below Carters Lake, an ethereal mist shrouds the hills surrounding the reregulation reservoir.

bench affords a view of an area designed to attract wood ducks. Nearly extinct at the start of the 20th century, the wood duck was protected by treaty in 1918. It has made a long, slow recovery in both Georgia and the nation as a whole. Today the bird is no longer protected, but the species is closely watched in Georgia because much of its native habitat is being destroyed by development. Continue past the bench to an artificial rock dam that formed the small lake, specifically designed as a wood-duck habitat. Turn around and return to the three-way intersection.

At the intersection, turn right on a gravel road covered with mulch. On the right is the Oostanaula River; on the left is a moderate ascent to an unnamed knob. Note the large trees, some of which are oaks, in the bottomland forest on the right. Two important ingredients in creating a wood-duck habitat are mature oaks (for food—wood ducks feed on acorns) and forested wetlands (for shelter).

The trees are a typical Blue Ridge Mountain mix, with post and white oaks; American beeches; some hickory trees, pin oaks, and red maples; occasional short-leaf and loblolly pines; and holly. As the fully shaded trail climbs through the forest, the valley on the right levels and widens. At 0.7 mile the gentle valley on the right ends, and a steep-sided valley forms immediately on the left. This area is a known buck scrape, so be careful here, especially during hunting season. Wear hunter's orange September–November.

The wide path is easy over the next 0.2 mile, and the path begins a moderate descent to an intersection with a trail that heads left. Bear right and continue to a second intersection, which marks the start of the overlook loop. Pine-beetle devastation is becoming overgrown here, and the trail slowly regains trees as it wends around to the west side of the mountain.

The forest soon opens, letting you see the reregulation pool directly in front of and beneath you. From this overlook, the rolling hills of Georgia's Valley and Ridge section not only create a beautiful scene but also represent a major geologic division of the state. You're standing on the Blue Ridge Mountains—metamorphic rock formed during an uplift some 350 million years ago, looking out on a much older formation of sedimentary rock, indicating that the region was once covered by a great inland sea.

Carters Lake, which reached its full level for the first time in 1977, destroyed some of the finest whitewater runs in the nation. It was here that outdoorsman and poet James Dickey had a real-life run-in with moonshiners that led him to write *Deliverance*. The reregulation dam was added to let water pass through the generators at peak hours and then be pumped back into the lake during off-peak hours, efficiently getting the maximum power out of every cubic foot of water.

From the overlook the path continues, curving left beside an open field and eventually returning to the start of the loop. Turn left to follow the path back to the starting point.

NEARBY ACTIVITIES

Add the nearby **Hidden Pond Songbird Trail** to this hike as a good cooldown. This bird habitat is an easy nearby hike of 0.6 mile. To reach the trailhead, return to GA 136; then turn right and drive 1 mile to old US 411. Turn right and travel 0.4 mile to Reregulation Dam Recreation Area (706-334-2248). Follow the road around to the parking area; a large brown sign marks the trailhead.

THREE FORKS LOOP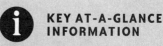

IN BRIEF

The Three Forks Loop combines portions of the Appalachian and Benton MacKaye Trails between the day-use parking lot on FS 42 and Three Forks.

DESCRIPTION

This rugged, remote trail is a great place to get away from it all, quite literally—there have been times when we've hiked here and haven't met a single person. Hunting is prohibited in the vicinity of the Appalachian Trail but is allowed along the Benton MacKaye, so wear hunter's orange September–November (hunting season). A deeply creviced rock designed to block motorized vehicles marks the start of the trail. The white rectangle–blazed Appalachian Trail is straight ahead and clearly marked. A level, grassy area to the right after the rock may be confused with the trail, but it's short and goes nowhere.

Directions ⟶

Take I-75 North to Exit 260 and merge onto I-575. At the northern border of Cherokee County (30.7 miles), limited-access I-575 becomes full-access GA 515. Drive a total of 55.7 miles on I-575/GA 515 to First Avenue, and turn left. Drive 0.1 mile and turn right on GA 52 East. Drive 3.7 miles and turn left on Big Creek Road, which becomes Doublehead Gap Road at 8.5 miles. Drive a total of 15.3 miles on Big Creek/Doublehead Gap and then turn right on FS 42, a gravel road; watch for Pleasant Hill Baptist Church on the left and the signed entrance to Blue Ridge Wildlife Management Area on the right. Drive 6.5 miles on FS 42 to the day-use parking area for the Appalachian Trail/Springer Mountain, on the left. To reach the trailhead, walk to the brown-roofed building in the northwest corner of the parking lot.

KEY AT-A-GLANCE INFORMATION

LENGTH: 6.6 miles

CONFIGURATION: Loop

DIFFICULTY: Moderate

SCENERY: Long-distance winter vistas

EXPOSURE: Full shade

TRAFFIC: Light

TRAIL SURFACE: Packed clay

WHEELCHAIR ACCESS: None

HIKING TIME: 3.5 hours

ACCESS: Daily, year-round, sunrise–sunset; free

MAPS: Fannin County Chamber of Commerce (800-899-6867), USGS *Noontootla*

MORE INFO: 770-297-3000; tinyurl.com/springermtn

FACILITIES: None

SPECIAL COMMENTS: The original Appalachian Trail, which was rerouted in the 1970s, is now known as the Benton MacKaye Trail in this area. You'll need to wear hunter's orange during deer season (September–November).

DISTANCE: 91 miles from I-75 North/I-285 Northwest

GPS INFORMATION

N34° 38.258' W84° 11.709'

Three Forks Loop

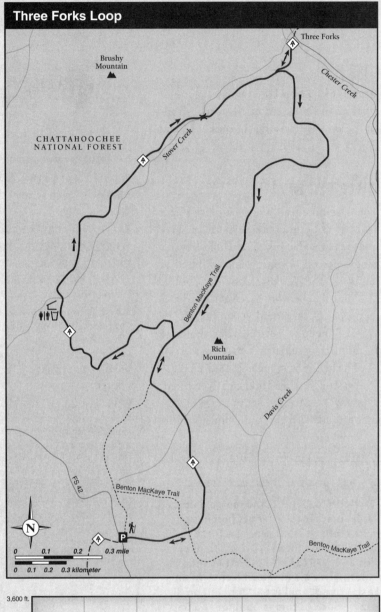

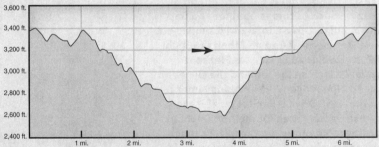

Immediately entering a second-growth forest where post, white, and pin oaks predominate, with red maples and the odd loblolly pine thrown in, you begin a long arc to the left around the top of a mountain. After you complete the arc, you'll see a large, moderately steep valley on your right. At just under 0.5 mile, you'll reach the first intersection with Benton MacKaye Trail. Go straight, following the Appalachian Trail (AT) through rhododendron thickets. These are known locally as laurel hells because the thickets are so dense that their common companion, mountain laurel, cannot grow. At times the rhododendron forms an arch over the footpath. After a rain, Davis Creek, a tributary of Chester Creek, can be heard nearby.

The path is well defined, continuing to curve around a mountain on your left. Davis Creek lies in front of you—a rooted, rocky, wet-footed crossing. About 25 feet after you cross Davis Creek, you'll reach a second creek, which runs after a heavy rainfall and which you may also have to ford.

Now the path meanders into a laurel thicket interspersed with tulip poplars and maturing evergreens. At 1 mile the AT again crosses Benton MacKaye Trail. This is the return point of the loop. Continue straight on the AT. Up to this point the footpath has been following near the top of a long ridge known as Rich Mountain. Now the AT comes off the ridge, falling, sometimes sharply, to the valley that holds Stover Creek.

As you descend the ridge, the sound of cascading water fills the air. In places, ferns indicate that the ground is regularly moist, and the trail becomes rooted and rocky. At 1.8 miles, winter hikers are treated to a panorama of the valley that the AT follows. The trail then descends a set of 10 rolled-log steps before bearing right to a marked T-intersection. The path briefly follows an old logging road before entering the forest, passing through a rhododendron thicket before steeply descending to Stover Creek. The trail to Stover Creek Shelter, a blue rectangle–blazed path, heads left at 1.9 miles.

After crossing Stover Creek (a wet-thigh crossing), the trail climbs the riverbank and reenters the forest, quickly reaching a right turn on a road with a sign pointing to Three Forks. Over the next 1.5 miles, the footpath continues downhill much more gradually, with the occasional few steep steps. During this portion of the trek to Three Forks, the AT parallels Stover Creek, which is never more than 100 feet away.

In the Stover Creek valley, both the pathway and nearby areas tend to be moist, and at one point a tributary cascades onto the trail. Finally crossing Stover Creek on a bridge with handrails (the old bridge, a large log with one flat side, lies to the left), the AT begins to follow an old logging road. Just past the bridge, a side trail heads left, and about 0.5 mile later Benton MacKaye Trail heads right, marked with a wooden sign. Bear left and continue 0.1 mile on the AT to Three Forks, where Stover, Chester, and Long Creeks form Noontootla Creek.

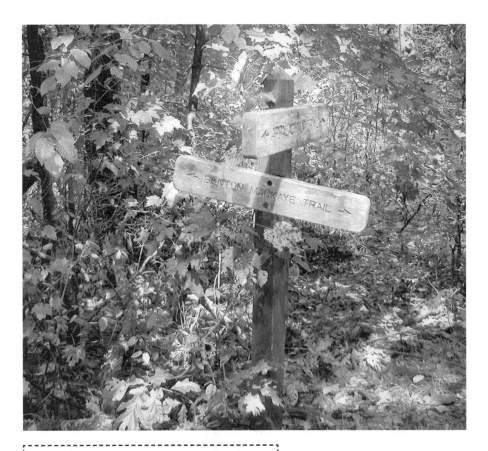

A signpost marks the convergence of two renowned trails.

This area sees heavy use, and the lack of significant undergrowth near the crossing is a concern that will have to be addressed in the future. Turn around and return to the intersection with Benton MacKaye Trail, and turn left.

Named for the man who conceived the Appalachian Trail, at least in this area, the Benton MacKaye Trail follows the AT's original path. MacKaye (rhymes with *eye*) parted ways with members of the Appalachian Trail Club after a dispute and formed the Wilderness Society with other conservationists. Today, the Benton MacKaye and Appalachian Trails form a loop of nearly 500 miles through Georgia, North Carolina, and Tennessee.

As you turn onto the Benton MacKaye, it almost immediately enters a forest composed of pine saplings and rhododendrons, with larger trees farther from the path. The trail begins an S-curve, climbing to an old road where it continues a moderate-to-difficult climb back to the top of Rich Mountain. On your left, a deep, steep-sided valley offers good winter views. The road circles the mountain as it climbs, finally leveling as it approaches the top of Rich Mountain, where the road is blocked and the path bears right, into the forest.

Unlike the AT some 600 feet below, the Benton MacKaye crosses no rivers and shows little sign of moisture. Along the ridgetop, the lightly used trail narrows where grass encroaches. Luckily, the Benton MacKaye is well blazed, and you rarely take more than a few steps before seeing another blue-rectangle blaze indicating a connector trail for AT access or a white-diamond blaze marking Benton MacKaye's own path (not to be confused with the white rectangle of the AT).

Curving gracefully to the right but still climbing, the trail circles near the top of an unnamed knob and then curves back to the left to continue its final ascent to Rich Mountain. At 4.6 miles you reach the mile-long ridge that is the top of the mountain. Along the ridgetop the ascent continues at an easy grade, with only the occasional short level or downhill stretches. Finally, at 5.4 miles you reach the pinnacle of Rich Mountain. Over the next 0.3 mile, the Benton MacKaye makes an easy descent to the intersection with the AT. Turn left on the AT and return to the day-use parking lot on FS 42.

NEARBY ACTIVITIES

On your way to the trail, stop by **Poole's Bar-B-Q** in East Ellijay (164 Craig St.; 706-635-4100; **www.poolesbarbq.com**) to fill up on classic Georgia barbecue and see the Pig Hill of Fame. The restaurant is open Thursday, 11 a.m.–7 p.m.; Friday and Saturday, 11 a.m.–8 p.m.; and Sunday, 11 a.m.–6 p.m. Retrace your route from the trailhead to the intersection of GA 52 West and GA 515 South. Turn left on GA 515 and drive 1 mile. Turn left on Maddox Drive, which becomes Yukon Road; then make an immediate left on Craig Street. Poole's is 0.2 mile ahead, on your left.

29   VICKERY CREEK TRAIL

KEY AT-A-GLANCE INFORMATION

LENGTH: 6.5 miles

CONFIGURATION: Loop

DIFFICULTY: Moderate

SCENERY: Views of creek, antebellum dam, covered bridge, and Roswell Mill

EXPOSURE: Partially shaded

TRAFFIC: Moderate

TRAIL SURFACE: Compacted dirt, some gravel

WHEELCHAIR ACCESS: None

HIKING TIME: 3 hours

ACCESS: Daily, year-round, sunrise–sunset. Although this trail is part of the Chattahoochee River National Recreation Area (CRNRA), there is no fee collection at the Oxbo Road parking area; you will, however, pass a CRNRA collection box along the trail where you pay the $3 day-use fee on the honor system.

MAPS: On kiosks throughout the hike, except for the portion near Roswell Mill; CRNRA Headquarters at Island Ford; USGS *Roswell*

MORE INFO: 678-538-1200; nps.gov/chat

FACILITIES: None

SPECIAL COMMENTS: This diverse hardwood forest is more typical of the Georgia mountains farther north. Vickery Creek is also known as Big Creek (see Hike 32, page 156).

DISTANCE: 8.7 miles from GA 400 North/I-285 North

GPS INFORMATION

N34° 1.0334' W84° 21.456'

IN BRIEF

This loop trail explores a low knoll north of the Chattahoochee River and east of the oxbow in Vickery Creek. The fast-moving creek supplied power to Roswell Mill, which you can also explore on this hike.

DESCRIPTION

Unlike most of the Chattahoochee River National Recreation Area (CRNRA) hikes, this one doesn't explore the floodplain of the Chattahoochee River, nor does it approach the Chattahoochee itself. Rather, the hike covers a small knoll north of the river, along Vickery Creek, twice dipping to the broad, full waterway that once powered Roswell Mill (which made cotton) and many other mills in the area.

This hike begins at the Oxbo Trail parking lot instead of the Vickery Creek Unit parking area—the small CRNRA lot is frequently full on weekends, and the single-lane entrance can be dangerous. Follow Vickery Creek, also known as Big Creek, 0.3 mile until it curves left and rises slightly. At the top of the rise, turn right and climb the stairs to the bridge over the creek. On your left, a dam-created waterfall is a pleasing sight at the start of the hike. On the far side of the bridge the path bears left, climbing stairs as it curves back

----

Directions ———————————→

Take GA 400/US 19 North to Exit 6/Northridge Road. Turn right on Northridge, cross back over GA 400, and then take the first right onto Dunwoody Place. Drive 1.2 miles and turn right on Roswell Road, which crosses the Chattahoochee River and becomes South Atlanta Street. Drive 1.3 miles and turn right on Oxbo Road. Drive 0.2 mile to the gravel parking lot, on your right.

Vickery Creek Trail

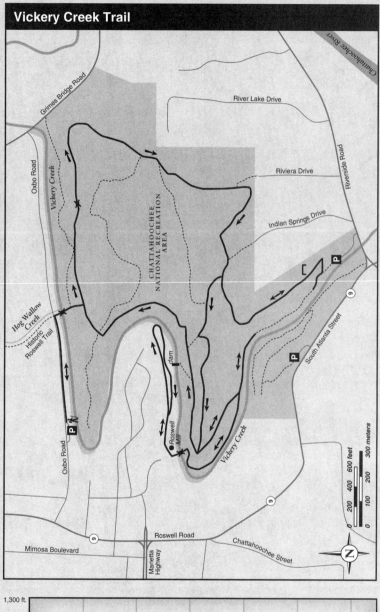

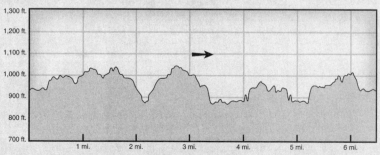

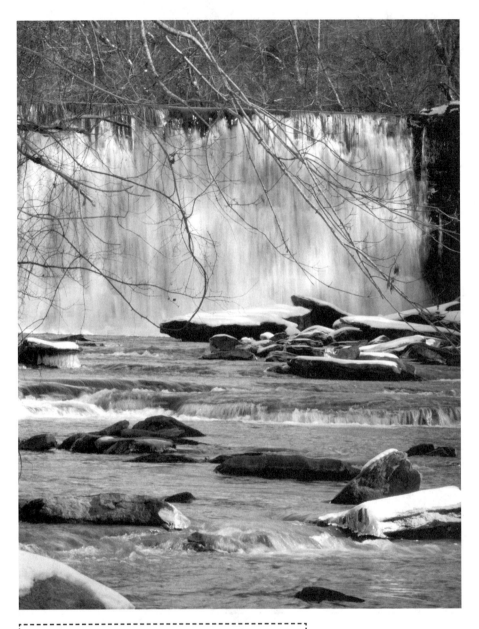

An antebellum dam created the millrace for historic Roswell Mill.

around to the right. The familiar CRNRA entrance kiosk is on the left, with a YOU ARE HERE map on a separate pedestal. Here is where you pay the $3 use fee; most of the money helps improve federal parks in the Atlanta area.

Initially the trail continues its climb through a mature second-growth hardwood forest composed of post and white oaks and, less frequently, pin and red oaks, intermixed with loblolly and/or shortleaf pines. American beeches, hickory trees, and sassafras are common in some areas. Red foxes, wild turkeys, beavers, otters, and tortoises are among the wildlife you may spot along the trail.

Arrive at a T-intersection near the top of the unnamed knoll, and turn left. The trail quickly begins an easy-to-moderate descent to a wet-footed crossing of a tributary of Vickery Creek. After a brief climb, the trail rolls through an area recovering from pine-beetle destruction to a second easy-to-moderate descent to the Grimes Bridge Road entrance kiosk, at 0.8 mile. Turn right and begin climbing, once again through an area recovering from pine-beetle destruction.

The first of two major crossover trails heads right at 1 mile; this is actually an old road that leads to Roswell Mill Dam (the road continues to the left, but this is not a path). As you continue on the main trail, notice that it too has become a road, covered with gravel in places. You can see houses to the left; the second crossover trail heads right at 1.1 miles. The footpath descends to a side trail on the left, and you soon reach an intrusive chain-link fence where the main trunk makes an abrupt right turn into a climb at 1.4 miles. The path then heads past another side trail to the housing development and the three-way intersection with the trail from the CRNRA parking area. Turn left and follow the trail for an easy descent, with the Vickery Creek gorge on the right. A side trail on the right once descended to the cliffs, but it's been closed for many years.

Now descending moderately, the footpath makes an unusual transition at 1.8 miles. The rocky path becomes rock-free and graded for the next 0.1 mile, after which an old road goes straight as the path bears right at a bench. Shortly past the bench the trail switches back and becomes steeper, finally dropping down a set of wooden steps at the entry to the river gorge. Down to the left is the CRNRA kiosk, and to the right is a brief path that quickly closes. Turn around and retrace your steps to the main trunk and turn left.

With the river valley occasionally visible on the left, the footpath continues to rise to a crossover trail at 2.6 miles, quickly followed by a three-way intersection 0.1 mile later. Turn left and begin an easy descent into the Vickery Creek gorge. As the footpath approaches a left turn at 3 miles, it becomes steeper but never more than moderate. When the trail reaches the river, turn left and follow Vickery Creek past a sewer pipe until a wire blocks access to the cliffs, at 3.4 miles. Turn around and follow the river to the bend, stepping up and over another sewer pipe. As the trail turns 90 degrees to the right, Georgia's newest covered bridge comes into view. The path leads you under the bridge, but don't try to climb uphill near the bridge—there's a much easier way to get there.

Return to the three-way intersection and turn left, climbing back to the second intersection. Bear right—don't take the hard right, the trail you came in on—and watch on the left for the trail a few steps up the path. The path drops steeply to the covered bridge, which spans Vickery Creek. On the far side, the trail climbs a gravel road, passing one of many buildings collectively known as Roswell Mill, today part of Old Mill Park.

As the road reaches a level section, bear right and follow the path down to the mill's powerhouse and dam. Just before you reach the powerhouse, turn right and descend to the riverbank; follow the trail to a wooden viewing deck just before the dam.

Return to the trail and turn right, following the footpath to a gravel road that sharply rises to King's Mill Court, a paved residential street. Turn left on Sloan Street. As Founder's Cemetery appears on the right, the entrance to an interpretive trail leading to Roswell Mill is on the left, just after a small streetside parking lot. Descending the stairs, you'll find signs telling the story of Roswell Mill. As you return to the riverbank, turn right and retrace your steps to the covered bridge, climbing to the Vickery Creek Trail complex after crossing the bridge. Turn left and follow the wide path as it climbs to a road on the left, at 5.5 miles. This road drops steadily to the milldam. This is a pleasant area for a break, with the roaring water of Vickery Creek tumbling over the massive dam.

Turn around, climb back to the top of the road, and turn right. The trail becomes a footpath through thickets of mountain laurels and rhododendrons. A three-way intersection is marked by a split rail fence on the left to prevent hikers from trying to climb down the steep, fragile embankment to the milldam. Continuing straight, the trail once again becomes a footpath through a sometimes dense forest. A stream with a couple of small waterfalls requires a wet-footed crossing at 5.9 miles as the footpath gently sweeps left. As Vickery Creek Trail curves back around to the right, it passes a crossover trail to the right at 6 miles. From this point the trail drops quickly to the start of the loop, where you turn left and return to your car.

NEARBY ACTIVITIES

Archibald Smith was an influential resident of Roswell. His 1840s **plantation home** (950 Forrest St. [GPS address]; 770-641-3978; **archibaldsmithplantation.org**), adjacent to the impressive Roswell City Hall, is open Monday–Saturday, with tours on the hour 10 a.m.–3 p.m., and Sunday, with tours on the hour 1–3 p.m. (closed major holidays). Admission (cash or check only) is $8 adults, $7 seniors age 65 and older, $6 kids ages 6–12 and students with valid ID, and free for kids age 5 and younger. According to the city of Roswell, which owns the site, the home features original furnishings and 12 outbuildings. Turn left out of the Oxbo parking lot, travel 0.1 mile to Roswell Road, turn right, and proceed two blocks to Hill Street. Make the first left into the Roswell City Hall parking lot and continue to the other side of the building. Watch for the signed entrance for the Smith Plantation, on the left. Also worth a look is the stunning **Faces of War Memorial**, in the city-hall parking lot.

WILDCAT CREEK TRAIL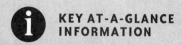

IN BRIEF

This trail climbs into the Amicalola Creek watershed along Wildcat Creek. Because the trail is in a remote area, it's possible to see a wide range of wildlife.

DESCRIPTION

Although this part of the Dawson Forest Wildlife Management Area is technically under the control of the Georgia Department of Natural Resources (DNR), it is the nonprofit Mountain Stewards who have developed the multiple-trail complex in this area. Wildcat Tract spans the forest from Monument Road to Steve Tate Highway, and the Mountain Stewards have developed Tobacco Pouch Trail, Fall Creek Trail, Rocky Ford Trail, Windy Ridge Trail, Turner Trail, and Wildcat Creek Trail—12 miles of trails in all. For this hike we chose Wildcat Creek Trail.

At the end of the Wildcat Campground, a brown hiker sign in front of the fast-flowing Amicalola Creek marks the trailhead. Follow

- -

Directions ⟶

Take I-75 North to Exit 260 and merge onto I-575. At the northern border of Cherokee County (30.7 miles), limited-access I-575 becomes full-access GA 515. Drive a total of 42.6 miles on I-575/GA 515 to GA 53, and turn right. Continue 8.5 miles and turn left on Steve Tate Road. Drive 7.2 miles and turn left on Wildcat Campground Road. Drive 0.8 mile, following the road to the far end of the campground, and park on either side. Or, from I-285 North, take GA 400/US 19 North 38 miles to GA 53. At the first traffic light after the outlet mall, turn left and drive 10.8 miles; then turn right on Steve Tate Road and follow the remaining directions to the campground.

KEY AT-A-GLANCE INFORMATION

LENGTH: 3 miles round-trip

CONFIGURATION: Out-and-back

DIFFICULTY: Easy–moderate

SCENERY: Views of Wildcat Creek

EXPOSURE: Mostly shaded

TRAFFIC: Light

TRAIL SURFACE: Packed dirt, gravel roads

WHEELCHAIR ACCESS: None

HIKING TIME: 1.5 hours

ACCESS: Daily, year-round, 24/7; Georgia Outdoor Recreation Pass required for visitors ages 16–64, $3.50/3 days or $19/year (buy online at georgiawildlife.com /recreational-licenses; transaction fees may apply)

MAPS: USGS *Amicalola, Nelson*

MORE INFO: 770-535-5700; mountainstewards.org

FACILITIES: None

SPECIAL COMMENTS: Although the trail is in a remote area of North Georgia, don't worry about wildcats— the name probably refers to the miners who sought alluvial gold.

DISTANCE: 60 miles from I-75 North/I-285 Northwest

GPS INFORMATION

N34° 29.732' W84° 16.920'

Wildcat Creek Trail

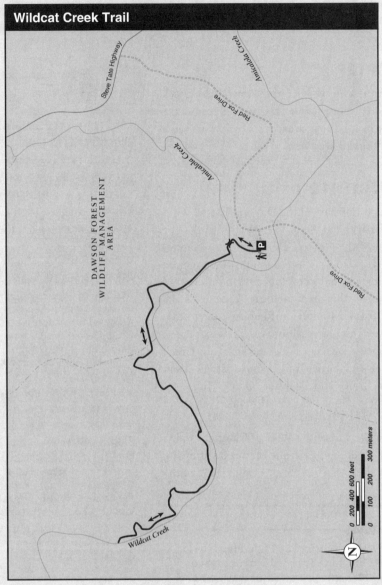

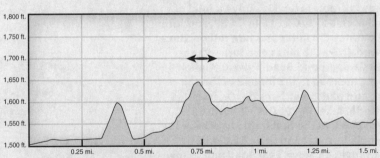

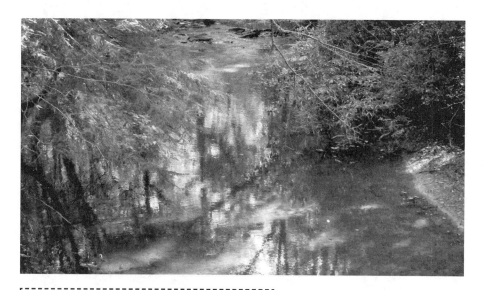

Reflected light dapples the calm waters of Wildcat Creek.

the creek 20 steps to the right to reach the first green blaze, which marks Wildcat Creek Trail. Walk 0.1 mile to reach a wooden bridge built by Mountain Stewards and the DNR. Take the bridge across the creek and hike over some soggy level ground to reach Wildcat Creek. Follow it upstream into the watershed of the Amicalola Creek. Rhododendrons are prevalent, as are hemlocks and shortleaf and longleaf pines. Oaks and dogwoods abound near the trail, which hugs a riverbank that drops sharply to the creek. Occasionally, side trails allow fishing access.

About 0.3 mile into the hike, the trail bears away from the creek and begins climbing a small hill rising some 80 feet above the water. The climb is relatively easy, but the path narrows at the top, so returning to the creek means a scramble down a steep, slippery, tree-rooted path with rock outcrops. As you return to the creek, rhododendrons and laurels battle for sunlight, and both the creek and trail make a 90-degree left turn about 0.5 mile into the hike.

Joining an old road at 0.6 mile, the trail bears right (away from the creek) and climbs into a mostly pine forest. Near the top of this hill, look left to see the creek, well below you. (On one hike as we climbed the third mountain, we heard the call of a hawk to our left. He flew away with dinner—a gray squirrel—in his grasp. A short time later, we spotted the squirrel carcass a few feet off the trail.) Leaving this hill, the trail returns to the creek at 1.4 miles, now more heavily covered with rhododendrons and requiring carefully maneuvering over slippery rocks. Finally, 0.1 mile later, the trail ends at Wildcat Creek. This is your turnaround point.

NEARBY ACTIVITIES

Any of the trails in the **Dawson Forest Wildlife Management Area** would make an excellent adjunct to this hike. For more information, visit **mountainstewards.org**.

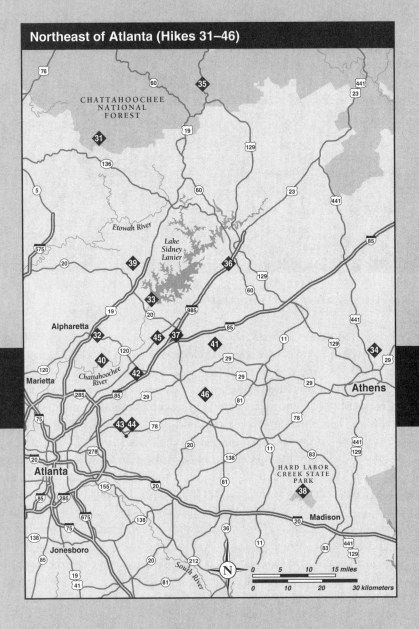

CHATTAHOOCHEE
NATIONAL
FOREST

Etowah River

Lake
Sidney
Lanier

Alpharetta

Marietta

Chattahoochee
River

Atlanta

Jonesboro

South River

Athens

HARD LABOR
CREEK STATE
PARK

Madison

N

| 0 | 5 | 10 | 15 miles |

| 0 | 10 | 20 | 30 kilometers |

NORTHEAST OF
ATLANTA

31 AMICALOLA FALLS LOOP

KEY AT-A-GLANCE INFORMATION

LENGTH: 2.8 miles

CONFIGURATION: Loop

DIFFICULTY: Hard

SCENERY: Waterfalls, mountains

EXPOSURE: Full sun at falls and visitor center and along the upper third of the East Ridge; shaded elsewhere

TRAFFIC: Heavy, especially during peak leaf season

TRAIL SURFACE: Compacted soil and gravel. The trail from the West Ridge Parking Lot to the falls is made of rubber tires.

WHEELCHAIR ACCESS: Limited

HIKING TIME: 2 hours

ACCESS: Daily, year-round, 7 a.m.– sunset; park office: daily, 8 a.m.– 5 p.m.; $5 state-park fee

MAPS: Available at visitor center; USGS *Amicalola, Nimblewill*

MORE INFO: 706-265-4703; gastateparks.org/amicalolafalls

FACILITIES: Restrooms, picnic tables, visitor center. Amicalola Falls is the only access point to the southern terminus of the Appalachian Trail with long-term parking for thru-hikers.

SPECIAL COMMENTS: The best views come after a winter rain, when there is no tree cover and the river is high.

DISTANCE: 59.3 miles from GA 400 North/I-285 North

GPS INFORMATION

N34° 34.037' W84° 14.563'
418 Amicalola State Park Rd.
Dawsonville, GA 30534

IN BRIEF

This trail explores the watershed of the Amicalola Creek in the area of Amicalola Falls.

DESCRIPTION

Tumbling 729 feet in a series of free falls and large cascades, Amicalola Falls is clearly the focus of this trail. The first written account of these falls at the southern end of the Blue Ridge Mountains appeared in 1832 when surveyor William Williamson wrote, "I discovered a Water Fall perhaps the greatest in the World." Williamson was surveying lots for the Sixth Georgia Land Lottery, which precipitated the Cherokee Trail of Tears.

When the Appalachian Trail (AT) was rerouted to end at Springer Mountain in 1959, Amicalola Falls became known as the southern terminus access for thru-hikers. A portion of the loop trail is actually part of the access trail, an 8-mile point-to-point path from Amicalola Falls to the Appalachian Trailhead on Springer Mountain.

Directions ———————————→

Take GA 400/US 19 North to GA 53. At the first traffic light after the outlet mall, turn left and drive 6.5 miles to a stop sign. Turn left and continue on GA 53, around Dawson County Courthouse and through downtown Dawsonville. Drive 2.6 miles and go right on Elliott Family Parkway/GA 183. Drive 10.4 miles to GA 52, following the traffic triangle to the right. Drive 1.5 miles to the entrance to Amicalola Falls State Park and pay the $5 entrance fee. Just more than 0.2 mile into the park, turn left onto Amicalola State Park Road and drive 1.1 miles to the parking area on the right. If the lot is full, you'll find overflow parking down the road, also on the right.

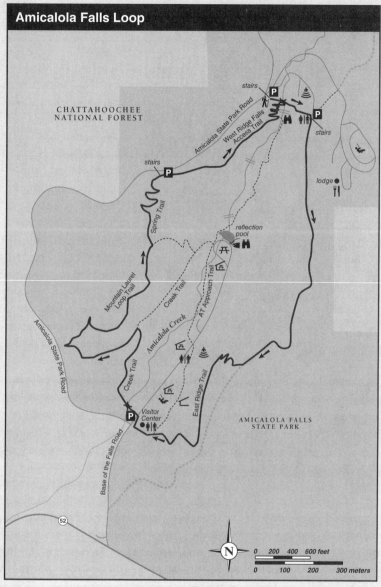

Amicalola Falls Loop

CHATTAHOOCHEE
NATIONAL FOREST

stairs

Amicalola State Park Road

West Ridge Falls
Access Trail

stairs

lodge

stairs

Spring Trail

reflection
pool

Mountain Laurel
Loop Trail

Creek Trail

AT Approach Trail

Amicalola Creek

Amicalola State Park Road

Creek Trail

East Ridge Trail

AMICALOLA FALLS
STATE PARK

Visitor
Center

Base of the Falls Road

52

N

0   200   400   600 feet

0   100   200   300 meters

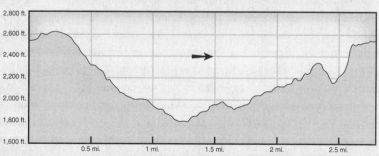

2,800 ft.

2,600 ft.

2,400 ft.

2,200 ft.

2,000 ft.

1,800 ft.

1,600 ft.

0.5 mi.   1 mi.   1.5 mi.   2 mi.   2.5 mi.

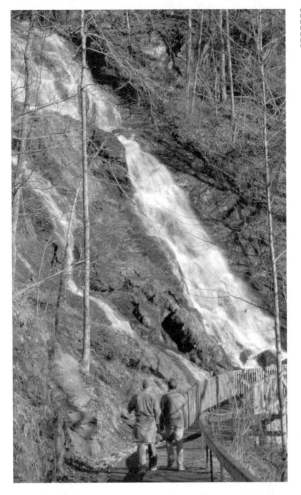

Descending a set of stone steps from the parking lot, on the left you'll see interpretive signs that discuss Hurricane Opal, which swept across the North Georgia mountains on October 4, 1995. As you continue, the concrete path turns to wood and then juts over the falls. The trees open to reward you with incredible views of the southern Blue Ridge foothills and the Amicalola Creek watershed. The stable flow of the Amicalola, combined with its high oxygen content, makes the creek an excellent fishing stream and provides habitat for a wide range of waterfowl and other animals downstream.

Continue across the bridge, climbing a set of railed concrete steps to the paved east overflow parking area. Turn right, descending to the gated entrance to the East Ridge Trail. On your right are concrete-block restrooms and vending machines. The upper portion of East Ridge Trail follows the original gravel road to the top of Amicalola Falls. The upper portion of the road is sunny, rocky, and heavily rutted in areas, but the view to the right, across the Georgia Piedmont, is simply stunning.

As the gravel road reenters the forest at 0.4 mile, the trail moderates. Now walking in partial shade through a mature second-growth hardwood forest, you'll find that the incline lessens and the road is less rutted. A double blaze indicates a turn ahead, which comes at 0.5 mile at a red visitor-center sign. The trail descends wooden steps into the full shade of a deciduous forest composed of oaks, native dogwoods, and mountain laurels. Entering a cove at 0.7 mile, the trail traverses a gully on a wooden boardwalk. Here the maturing hardwoods are beginning to take on the appearance of an old-growth forest.

East Ridge Trail descends fieldstone steps at 1.1 miles into the opening for the visitor center. On the left is a stone in the shape of the state of Georgia, inscribed with MAINE TO GEORGIA, the slogan for the AT. Just past the stone are a stone bridge and an arch. You can walk around the building to the left (restrooms are here) or enter the visitor center, with displays on the natural history of the area along with an excellent bookstore. Rangers frequently lead interpretive sessions at the center as well.

Cross the paved road to a small parking lot. At the far end of the lot, a wooden bridge crosses Amicalola Creek. On the far side of the bridge, the trail turns right and begins a steady, moderate climb; some 150 feet above the creek, there are occasional streamside views. At 1.5 miles, turn left onto Mountain Laurel Loop Trail at the signed three-way intersection. Gradually climbing a gravel road for 0.2 mile, the trail bears right, returning to a forest of pines mixed with young oaks. As the green-blazed trail rises, it comes to a confusing three-way intersection at 1.7 miles—all the trails sport a green blaze. Turn right here and continue your easy climb through a thicket of mountain laurels, which sometimes form a canopy over the path.

Take the yellow-blazed Spring Trail, which heads left at 2 miles and begins a steady, moderate climb to the West Ridge parking area. The trail switchbacks a couple of times to ease the climb; at 2.2 miles, it climbs a set of stairs, turns right, and then makes a left, following a grade to the embankment of the modern road. For a few steps, the pathway climbs the embankment; then it switches back and returns to compacted soil.

Spring Trail ascends a set of stairs to the West Ridge parking lot. In the lot, turn right and continue to the West Ridge Falls Access Trail. Only 0.2 mile long, this easy, level trail allows wheelchair access to the Lower Falls. At the end of this trail, a wooden bridge crosses in front of the falls, giving visitors an unrivaled view of Amicalola Creek tumbling down the mountain. Return 0.1 mile to the metal-grate stairs, on your left.

The final ascent of the face of the falls requires a hike of more than 300 steps, but along the route are wide areas with benches if you need a breather. At the top of the stairs, turn right to return to the first long-distance view over the falls, or turn left to return to your car.

NEARBY ACTIVITIES

Day hikers can visit the **Len Foote Hike Inn** (800-581-8032; **hike-inn.com**) via an easy-to-moderate 5-mile hike over 2–4 hours (reserve a room by phone if you want to spend the night). For seasonal fun in the fall, try **Burt's Pumpkin Farm**, across the street from the entrance to Amicalola Falls (5 Burt's Pumpkin Farm Rd., Dawsonville; 800-600-2878 or 706-265-3701; **burtsfarm.com**). Kids will love choosing their Halloween pumpkin, and Mom and Dad will have a good time creating memories.

32   BIG CREEK GREENWAY: NORTH POINT

KEY AT-A-GLANCE INFORMATION

LENGTH: 12.5 miles round-trip

CONFIGURATION: Out-and-back with a small balloon at the end

DIFFICULTY: Moderate

SCENERY: Creekside views, forested wetlands

EXPOSURE: Partly shaded

TRAFFIC: Heavy; multiuse trail

TRAIL SURFACE: Concrete pavement, except for a section of boardwalk on the balloon at the end

WHEELCHAIR ACCESS: Yes, although access is probably easiest from the greenway parking area, which you enter on a driveway that adjoins the Ethan Allen parking lot at 6800 North Point Pkwy., Alpharetta.

HIKING TIME: 5 hours

ACCESS: Daily, year-round, sunrise–sunset; free

MAPS: Brochure at trailhead (sometimes); USGS *Roswell*

MORE INFO: georgiatrails.com/gt /big_creek_greenway_(north_point); bigcreekgreenway.com

FACILITIES: Restrooms at Mansell Road

SPECIAL COMMENTS: Atlanta's most cosmopolitan trail—it's possible to hear a wide variety of languages as you hike this trail with people from around the world, due to local businesses with international hiring practices.

DISTANCE: 13.8 miles from GA 400 North/I-285 North

GPS INFORMATION

N34° 4.182' W84° 15.218'

IN BRIEF

This portion of the multiuse Big Creek Greenway explores the floodplain of Big Creek, also known as Vickery Creek (see Hike 29, page 142), from Webb Bridge Road to Mansell Road.

DESCRIPTION

Rob Warrilow got the idea for the Big Creek Greenway when he was visiting his son at college in Colorado, where a similar trail existed. Warrilow, an engineer for the city of Alpharetta, knew that an easement in the hundred-year floodplain of Big Creek would be a great place to build the same kind of trail. He walked the Colorado trail with his video camera and returned home to show the trail to the Alpharetta city council as he discussed plans for the floodplain. With the council's support, Warrilow secured funding, and work on the trail began. The north and south ends were completed first. In 2001 the city completed the connection, creating a 6.2-mile-long park. Plans to extend the trail from Forsyth County to Cobb County (a total of 26 miles) were announced in 2005 and later expanded to 40 miles; the first 7 miles in Forsyth County are now complete. The city of Roswell has also extended the trail south of Mansell Road.

Directions

Take GA 400/US 19 North to Exit 10/Old Milton Highway. Turn right at the end of the ramp and move to the left lane. At 0.5 mile turn left on North Point Parkway; drive 0.4 mile and make a right on Preston Ridge Road. On-road parking is 0.1 mile ahead, on the right. You'll find more parking at North Point Mall and on Haynes Bridge Road, next to the mall.

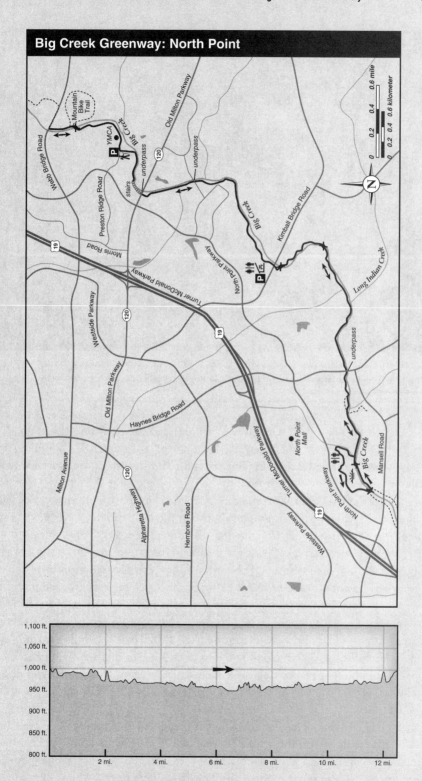

Big Creek Greenway: North Point

Mountain Bike Trail

Big Creek

YMCA

Webb Bridge Road

Preston Ridge Road

Old Milton Parkway

underpass

underpass

(120)

stairs

Morris Road

19

Big Creek

Kimball Bridge Road

Long Indian Creek

Turner McDonald Parkway

North Point Parkway

Westside Parkway

(120)

19

underpass

Old Milton Parkway

Haynes Bridge Road

North Point Mall

Big Creek

Mansell Road

Milton Avenue

(120)

Alpharetta Highway

Hembree Road

Turner McDonald Parkway

Westside Parkway

North Point Parkway

19

0.6 mile
0.4
0.2
0
0.2 0.4 0.6 kilometer

N

1,100 ft.
1,050 ft.
1,000 ft.
950 ft.
900 ft.
850 ft.
800 ft.

2 mi.   4 mi.   6 mi.   8 mi.   10 mi.   12 mi.

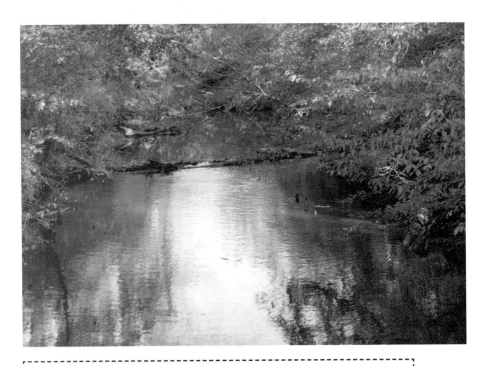

This hike takes in the languid waters of Big Creek. During heavy rains, the creek sometimes overflows its banks and floods the trail.

From the Big Creek Greenway parking area on Preston Ridge Road in Alpharetta, turn left on the sidewalk, heading toward the YMCA building, and cross a side street that leads to parking for the YMCA youth camp. On the far side of the street, the path slowly drops into the surprisingly large Big Creek floodplain. On the left, the modern YMCA building rises well above the path. Post oaks, river birches, and sycamores fill in the area between the trail and the river on the right side of the path. Just under 0.5 mile into the hike, Big Creek comes into view for the first time. Wide and fast-flowing, its water is frequently muddy because of erosion, which is of some concern. Urban runoff has also become a problem for the river, which provides some of the drinking water for communities along it.

A few steps farther on, the pathway curves right, crosses its first bridge—concrete with metal railings—and curves left. On the right, a dirt path leads to a hiking/biking trail that adds 1 mile to the trip. At 0.8 mile the multiuse trail turns right at Webb Bridge Road, crossing the road in 0.2 mile and following Big Creek north to a parking area on Marconi Drive, off Windward Parkway. If you decide to add this stretch to your hike, the total mileage jumps to 14.5 miles.

Turn around and retrace your route to the entrance, but as you cross the asphalt road, make a left. The YMCA youth camp is on the left—the trail runs beside it as it drops gently before curving right. Be careful here: you can't see around the corner, and cyclists occasionally exceed the posted 15-mile-per-hour speed limit. The trail runs next to apartments from here to Old Milton Parkway. At

1.8 miles you'll see a small falls along the creek to your left. Just over 2 miles into the hike, Big Creek Greenway makes an S-curve as a concrete stairway rises to Old Milton on the right. After the stairway, the trail curves left under the Old Milton overpass, affording some good views of the creek at a metal railing.

A second bridge carries you across a tributary at 2.5 miles, where you'll see commercial buildings on the right, homes on the left, and a bridge crossing the trail that eases traffic congestion in the office park. From this point on, you can sometimes see homes from the trail. As the trail curves right at 3 miles, a forested wetlands appears on the right. A bridge over a tributary at 3.4 miles is followed by a concrete path heading right, leading in 0.5 mile to more commercial buildings. Here we once spotted a pair of owls who joined us for part of the southbound walk. The original path makes a hard right and climbs to Rock Mill Park and Kimball Bridge Road. A new trail follows Big Creek's floodplain past an environmentally sensitive wetlands and goes under Kimball Bridge Road, rejoining the original trail just before the first bridge south of the underpass. With Big Creek again on your left, the path sweeps right and changes from a north–south trail to an east–west one. At 5.1 miles a trail on the right leads to a housing development, and then Big Creek Greenway arrives at the Haynes Bridge Road overpass 0.4 mile later. On the right is a trail to a parking area.

Splitting at 5.8 miles, the two paths come together 0.1 mile later. You'll soon reach a side path on the left that crosses Big Creek on a bridge and ends in a commercial area. At a four-way intersection at 6.3 miles, take the trail on the right, 0.2 mile from the restrooms. Just before the restrooms, a wood chip–covered path heads left, entering a mostly pine forest at the start of an extensive forested wetlands area. The trail turns left after a bridge at 6.7 miles, running beside North Point Mall a short distance. As the trail curves back to the right, you'll come to a frequently muddy area, followed by a side trail to another shopping area. At 7 miles the pathway turns into a boardwalk leading to a bridge over a creek. A trail heads right as you step off the bridge—continue straight. The footpath climbs concrete steps up to the greenway. At the intersection you can go straight or left—both trails return you to the previous four-way. We prefer the path on the left, which combines paved path, railed boardwalk, and an excellent scenic view into the forested wetlands to create a pleasant walk back to the intersection. At the four-way, take a few moments to view Big Creek from the bridge on your right. Return to the main trail, turn right, and retrace your steps to your car.

NEARBY ACTIVITIES

The Forsyth County portion of Big Creek, beginning at McFarland Road and ending at Bethelview Road, is 6.3 miles long. Plans call for the greenway to continue to **Sawnee Mountain Preserve,** home of the Indian Seats Trail (see Hike 39, page 187).

33 BOWMANS ISLAND TRAIL

KEY AT-A-GLANCE INFORMATION

LENGTH: 3.5 miles

CONFIGURATION: Double loop

DIFFICULTY: Easy

SCENERY: Some winter views of the Chattahoochee River

EXPOSURE: Full sun at start, then mostly shaded

TRAFFIC: Low; horseback riding allowed

TRAIL SURFACE: Mostly old gravel roads connected by compacted dirt

WHEELCHAIR ACCESS: None

HIKING TIME: 1.5 hours

ACCESS: Trail: daily, year-round, sunrise–sunset; headquarters: daily, year-round, 9 a.m.–5 p.m., except December 25; $3 day-use fee

MAPS: At trailhead kiosk; USGS *Buford Dam*

MORE INFO: 678-538-1200; nps.gov/chat/planyourvisit /bowmansisland.htm

FACILITIES: Restrooms and picnicking nearby

SPECIAL COMMENTS: Dogs are prohibited in both the Bowman Island Unit of the Chattahoochee River National Recreation Area and in Buford Dam Park. This hike doesn't cross onto Bowmans Island.

DISTANCE: 30.1 miles from GA 400 North/I-285 North

GPS INFORMATION

N34° 9.404' W84° 4.807'

IN BRIEF

This double loop in the Bowman Island Unit of the Chattahoochee River National Recreation Area circles just below the crest of two hills south of the Buford Dam. Horseback riding is allowed, but this section of the trail is only lightly used.

DESCRIPTION

At the south end of the first parking lot, a modular bridge spans Haw Creek. After crossing the creek, the pathway bears left, crossing a wide, level field that was once part of the Chattahoochee River floodplain. At 0.2 mile a second path heads right, almost doubling back on the trail as it begins an easy-to-moderate climb to an old road that circles the top of a low hill. Once on this road, you'll notice some elevation change as the pathway climbs and falls, in and out of coves. Much of the pine cover has fallen prey to the pine borer, but there are still some good stands of longleaf. A few homes are visible behind the trees, but for the most part they aren't obtrusive.

At a three-way intersection at 0.8 mile, take the pathway that bears left and climbs to the top of the ridge. From here the path drops

----

Directions

Take GA 400/US 19 North to Exit 20/Buford Road; turn right. Drive 2 miles to Samples Road and turn left. Drive 2.3 miles to Buford Dam Road; turn right. Drive 1.6 miles until Buford Dam Road turns 90 degrees to the left; Little Mill Road (which looks like a wide driveway) is straight ahead. As you enter the apron, a LOWER POOL PARK sign is almost straight ahead. Continue on this dirt road 0.2 mile to the first lot on the right. The trailhead is at the west end of the lot.

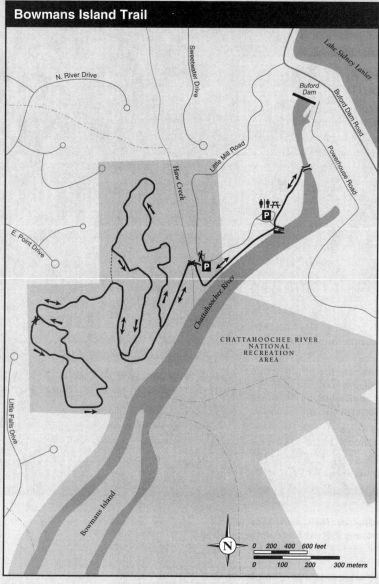

Bowmans Island Trail

N. River Drive

Sweetwater Drive

Lake Sidney Lanier

Buford Dam

Buford Dam Road

Little Mill Road

Haw Creek

E. Point Drive

Powerhouse Road

Chattahoochee River

CHATTAHOOCHEE RIVER
NATIONAL
RECREATION
AREA

Little Falls Drive

Bowmans Island

N

| 0 | 200 | 400 | 600 feet |

| 0 | 100 | 200 | 300 meters |

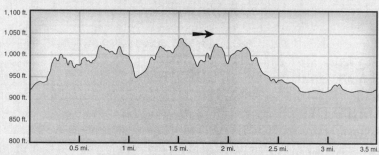

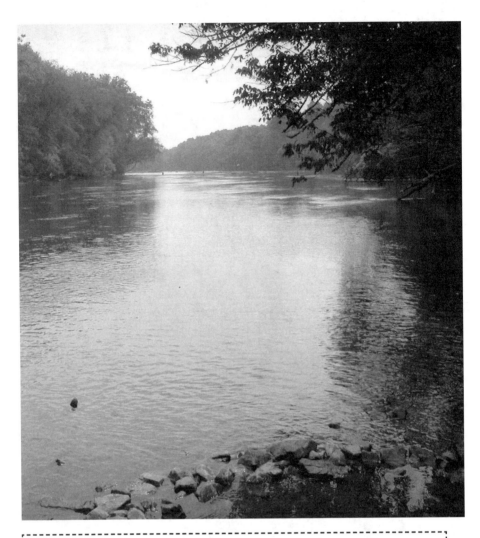

Just below Buford Dam, which forms Lake Sidney Lanier, the Chattahoochee River flows in a southwesterly direction toward Bowmans Island.

rapidly but not steeply, finally curving hard to the right and dropping to a wide road 0.3 mile later. Continue straight, following the gravel road as it climbs to another three-way intersection 0.1 mile ahead. The trail turns left, joining the second loop 0.3 mile later. Turn right and cross a shallow creek on a wooden bridge 1.5 miles into the hike. Dammed downstream, the river forms a small lake to the left of the path. You can also see homes ahead and on the right.

As the trail follows an old road through a mostly hardwood forest, watch for the occasionally large beech trees throughout the hike. The barrage of oak trees, including red, white, and pin oaks with the occasional maple, is typical of a Georgia Piedmont forest. The trail drops, and off to the right you can hear the rush of water. In some places you can spot the wide Chattahoochee River, especially in the winter. As the trail circles left, it moves away from the river and climbs back to the intersection with the trail from the first loop. Turn right, then right again, and follow the road back to the parking lot.

After crossing the bridge at the start of the trail, turn right and follow the creek to the Chattahoochee. As the trail turns left at the riverbank, you can usually see the shoals in center; waterfowl are frequently found on or near them, even if a trout fisherman is nearby. Follow the trail to the left, past a "blooper" siren that warns of an imminent release from Buford Dam. Continue on, moving slightly inland and crossing a boat ramp and picnic area to a prefabricated bridge over the powerhouse channel. Part of the powerhouse is visible from the left side of the bridge. Turn around and retrace your steps to the parking lot.

NEARBY ACTIVITIES

The visitor center at the US Army Corps of Engineers' **Lake Lanier Resource Management Office** (1050 Buford Dam Rd., Buford; 770-945-9531) provides information on the creation of Buford Dam, facts about Lake Lanier, and a general history of the area around the lake. The **Laurel Ridge Trail,** a 3.4-mile loop that explores the valley of the Chattahoochee and several Corps of Engineers–managed parks along Lake Lanier, starts in Buford Dam Park (1200 Buford Dam Rd., 770-945-9531; $4 vehicles, $1 pedestrians).

34 COOK'S GREENWAY TRAIL

KEY AT-A-GLANCE INFORMATION

LENGTH: 8.4 miles round-trip

CONFIGURATION: Out-and-back

DIFFICULTY: Moderate

SCENERY: Creekside views of Sandy Creek, wetlands, and small lakes

EXPOSURE: Partial shade

TRAFFIC: Moderate

TRAIL SURFACE: Moist dirt that is heavily rooted at times; boardwalks over wet areas

WHEELCHAIR ACCESS: None

HIKING TIME: 4.5 hours

ACCESS: Daily, year-round, sunrise–sunset; free

MAPS: Available at Sandy Creek Nature Center; Sandy Creek Park; USGS *Athens East, Athens West, Hull, Nicholson*

MORE INFO: 706-613-3800; tinyurl.com/clarkecountyparks

FACILITIES: Restrooms at both ends of the trail

SPECIAL COMMENTS: Cook's Greenway Trail can be combined with the adjacent Lakeside Trail to create a 13-mile round-trip hike.

DISTANCE: 63 miles from I-85 North/I-285 Northeast

GPS INFORMATION

N34° 1.548' W83° 22.518'

Sandy Creek Park: 400 Bob Holman Rd. Athens, GA 30607

IN BRIEF

Cook's Greenway Trail follows the floodplain of Sandy Creek from Lake Chapman in Sandy Creek Park to Sandy Creek Nature Center.

DESCRIPTION

Conceived and developed by Walter L. Cook Jr., a retired University of Georgia forestry professor, Cook's Greenway Trail is an extension of the North Oconee River Greenway, a 3-mile-long paved park that connects Sandy Creek Nature Center to The University of Georgia on the south and Lakeside Trail on the north. The trail follows Sandy Creek from Sandy Creek Park to Sandy Creek Nature Center, which Cook also founded.

The development of the trail actually began at about the time work was being completed on Lake Chapman in the early 1970s, when the U.S. Soil Conservation Service wanted to channelize Sandy Creek to control erosion. UGA landscape-architecture professor Charles Aguar led the battle to preserve the natural setting. Cook pushed the concept

---

Directions ————————————➤

Take I-85 North to Exit 106 and merge onto GA 316. Drive 39.7 miles until you see a sign that says GA 316 ENDS. Follow the signs for GA 10 Loop North and take the road 4.6 miles to Exit 12/US 441 North/GA 15/MLK Parkway/Commerce. At the end of the ramp, turn left and drive 3 miles. Turn right on Bob Holman Road and proceed 0.7 mile; then make a right into Sandy Creek Park. At the pay booth and information kiosk, ask for the map to Cook's Greenway Trail. Continue 0.1 mile, turning right at a stop sign. The road curves back to the left and Campsite Drive heads right. Cross the dam and park in the first parking area.

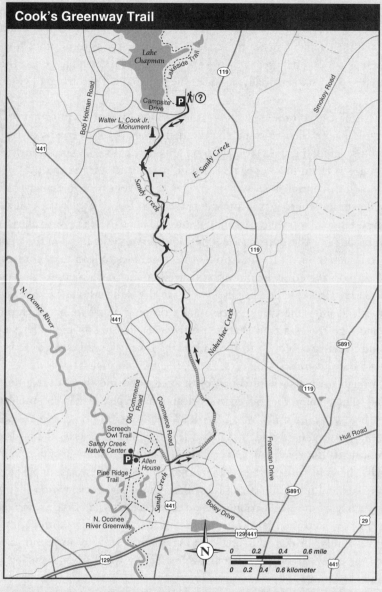

Cook's Greenway Trail

Lake Chapman

Lakeside Trail

119

Bob Holman Road

Smokey Road

Campsite Drive

P

Walter L. Cook Jr. Monument

441

E. Sandy Creek

Sandy Creek

119

441

N. Oconee River

119

Nobetchee Creek

S891

Old Commerce Road

Commerce Road

119

Screech Owl Trail

Sandy Creek Nature Center

P

Allen House

Pine Ridge Trail

Freeman Drive

Hull Road

S891

Sandy Creek

441

Boley Drive

29

N. Oconee River Greenway

129 441

441

129

N

| 0 | 0.2 | 0.4 | 0.6 mile |

| 0 | 0.2 | 0.4 | 0.6 kilometer |

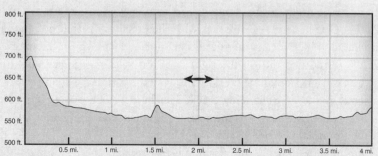

800 ft.
750 ft.
700 ft.
650 ft.
600 ft.
550 ft.
500 ft.

0.5 mi.   1 mi.   1.5 mi.   2 mi.   2.5 mi.   3 mi.   3.5 mi.   4 mi.

of a nature center, not only to preserve the area near the confluence of Sandy Creek and the Oconee River but also to educate people about the importance of forests and their inhabitants in the cycle of life. After the nature center was completed, Cook proposed a greenway to connect it to Lake Chapman. Once the land was purchased, Cook personally designed the trail and led the group of volunteers who built it.

The trailhead, on the east side of the parking lot, has an information kiosk and a three-page welcome stand that contains a map, an overview of the trail, and trail-use guidelines. As you descend through a loblolly-and-shortleaf-pine forest, a green chain-link fence at 0.2 mile marks the start of the trail. Cook's Greenway Trail continues an easy-to-moderate descent to a three-way intersection at 0.4 mile, where a trail provides access to Sandy Creek Park's Lakeside Trail. Turn left and continue descending into the Sandy Creek river valley. As the descent moderates, the trail starts a long, slow curve to the left. On the right side of the trail, a monument to Dr. Cook—who continues to lead local conservation efforts—honors the effort he put into this trail. You also get a good "above it all" view of Sandy Creek, which lies in a valley on the right. About 0.6 mile into the hike, the trail joins the creek, occasionally running along its banks. From this point, the hike traces a trail that is mostly level, frequently moist (wet after a rain), and heavily rooted. Until the end of the hike, the trail is never more than 100 feet from the creek.

Through a diverse hardwood forest composed mostly of white and post oaks and some maples, the trail enters a cleared gas-pipeline field and then crosses the first bridge, at 0.8 mile. When Cook's Greenway Trail reaches a tributary of the creek, it normally turns left, heads a few feet inland, crosses the bridge, and then returns to the riverbank. After crossing another tributary and a couple of wetlands, the trail turns left and then right across its first major bridge, with wooden slats and iron railings, at 1.2 miles. This clear creek, with a high water volume, is one of the larger tributaries on the hike. After crossing the bridge, the trail turns right and then left as it rejoins the river. Less than 0.3 mile later you come to a similar bridge, this one crossing Sandy Creek to an island and then crossing the creek to the far riverbank. Now Sandy Creek is on your left as the trail gradually climbs.

An intrusive green-roofed home comes into view as the treadway curves left, at 1.8 miles. One issue that Cook sees with the greenway is that not enough land was purchased, which means that development can encroach on the hike's serene beauty. A forested wetland on the right contrasts with the green-roofed house's backyard on the left, across the creek. Following the forested wetlands is an oxbow lake, created by the ever-changing creek. This lake was once a curve in the river, but it was eventually bypassed as the river straightened and the oxbow lake became part of the floodplain. When Sandy Creek runs high, the oxbow lake floods, preventing too much sediment from flowing downstream.

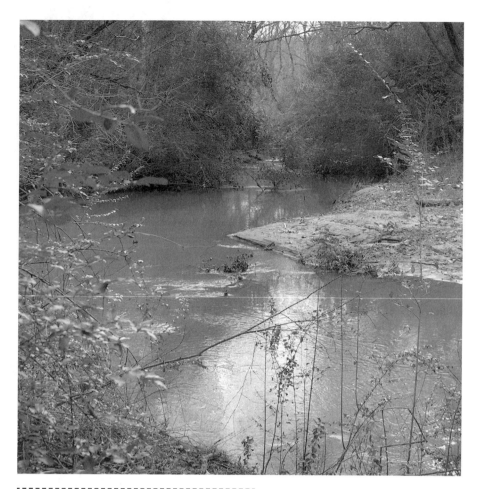

Sandy Creek, an environmentally sensitive waterway

Not very far after you pass a trail on the right, the path turns and crosses Sandy Creek again, quickly entering a heavily rooted, muddy area. Just after 2.6 miles, the path begins to run on a long elevated walkway as the creek spreads out to form a wetland. Segments of boardwalk are interspersed with short sections of normally moist, rooted, occasionally muddy track. Unfortunately, houses once again intrude on pristine nature.

Over the next 0.6 mile, the trail circles a large wetland area to the east and south of Sandy Creek before rejoining a wider, fuller creek at 3.6 miles. Shortly after rejoining the stream, the pathway turns right, crosses a wooden-planked iron bridge, and then turns left at the far side of the creek and passes under US 441. After exiting the bridge, the treadway parallels the road, heading north to the signed entrance to Sandy Creek Nature Center, at 3.9 miles. The trail sweeps to the left, joining Pine Ridge Trail after the marked Screech Owl Trail leaves to the

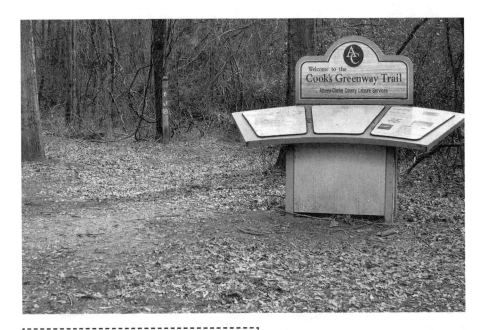

A wealth of information is displayed at the trailhead.

right from Cook's Greenway Trail. After Screech Owl appears on the right a second time, continue straight to a T-intersection. Turn right and follow the trail to the Allen House (circa 1900), at the nature-center trailhead. After visiting the nature center, retrace your route back to your car.

NEARBY ACTIVITIES

Sandy Creek Nature Center's **ENSAT (Environment, Natural Science, and Appropriate Technology) Center,** a regionally focused environmental-education center, demonstrates ways to incorporate modern technological advances into construction projects to reduce their impact on the environment. Two exhibits highlight the coastal community and the wetlands community, including life-cycle information on endangered loggerhead turtles, along with a 1,500-gallon aquarium and 500-gallon feeding tank. Miles of hiking trails crisscross the nature center, which lies at the northern end of the **North Oconee Greenway,** a 3.75-mile, concrete-paved multiuse trail that connects to the University of Georgia trail system. For more information, call 706-613-3615 or visit **tinyurl.com/sandycreeknaturecenter.**

At the north end of Cook's Greenway Trail, the **Lakeside Trail** (706-613-3631; **tinyurl.com/sandycreekpark**) explores the eastern shore of this 782-acre lake. For a complete hike profile, see the second edition of this book.

DeSoto Falls Trail 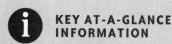 35

IN BRIEF

This is a wonderful waterfalls walk with a nearby babbling brook in the North Georgia mountains. Plan on spending the whole day hiking your choice of the multiple short trails listed in "Nearby Activities."

DESCRIPTION

Hernando de Soto explored Georgia—from the extreme southwest corner near Bainbridge across to Augusta and back over to the northwest—in search of gold in 1540 and 1541. In the 1880s a Spanish breastplate was found near the falls, giving DeSoto Falls its name and lasting legacy. Many scholars didn't even think that finding a breastplate intact more than 300 years later was possible until a 1540s-era Spanish sword was discovered intact near Rome in 1983.

At the entrance to the trail's parking lot is a brown-roofed trailhead kiosk where you pay the $3 US Forest Service fee. The pathway, left of the kiosk, is covered with pea-sized gravel and curves left as it falls to a picnic area within the park. As the trail levels, it turns right and runs along Frogtown Creek. Frogtown was the

---

Directions ———————————➤

Take GA 400/US 19 North to its end. Turn left on US 19/GA 60; look for a Shell station, Waffle House, and Home Depot at this intersection. Continue 5.1 miles and then turn right on US 19/GA 60/GA 9. Drive 8.2 miles and, where GA 60 goes straight at US 19/GA 9, curve right at Stone Pile Gap Road. Continue on this road another 5.3 miles to Turner's Corner. Turn left on US 19/129 and drive 5.3 miles to DeSoto Falls Recreation Area, on the left. Parking is in the first lot on the left; walk to the trailhead kiosk next to the restrooms.

KEY AT-A-GLANCE INFORMATION

LENGTH: 2.5 miles round-trip

CONFIGURATION: 2 out-and-back trails

DIFFICULTY: Easy; climb to Lower Falls is easy–moderate

SCENERY: Mountain streams, 2 waterfalls

EXPOSURE: Full shade

TRAFFIC: Moderate

TRAIL SURFACE: Compacted soil, dirt road

WHEELCHAIR ACCESS: None

HIKING TIME: 1.25 hours

ACCESS: Daily, year-round, 7 a.m.– 10 p.m.; $3 day-use fee

MAPS: USGS *Neels Gap*

MORE INFO: 706-745-6928; tinyurl.com/desotofalls; georgiatrails. com/gt/desoto_falls_trail

FACILITIES: Restrooms, picnic tables with grills; camping early May–November

SPECIAL COMMENTS: Many of the unusual names in this area are Cherokee in origin. In 1838 the Cherokee were forcibly removed by the state of Georgia in a tragedy known as the Trail of Tears.

DISTANCE: 69.8 miles from GA 400 North/I-285 North

GPS INFORMATION

N34° 42.388' W83° 54.898'

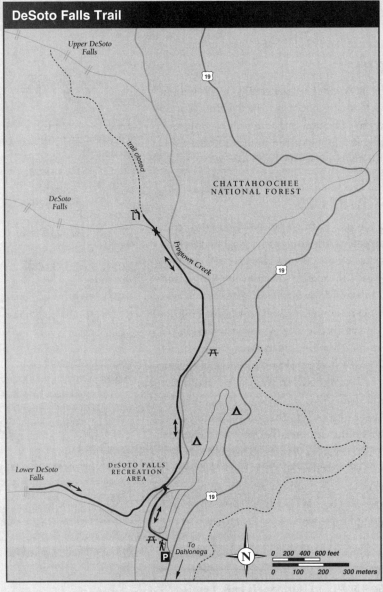

DeSoto Falls Trail

Upper DeSoto Falls

trail closed

CHATTAHOOCHEE NATIONAL FOREST

DeSoto Falls

Frogtown Creek

Lower DeSoto Falls

DeSOTO FALLS RECREATION AREA

To Dahlonega

19

19

19

N

0   200   400   600 feet
0   100   200   300 meters

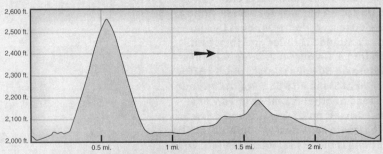

settlers' name for the Cherokee village of Walasi-yi, near the creek. According to Cherokee lore, a giant frog named Walasi lived in the gap above the creek (*Walasi-yi* means "place of the great frog"). In 1946 the Appalachian Trail Conference changed the name of Frogtown Gap to Neels Gap. Only the stone building at the top of the mountain, Mountain Crossings at Walasi-yi (see "Nearby Activities," below), honors the Cherokees by preserving their name for the area.

After you turn left on an asphalt road, you'll see a path to the left, just past the camp host's site, crossing Frogtown Creek on a wooden bridge. A sign on the far side of the bridge tells the story of DeSoto Falls. Turn left to follow the trail along Frogtown Creek, and then make a hard right as the path begins an easy-to-moderate switchback climb to the Lower Falls. Just past a large rock outcrop, the path turns right, rising to a viewing platform directly in front of the 35-foot-tall Lower Falls. Typical of a North Georgia waterfall, the water drops off a ledge and cascades a few feet to a second ledge, where it free-falls to a second cascade and then to a third ledge-cascade combination. After visiting a few minutes, retrace your steps to the bridge over Frogtown Creek.

As you pass the sign at the bridge, the footpath enters a wide, level floodplain of the river in a diverse pine and hardwood forest typical of the North Georgia mountains. The canopy of trees contains white and chestnut oaks, loblolly pines, tulip poplars, and sweet gums. Occasionally, hickory trees, red oaks, and pin oaks can be found. After reaching the confluence of Frogtown Creek and an unnamed tributary, the footpath climbs and descends three short hills near the creek. After you cross a wooden bridge, a sign informs you that the trail to Upper DeSoto Falls is closed for now. Beginning in 1993 with a snowstorm commonly called the Storm of the Century, and followed by 1994's Palm Sunday killer tornadoes and Hurricane Juan in 1995, the North Georgia mountains were repeatedly raked by damaging storms. Downed trees make ascending to the Upper Falls very difficult, but don't worry—the middle falls are spectacular.

Turn left and climb to the viewing platform. Coming off Blood Mountain, a narrow stream of water drops to a ledge, where the stream widens and cascades down to a second ledge. From here the falls make a brief drop to a third shelf that juts over a large rock. At the bottom of the falls, a small pool with a number of larger rocks makes for an excellent photo op. To get the best pictures, plan to be here in the morning of the first sunny day after a rain, when the falls are at their fullest.

NEARBY ACTIVITIES

Turn left out of the park and climb Blood Mountain to **Neels Gap**. On the right is a stone lodge built by the Civilian Conservation Corps in 1937. The building—through which the Appalachian Trail actually passes—now houses **Mountain Crossings at Walasi-yi,** an outdoors shop beloved by scores of AT thru-hikers (9710 Gainesville Hwy., Blairsville; 706-745-6095; **mountaincrossings.com**). Turn right out of Neels Gap and drive 0.25 mile to the **Byron Herbert Reece Memorial Trail**

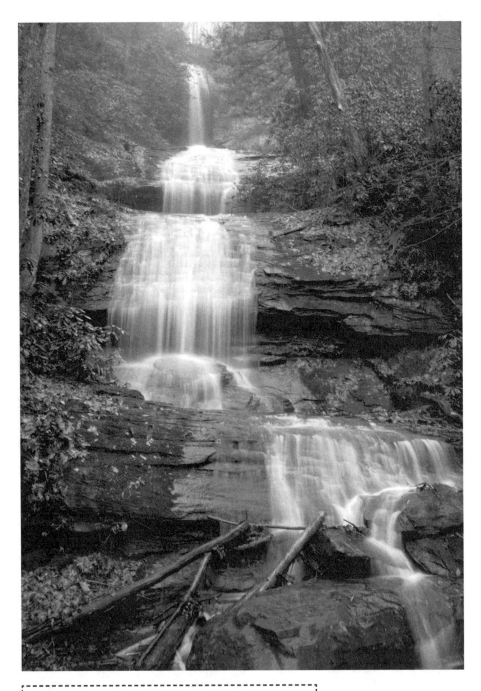

Picture-perfect DeSoto Falls comprises a series of smaller cascades.

parking lot, on the left. This access trail climbs steeply to the AT on Blood Mountain (706-745-6928; **tinyurl.com/reecetrail**; free). Farther down the mountain, **Vogel State Park** is home of the Bear Hair Trail (5 miles) and Coosa Bald Trail (11 miles), along with camping and cabins (706-745-2628; **gastateparks.org/vogelstate park**; $5 state-park fee). Watch for **Spillway Falls** on the left, after the entrance. Turn left on GA 180, climbing to **Sosebee Cove** (706-745-6928; **tinyurl.com/sosebeecove**; free). This 0.3-mile hike is great between mid-April and late September, when the wildflowers are in bloom.

Farther down GA 180 on the left, **Lake Winfield Scott** has additional AT access (706-745-6928; **tinyurl.com/lakewinfieldscott**; $5 use fee). In Suches, turn left on GA 60. After passing through Woody Gap, the road descends to Stonepile Gap. Go straight ahead on US 19 to **Dahlonega**, site of America's first gold rush. The state of Georgia established the **Dahlonega Gold Museum Historic Site** in the old county courthouse in 1965 (1 Public Square; hours and admission info: 706-864-2257 or **gastateparks.org/dahlonegagoldmuseum**). **The Smith House**, one of the best family-style restaurants in the Southeast, is one block south of the museum, at 84 S. Chestatee St. (800-852-9577 or 706-867-7000; **smithhouse.com**; hours vary).

36 EAST AND WEST LAKE TRAILS

KEY AT-A-GLANCE INFORMATION

LENGTH: 4.5 miles

CONFIGURATION: Loop

DIFFICULTY: Moderate

SCENERY: Long-distance and water views (lakeside and creekside)

EXPOSURE: Full sun in the area around Chicopee Lake, mostly shaded along the rest of the trail

TRAFFIC: Light, except in the vicinity of the lake, where traffic is moderate

TRAIL SURFACE: Gravel, compacted soil, concrete in the interpretive area of the lakeshore

WHEELCHAIR ACCESS: None

HIKING TIME: 3 hours

ACCESS: Daily, year-round, 8 a.m.–sunset; dogs prohibited Monday–Friday, 9 a.m.–3 p.m. Free.

MAPS: Available at Elachee Nature Science Center; USGS *Chestnut Mountain*

MORE INFO: 770-535-1976; elachee.org

FACILITIES: Restrooms available Monday–Saturday at Elachee Nature Science Center and Chicopee Lake

SPECIAL COMMENTS: The 1,500-acre Chicopee Woods Nature Preserve has 13 miles of trails. The Elachee Nature Science Center offers programs that promote environmental education.

DISTANCE: 36.5 miles from I-85 North/I-285 Northeast

GPS INFORMATION

N34° 14.778' W83° 49.927'

2125 Elachee Dr.
Gainesville, GA 30504

IN BRIEF

This loop trail explores the foothills of the Blue Ridge Mountains, traversing a typical hardwood forest from the Elachee Nature Science Center to the Chicopee Aquatic Studies Center at Chicopee Lake.

DESCRIPTION

First following a developed dirt road (notice the runoff ditches on either side) that ascends 0.1 mile, the trail then begins to descend at an easy-to-moderate pace over the next 0.3 mile. After a four-way intersection at the top of the hill, the road becomes very rocky. Tree limbs cover the road as it bears left at 0.4 mile, while the trail bears right and enters the woods. Briefly, the orange-blazed trail becomes loamy and is covered by sand. As you begin walking downhill along a low ridge, the forest is made up mostly of post and white oaks, American beeches, and native dogwoods. Crossing a wooden bridge over a normally dry gully at 0.5 mile, the trail quickly crosses a second bridge, just after a large post oak.

After the second bridge, the trail narrows and follows the riverbank downhill through an old-growth forest. After climbing away from the riverbank, the trail begins a rapid

----

Directions ⟶

Take I-85 North to Exit 113/I-985 North. Drive 16 miles to Exit 17/Atlanta Highway/GA 13 North, and turn left. Drive 1.8 miles and turn right onto G Avenue at Chicopee Baptist Church. Make a hard right onto A Avenue, which becomes Elachee Drive, and in 0.8 mile you'll see trailhead parking straight ahead, just across a bridge over I-985. Walk to a brown kiosk at the east end of the parking lot.

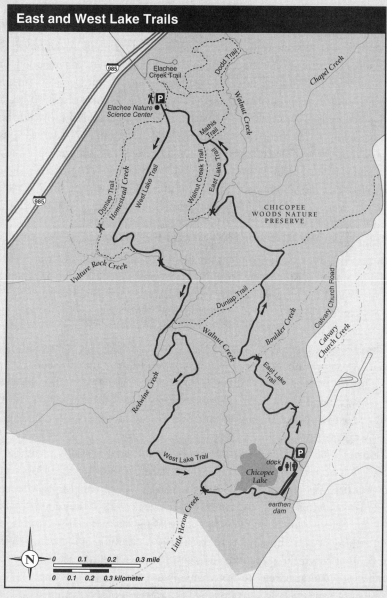

East and West Lake Trails

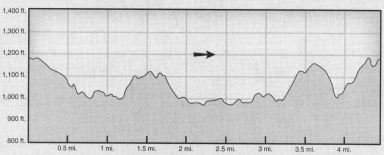

switchback descent until it bears right and descends stairs. At this point, West Lake Trail turns left, joining Dunlap Trail along Vulture Rock Creek, a wide, well-defined waterway to your right. Side trails lead down to and cross the creek, but you should continue along the riverbank until you come to a wooden bridge. Cross the bridge and, on the far side, you'll come to a T-intersection. Turn left.

West Lake Trail briefly follows the river before making a hard right and climbing a rooted, occasionally rocky pathway through a second-growth forest. As you move away from the river, the number of ferns quickly decreases; as you climb, the number of pines increases. At 1.1 miles the trail joins an old road, soon making another hard right to leave this road. Now the trail begins a zigzag climb, joining another road about halfway up the hill. At the top of the hill, the trail turns left at a map stand. A small hand-painted sign reads 1.4 MILES, the distance to Chicopee Lake.

Falling to a dry creek at 1.6 miles, West Lake Trail crosses the creek, turns left, and then curves back around as it begins to climb. Making a moderate-to-difficult climb up a steep-sided hill, the footpath turns left at another hand-painted sign and begins a somewhat easier descent to the first view of Chicopee Lake, at 2 miles. Make a note of the kiosk to your right and then explore the several viewing areas.

The lake is a diverse ecosystem that attracts a wide variety of animals. On one visit, we saw a snowy egret foraging for food in the marshy wetlands where the lake forms, while a family of otters churned the water along the distant lakeshore. Geese landed in the lake, taking a rest on their long journey south. Above, a red-tailed hawk soared on the thermals—perhaps looking for food, or perhaps just enjoying the ride.

Return to the kiosk and, with it on your right, walk straight ahead, as if you had taken a hard right from the trail coming into the viewing area. A brown sign quickly confirms that you're on West Lake Trail. Over the next mile, the trail circles the lake, moving inland and up to a boardwalk that crosses a small wetlands and stream before returning lakeside and heading down to the lakeshore and a popular fishing area. Follow the trail to the right, climbing and circling to the left before coming down the steps into full sun as you walk across the top of the dam that impounds Walnut Creek to form Chicopee Lake.

The dam yields scenic views of the lake to the left and Walnut Creek to the right. At a mailbox the trail bears slightly left, toward a white building with restrooms and interpretive information. Walk around the building, turn right, and walk toward a white fence near a main road. An interpretive sign describes the flowers in the dry meadow before you. Turn around, keeping the parking lot on your right, and follow the sidewalk to a cement path on the left, down to the boardwalk-style dock on the lake. This area is also signed and indicates that the lake is home to both ospreys and bald eagles in addition to a wide variety of smaller animals, waterfowl, and fish.

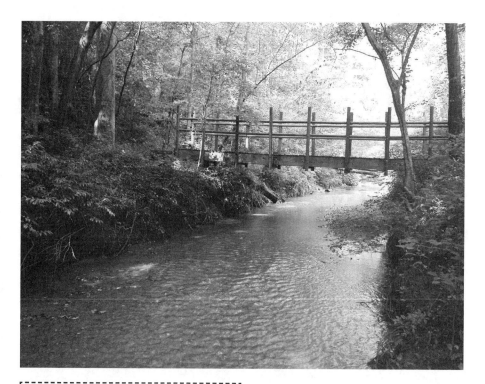

You'll cross Vulture Rock Creek on this footbridge.

Return to the parking lot and turn left on the sidewalk. Continue to an unmarked but well-worn path to the left, just before the ranger's cottage, and head into a forest of red maples and white oaks mixed with pines. Fully shaded and now called East Lake Trail, the path joins Calvary Church Creek at 3.2 miles, soon making a hard left turn into the creek and up the bank on the other side. The trail crosses creeks three times over the next 0.2 mile and then climbs a hill. Near the top, at 3.4 miles, the trail turns right and joins an old road before quickly turning left to leave the roadbed.

East Lake Trail makes an easy descent to a bridge over a boulder-strewn creek. After the bridge, the trail turns left and briefly levels before beginning an extended climb to a hilltop. Difficult at first, the climb moderates as it rises, becoming easier near the top. At a kiosk near the top of the hill, East Lake Trail joins Dunlap Trail and bears right.

Coming to the top of a hill at 3.6 miles, the combined East Lake/Dunlap Trail makes a hard left, although an unmarked path continues straight ahead. Now falling at a moderate-to-difficult grade over the next 0.2 mile, the pathway makes another hard left as it starts to run adjacent to a wetland near Walnut Creek. After crossing a bridge, the trail turns right and combines switchbacks and stairs to

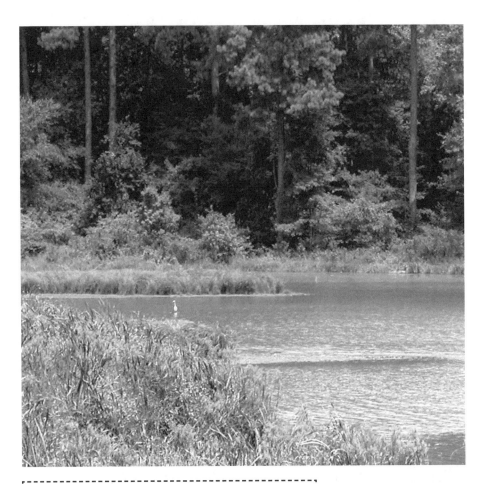

A lone egret enjoys acres of fishing grounds in this scenic reservoir.

quickly ascend from the river valley. East Lake Trail ends at a T-intersection with Mathis Trail. Turn left on Mathis Trail to return to your car.

Mathis Trail is well marked. At Walnut Creek Trail, Mathis Trail turns right and then bears right at a small rain shelter. Just over 0.1 mile after the shelter, a short trail on the left returns you to the trailhead.

GWINNETT ENVIRONMENTAL AND HERITAGE CENTER TRAIL

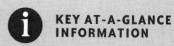

IN BRIEF

Nine short trails, none more than a mile long, can be combined for a fun exploration of an ecology- and history-based attraction in northeast Georgia.

DESCRIPTION

With 5.4 miles of trails, not including the 4.8-mile (round-trip) Ivy Creek Greenway and the Greenway Spur, the 233-acre, mostly forested site of the Gwinnett Environment and Heritage Center (GEHC) is home to a wide range of hikes that can be combined for a number of different adventures. The center was completed in August 2006, and the building has received LEED Gold certification from the U.S. Green Building Council. Treetop Quest, opened in September 2011, offers about 2.5 hours of "treetop hiking" for those who pass a training course.

The trailhead kiosk is at the east end of the parking lot, at the entrance to Treetop Quest. Follow the paved Cherokee Trail as it climbs, crossing the entrance road, Clean Water Drive; then continue climbing to a T at 0.1 mile. This is the highest point on the hike. Turn left and continue 0.2 mile to Woodward Mill Road, the center's service road. Turn left and keep an eye out on the right for the entrance to the gravel-paved, blue-blazed Creekside Trail.

Directions

Take I-85 North to Exit 113/I-985. Continue on I-985 for 3.5 miles to Exit 4/Buford Drive. At the end of the ramp, turn right and continue on Buford Drive 0.4 mile. Turn right on Plunketts Road and drive 1.6 miles. Turn left on Clean Water Drive into the Gwinnett Environmental and Heritage Center.

KEY AT-A-GLANCE INFORMATION

LENGTH: 3.4 miles
CONFIGURATION: Double loop
DIFFICULTY: Easy
SCENERY: Streams, creeks, gullies
EXPOSURE: Full shade–full sun
TRAFFIC: Light
TRAIL SURFACE: Gravel
HIKING TIME: 2.2 hours
ACCESS: Daily, year-round, sunrise–sunset, except for major holidays. Admission, Gwinnett County residents: $7.50 ages 13–54, $5.50 seniors age 55 and older and students ages 13–22 with valid ID, $3.50 kids ages 3–12. Non–Gwinnett County residents pay $3 in addition to the previous fees. Kids age 2 and younger and GEHC members are admitted free.
MAPS: Handout at trailhead, USGS *Suwanee*
MORE INFO: 770-904-3500; gwinnettehc.org
FACILITIES: Restrooms
SPECIAL COMMENTS: Hikers get valuable lessons in the importance of clean water and how water shaped the history of Gwinnett County.
DISTANCE: 23 miles from I-85 North/I-285 Northeast

GPS INFORMATION
N34° 3.878' W84° 0.264'
2020 Clean Water Dr.
Buford, GA 30519

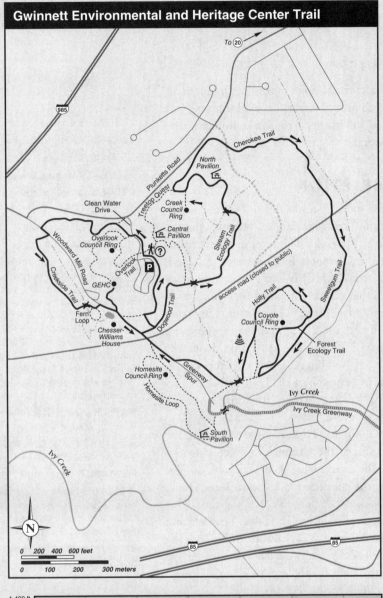

Gwinnett Environmental and Heritage Center Trail

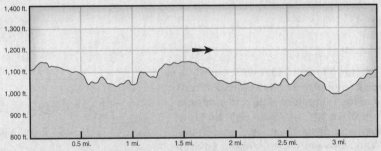

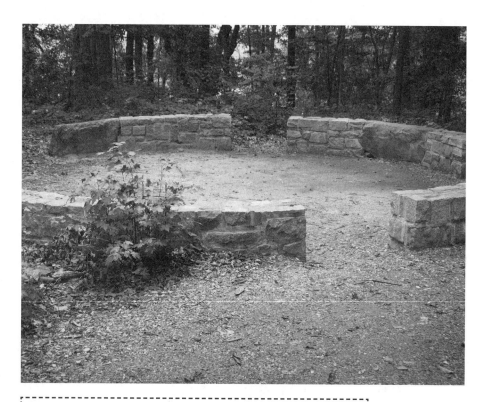

The stone seating of a "council ring" provides a peaceful place to rest a moment.

The wide gravel road crosses the headwaters of a small creek, and then the blue-blazed trail turns left. Quickly on your left a creek forms, and as you descend on the path, erosion wears a deeper valley for the creek. At 0.5 mile into the hike, the creek has become a gully running some 30 feet below the trail. The trail do-si-dos down to the creek, crosses it on a bridge, and rises to the Fern Loop, a 0.1-mile exploration of a moist woodland area that is conducive to ferns.

After the loop, turn right on the first trail and return to the paved road. In front of you is the Gwinnett Environmental and Heritage Center. Turn right and walk past a retention pond on the right. On your right is the Chesser-Williams House, one of Gwinnett County's oldest surviving homes; built in the 1850s, it was moved to the GEHC campus in late 2012 and is expected to open to the public in late 2013. On the left is a trail that quickly Ys as it climbs to the center. Ignore the steps on the right, and follow a trail on the left that crosses a bridge and rises to a self-contained water system, which creates a river that runs through the center. This area is fun to explore, and photographers will find some good shots here. Return to the Greenway Spur, turn left, and descend toward a road crossing. Just before this crossing, the gray-blazed Dogwood Trail comes off to the left at 0.8 mile. Follow it straight ahead for 0.1 mile to the Stream Ecology Trail and turn right, immediately crossing a bridge.

The Stream Ecology Trail rises and falls as it explores the forest surrounding a tributary of Ivy Creek, itself a tributary of Suwanee Creek. At 1.2 miles the trail veers left, drops quickly to cross a bridge, and then rises. At 1.4 miles turn right and take a short path up to the paved Cherokee Trail. Turn right and follow the trail to the marked entrance to the Sweetgum Trail, on the right at 1.6 miles. This trail lies in full sun and parallels a massive earthen berm to an access road maintained by the center at 2 miles. After passing the access road, the Sweetgum Trail connects to the Forest Ecology Trail, on the right at 2.3 miles.

As you enter the forest, keep right and make an easy-to-moderate climb through a second-growth hardwood forest to the Coyote Council Ring, used to interpret the importance of the surrounding forest for young children. At the ring, follow the trail right and continue to the balloon portion of the Holly Trail, less than 0.1 mile farther on. Instead of turning left at the T onto the inner portion of the loop, keep straight and then bear left after the intersection to hike around the outer portion of the loop and climb into the Ivy Creek watershed.

The Holly Trail climbs and falls, briefly rejoining the Sweetgum Trail to the left before ending at the Greenway Spur 2.9 miles into the hike. Turn right, climbing easily to an intersection. Just past the intersection, turn right on the Dogwood Trail and then turn left a few steps later to return the parking area.

NEARBY ACTIVITIES

The GEHC's main building comprises five areas covering the impact of water on local history and everyday lives through interactive displays. **Treetop Quest** is a supervised adventure course where visitors can "hike" safely in the trees; buy tickets at **treetopquest.com** or call 770-904-3547 for more information.

HARD LABOR CREEK TRAIL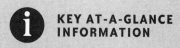

IN BRIEF

Consisting of the Brantley and Beaverpond Nature Trails, Hard Labor Creek Trail follows various creeks and explores ridges within Hard Labor Creek State Park.

DESCRIPTION

So how did Hard Labor Creek get its name? Some say that it comes from the travails of slaves who had to clear the rocky ground here. Others say that local American Indians named the creek for the difficulty of crossing it in wet weather. Adding to the speculation, the Civilian Conservation Corps (CCC) operated a rock quarry in the park during the 1930s.

To get to the trailhead from the parking area, walk back toward the trading post, turning right on the road that leads to the comfort station. Hard Labor Creek Trail is on the left, in the woods behind an open picnic area. A brown pole with trail names and distances marks the start of the trail. Two loops, the Brantley and Beaverpond Nature Trails, make up Hard Labor Creek Trail.

Beginning on the yellow-blazed Brantley Nature Trail, the hike leads through a typical Georgia Piedmont pine forest. Leaves and pine needles cover the relatively level ground, which was once home to antebellum plantations. Shortly after the hike starts, the trail

KEY AT-A-GLANCE INFORMATION

LENGTH: 2.1 miles

CONFIGURATION: Double loop—almost a figure eight

DIFFICULTY: Moderate

SCENERY: Cascades, deep ravines, long-distance view of small lake

EXPOSURE: Generally shaded

TRAFFIC: Light

TRAIL SURFACE: Compacted dirt that becomes rocky and heavily rooted at times

WHEELCHAIR ACCESS: None

HIKING TIME: 1.5 hours

ACCESS: Daily, year-round, 7 a.m.–sunset, except Thanksgiving and December 25; $5 state-park fee

MAPS: Available at park office; USGS *Rutledge North*

MORE INFO: 706-557-3001; gastateparks.org/hardlaborcreek

FACILITIES: Restrooms at trailhead, picnic tables nearby

SPECIAL COMMENTS: Lake Brantley is visible only occasionally from the trail. Hard Labor Creek State Park has 24 miles of trails for hikers and horseback riders. The park also offers camping, golf, and swimming (seasonal).

DISTANCE: 41 miles from I-20 East/I-285 East

Directions

Take I-20 East to Exit 101/US 278, and turn left. Drive 4 miles and turn left on Old Mill Road. Drive 3.1 miles and turn left on Fairplay Road. Drive 0.5 mile and turn left on Knox Chapel Road. Drive 0.4 mile and turn right on Hard Labor Creek Road. Drive past the trading post; parking is on the left.

GPS INFORMATION

N33° 39.841' W83° 36.375'

5 Hard Labor Creek Rd.
Rutledge, GA 30663

Hard Labor Creek Trail

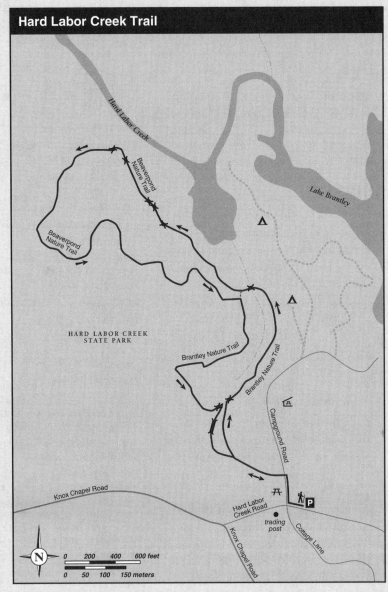

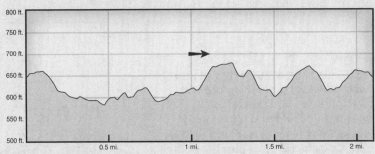

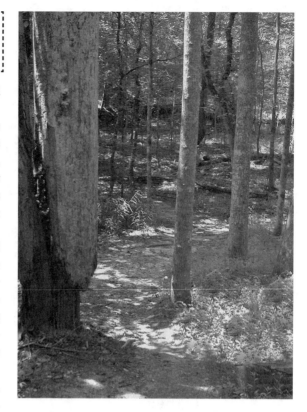

Hard Labor Creek State Park offers more than 24 miles of trails for hikers and horseback riders.

begins to descend and curves right.

Azaleas bloom in the early spring along the path—which, unfortunately, also harbors a large number of ticks. See page 11 for tips on protecting yourself from these pests.

At 0.1 mile the trail climbs a granite outcrop and then descends over rocks and roots to a wood-and-dirt stairway leading deep into a ravine. Completely shaded, the path has a wooden rail on the left. Large gopher holes and a downed tree make this area somewhat difficult to navigate. At 0.2 mile the trail splits at two wooden bridges. Take the bridge directly in front of you.

As you cross the bridge, look to the right into a large ravine created by a tributary. Shortly after the bridge, you come to a tree ravaged by woodpeckers and termites; walk around it. Next, a path to the right leads to a campground, which you'll see is just behind a stand of trees. Falling to the creek bed, the trail levels and becomes heavily rooted.

At 0.4 mile you come to another wooden bridge, this one built by the Young Adult Conservation Corps (YACC). Conceived during President Jimmy Carter's administration and loosely based on the CCC of the 1930s, this program provided employment to disadvantaged youth in the late 1970s, putting them to work on public-land projects throughout the United States. After the bridge the trail climbs to the start of the red-blazed Beaverpond Nature Trail, which heads right and splits shortly after the turn. Take the trail straight ahead.

As you descend toward a creek bed, notice how the size of the trees starts to increase. Some of the trees measure 12–13 feet around, indicating that this is an older-growth forest. Beaverpond Nature Trail climbs to the middle of a low ridge. Soon the path falls to a wooden bridge over a deep gully. After descending a few stairs at the end of the bridge, the path bears right. Two more bridges follow in rapid succession, and then the path falls to the wide, level plain of the creek, which it follows briefly.

As Beaverpond Nature Trail turns left at 0.8 mile, it begins to climb alongside another stream and takes on a different personality. Now rocky and heavily rooted, the path climbs along a creek that cascades in spots. Finally, just short of a mile into the journey, the footpath leaves the stream, enters heavily shaded forest, and begins to climb to a ridgetop covered with maple, oak, and beech trees.

From the ridge, the trail begins to switchback, sometimes descending steeply back to the start of the loop. As you reach the short return path to Brantley Nature Trail, turn right. You'll take just a few steps before the red blazes of Beaverpond Nature Trail are almost seamlessly replaced by the yellow blazes of Brantley Nature Trail. At the intersection, Brantley Nature Trail bears right and then, a few steps up the trail, begins to make a harder right turn.

The trail begins a moderate climb through a partially sunny hardwood forest as you double back to the trailhead on the other side of the valley. From this peak the footpath begins to descend into the basin, toward the start of the loop. At 1.8 miles Brantley Nature Trail crosses the longest bridge of the hike, returning to the start of the loop trail. Turn right to return to the trailhead.

NEARBY ACTIVITIES

Historic **Madison, Georgia,** is the town that General Sherman *didn't* burn. For more information, call 800-709-7406, go to **madisonga.org,** or visit the Welcome Center on 115 E. Jefferson St., Monday–Friday, 9 a.m.–4:30 p.m., Saturday, 10 a.m.–5 p.m., and Sunday, 1–4 p.m.; closed Thanksgiving and December 24 and 25. **Rock Eagle Mound (rockeagle4h.org/about.html#location)**, a large stone effigy shaped like a prone bird and believed to have been built by American Indians about 2,000 years ago, is in nearby Eatonton at the UGA Rock Eagle 4-H Center.

INDIAN SEATS TRAIL 39

IN BRIEF

Climb to the top of Sawnee Mountain, west of Cumming, for prime long-distance views of Georgia's Blue Ridge Mountains.

DESCRIPTION

Sawnee Mountain is a monadnock, or knob, rising some 400 feet above the surrounding land in Forsyth County. Named for a Cherokee chief who lived near the headwaters of Vickery Creek, Sawnee Mountain has long been rumored to hold the chief's gold as well as his body. Although no one has found the latter, the former was discovered in 1895 but mined unsuccessfully.

As you approach the visitor center, the treetop Canopy Walk, on your right, is worth a look. After completing a training course, visitors can explore a hardwood forest from a suspended bridge (call 770-781-2217 for more information).

The Indian Seats Trail begins behind the visitor center. The 0.2-mile Laurel Trail Spur takes you past the Tree House (a kids' play area) to the trailhead. Clockwise is the easier direction in which to hike, so take the trail on the left. Rising along a gravel road through a mostly hardwood forest of maples, white oaks, post oaks, and the occasional hickory, the roadbed curves right and then left before making a hard right just before 0.4 mile.

Directions

Take GA 400/US 19 North to Exit 17/Keith Bridge Road/GA 306. Turn left and follow GA 306 for 1.2 miles to Dahlonega Highway/GA 9. Turn right on GA 9, drive 0.9 mile, and turn left on Spot Road. Drive 1.5 miles and turn left into Sawnee Mountain Preserve.

KEY AT-A-GLANCE INFORMATION

LENGTH: 3.75 miles

CONFIGURATION: Loop

DIFFICULTY: Moderate when hiked clockwise, hard when hiked counterclockwise

SCENERY: Vistas along the hike to the top of Sawnee Mountain, excellent long-distance views of the North Georgia mountains from the Indian Seats at the top

EXPOSURE: Full sun at Indian Seats, full shade elsewhere

TRAFFIC: Moderate

TRAIL SURFACE: Gravel

HIKING TIME: 1.5 hours

ACCESS: Daily, year-round, 8 a.m.–sunset; free to hike (fees charged for adventure programs and facilities rentals)

MAPS: Sawnee Mountain Preserve, USGS *Cumming*

MORE INFO: 770-781-2217; sawneemountain.org

FACILITIES: Restrooms and visitor center at trailhead

SPECIAL COMMENTS: Dogs are prohibited within the preserve, but rock climbing is allowed with a 10-day permit. According to the official map, the trail is 2.6 miles long—considerably shorter than the hike featured here.

DISTANCE: 33.1 miles from GA 400 North/I-285 North

GPS INFORMATION

N34° 15.289' W84° 8.323'

4075 Spot Rd.
Cumming, GA 30040

Indian Seats Trail

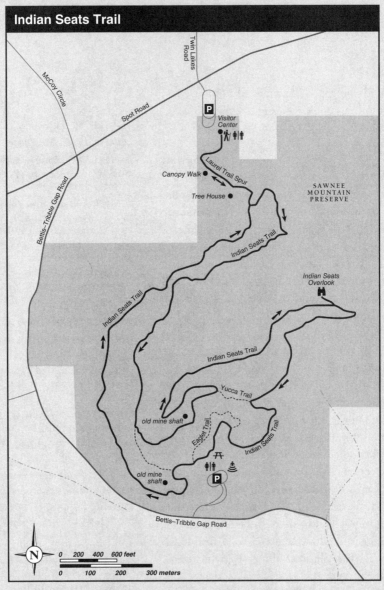

Twin Lakes Road

McCoy Circle

Spot Road

Bettis–Tribble Gap Road

P

Visitor Center

Laurel Trail Spur

Canopy Walk

Tree House

SAWNEE MOUNTAIN PRESERVE

Indian Seats Trail

Indian Seats Trail

Indian Seats Overlook

Indian Seats Trail

Yucca Trail

old mine shaft

Eagles Trail

Indian Seats Trail

old mine shaft

P

Bettis–Tribble Gap Road

N

0   200   400   600 feet

0   100   200   300 meters

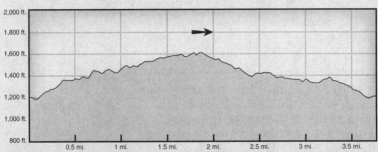

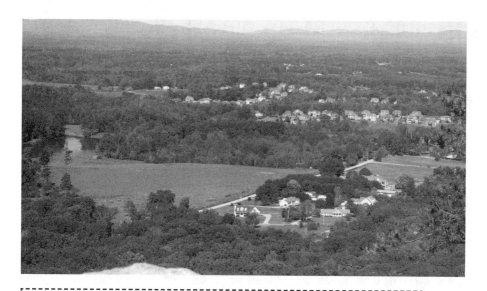

The Indian Seats Overlook yields 180-degree views of North Georgia's Blue Ridge Mountains.

At 0.7 mile the steady increase in elevation becomes an up-and-down affair, with some good views to the right until 1.2 miles, when a covered mine shaft on the left and the Yucca Trail on the right indicate the final approach to the top of Sawnee Mountain. The slope increases following the Yucca Trail intersection, and the pathway switches back a couple of times until it joins a ridge running just below the top of Sawnee Mountain. In this area, a number of old trails to the top have been covered.

Finally, at 1.8 miles, the Indian Seats Trail breaks into full sun, and only a few easy steps up some rocks bring you to a 180-degree long-distance view of the mountains of northern and northeastern Georgia. Feel free to explore your surroundings, but parents will want to keep kids away from steep drop-offs and be mindful of occasionally slippery conditions.

Once you're done exploring, find the Indian Seats Trail just below the ridge, and continue as it begins to descend sharply. A sharp left turn comes at the intersection with the Yucca Trail at 2.3 miles. At 2.6 miles, the descent eases and you enter an interpretive area where alluvial gold was taken from the ground in the 1890s. One-fifth of a mile later, the trail enters a day-use picnic area with restrooms.

The trail continues to run mostly level until 3.4 miles, when it begins an easy-to-moderate descent to the end of the loop portion. Return on the Laurel Trail Spur to the visitor center.

NEARBY ACTIVITIES

Balloons Over Georgia (678-283-4033; **balloonsovergeorgia.com**) is a unique way to see the area after you've seen it from Sawnee Mountain.

40 JONES BRIDGE TRAIL

KEY AT-A-GLANCE INFORMATION

LENGTH: 5 miles

CONFIGURATION: Loop

DIFFICULTY: Easy

SCENERY: Historical bridge, riverside views

EXPOSURE: Full sun in the vicinity of the historic bridge, full shade elsewhere

TRAFFIC: Heavy near the bridge, moderate down to the boat launch, and light south of the launch

TRAIL SURFACE: Compacted soil

WHEELCHAIR ACCESS: None

HIKING TIME: 2 hours

ACCESS: Trail: daily, year-round, sunrise–sunset; headquarters: daily, year-round, 9 a.m.–5 p.m., except December 25; $3 day-use fee

MAPS: Available at Island Ford headquarters (see page 32); USGS *Chamblee, Duluth, Norcross*

MORE INFO: 678-538-1200; nps.gov/chat

FACILITIES: Restrooms, boat launch, some picnic tables, fishing dock

SPECIAL COMMENTS: Jones Bridge was a privately owned tollway that was built in 1904 and ceased operation in 1922. Before that time, a ferry crossed the river at roughly the same spot.

DISTANCE: 8.4 miles from GA 141/I-285 Northeast

GPS INFORMATION

N34° 0.052' W84° 14.357'

IN BRIEF

This hike explores Jones Bridge, climbs into nearby hills that yield long-distance views of some of Atlanta's most expensive homes, and then follows the floodplain of the Chattahoochee, climbs to explore a ridge, and returns to loop around a second floodplain.

DESCRIPTION

Ferries were the first privately owned businesses to span Georgia's mighty rivers. With competition from railroads increasing, ferry owners began to build bridges and charge a toll to cross them. As the state and federal governments began building roads in the 1920s, many of the old bridges quickly became obsolete. Jones Bridge's usefulness (in the mind of its owner) came to an end in the early 1920s, when it was abandoned, although farmers did continue to use it until the wooden planking rotted. In 1940 World War II sent scrap-metal prices soaring, even though the United States had not yet entered the war. A group of

----

Directions ⟶

Take Peachtree Industrial Boulevard/GA 141 to Peachtree Corners Circle, and turn left. Drive 1.5 miles and turn left on Holcomb Bridge Road. Drive 2.3 miles and turn right on Barnwell Road (you'll see a CVS drugstore and a SunTrust Bank on the corner). Ignore the first brown sign, which marks the entrance to the Environmental Center. At 1.5 miles, turn right at the JONES BRIDGE UNIT sign. Follow the road as it curves around and switches back, passing a small parking lot on the right for cars with fishing boats. At 1.2 miles the main parking lot comes into view. Turn left, park, and walk to the trailhead kiosk, at the south end of the parking lot.

Jones Bridge Trail

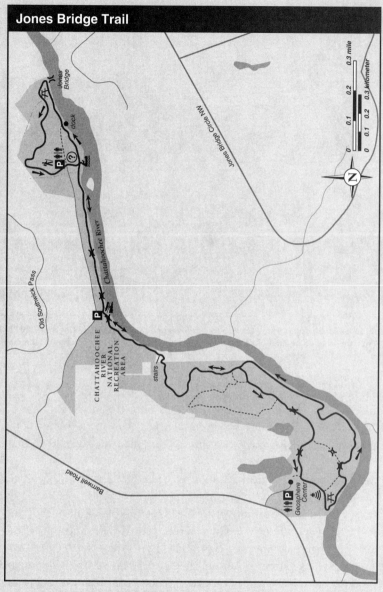

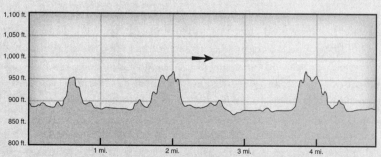

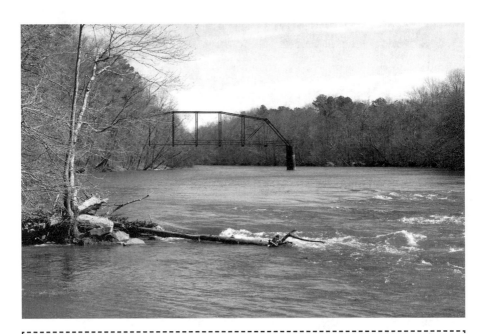

Historical Jones Bridge spanned the Chattahoochee River and was used for crossing from 1904 to 1922. In 1940 half the span of the then-abandoned bridge was stolen, and this section is all that remains.

workmen began dismantling the southern end of Jones Bridge, working in plain sight one day. People didn't ask any questions until the men didn't show up the second day. Then folks realized that the workers had made off with the scrap metal, probably selling it a piece at a time so that their theft would go undetected in the lucrative Atlanta market.

From the trailhead kiosk, follow a wide dirt road and descend easily through a diverse hardwood forest to a four-way intersection, 200 feet from the start. Take a minute to walk down to the riverbank, straight ahead, and enjoy the view of the Chattahoochee. On returning, turn right and follow the riverbank, keeping the river on your right. The trail runs some 20 feet inside the bank, and large rock outcrops tell the river's story. As you pass the outcrops on the left, take a close look at the waterworn edges and eroded strata in the rock. Before the river was controlled by Buford Dam—20 miles north as the river flows—water levels would fluctuate much more than they do today. The rock, which would be covered only in an unusual circumstance today, routinely flooded before 1953. As you continue along the trail, the floodplain opens into a park; a dock for both fishing and viewing extends onto the river, on your right. In the distance, the half-span of Jones Bridge waits for another crew to finish the job begun in 1940.

Continue straight toward the bridge, past a trail on the left and over a wooden bridge that crosses a stream. Finally, as you approach an intrusive chain-link fence, you'll reach the bridge, which juts into the Chattahoochee. Jones Bridge Road,

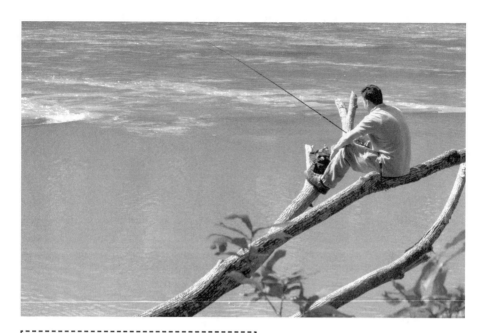

A natural perch furnishes easy access for this angler.

which is still a major road in north Fulton County, ran to this point, crossed the river on the bridge, and continued on the south side of the Chattahoochee. A number of large pines stand in the area. The trail continues a short way along the riverbank, next to the fence.

From the bridge, turn around and begin walking the inside of the open field, toward a creek crossing and map stand. After you make a wet-footed crossing, the path joins a road that bears right and begins to climb into the forest. As the trail begins a moderate ascent, it curves away from the riverbank. At 0.6 mile the climb eases as the roadway runs nearly level at the ridgetop. An easy descent returns you to the north end of the parking lot. Continue to the trailhead, but turn right and follow the riverbank, keeping the Chattahoochee to your left. Here the floodplain is wider, unconstrained by the hills adjacent to the river. We once flushed a blue heron at the first bridge, just after the turn.

Crossing another wooden bridge at 1.3 miles, the pathway takes you to a third bridge and, 0.1 mile later, the fishing-ramp parking area. Walk straight across the lot—the path continues, almost immediately crossing another bridge. Turning inland at 1.8 miles at a flight of wooden steps, the trail begins another moderate climb into the Chattahoochee watershed, dropping to a gravel road and then climbing again. Notice the American beech trees at the top of the mountain, some 0.2 mile after the start of the climb. Four or five massive beeches and many smaller ones inhabit the nearby forest. As the pathway begins to descend, you'll see a home on the left, between the trail and the river.

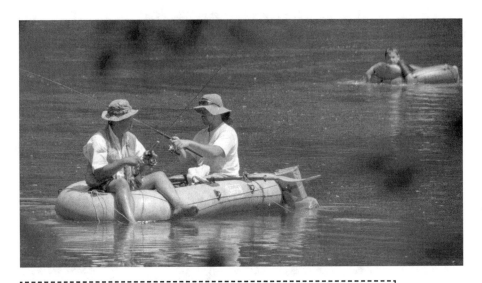

> **The Chattahoochee River is a recreational paradise; rafting and fishing are two of its most visibly popular pastimes.**

Come to a three-way intersection with a map stand at 2.1 miles. Turn left to continue on an easy descent toward the river, coming to a second intersection a couple hundred feet later. Take the trail on the right, which runs fairly level down to a wooden bridge at 2.5 miles. The footpath curves gently right, and a crossover trail heads left. Just past the crossover trail is an intersection where the trail bears left; then come to a bridge as you enter an open field near the Geosphere Center. At a grassy road leading to the center, turn left; the trail makes an easy descent, curving right at a map stand at 2.7 miles, then making a hard left less than 0.1 mile later.

After following the riverbank another 0.1 mile, the footpath curves left, away from the bank, to make a right turn at a three-way intersection. It next crosses a bridge and turns right, rejoining the river, at 3.2 miles. After passing two crossover trails on the left, take a few steps up to a low ridge in an area of large trees. The trail bears left, following the curve of the river and then leaving the riverbank to cross a tributary of the Chattahoochee. Returning to the riverbank, the path makes a hard left. At 3.9 miles the pathway crosscuts a historic road; look for a map stand 100 feet to the left, and follow the trail to it. Turn right and retrace your steps to the car.

NEARBY ACTIVITIES

Autrey Mill Nature Preserve and Heritage Center (9770 Autrey Mill Rd., Johns Creek; 678-366-3511; **autreymill.org**; free) features historic buildings as well as 2 miles of mulched trails through hardwood and pine forests. Turn right on Barnwell Road as you leave Jones Bridge, and after 0.95 mile curve around to Jones Bridge Road. In 0.66 mile turn right on Old Alabama Road. Drive 1.5 miles and turn left on Autrey Mill Road. The preserve is 0.45 mile ahead on your left, just before the road dead-ends.

LITTLE MULBERRY TRAIL 41

IN BRIEF

This combined multiuse and pedestrian trail offers a 2-mile hike through an old-growth forest to unspoiled Table Rock Falls and then explores the adjacent river valley. Some long-distance scenic views make the multiuse section of the trail pleasing.

DESCRIPTION

Little Mulberry Park in Auburn is part of a major park-building program that Gwinnett County began in the late 1990s. Among the other parks built are McDaniel Farm (see page 199), Tribble Mill (see page 219), Yellow River, Freeman's Mill, and Harbins.

From the trailhead kiosk, turn right on the Pond Trail, a paved multiuse trail that encircles a small pond. This is the smallest of the four distinct loops that make up the park's trails. Pass a side trail to the parking lot; the trail begins to wind as it drops to the bed of the creek that forms the lake, crossing it on a wooden bridge. Just past the bridge is the spillway of the earthen dam. The trail begins an easy climb past a dock overlooking the lake. As the trail curves left, it passes picnic tables and a playground.

Watch for a connector trail on the right, just past the playground. This rises to the second loop, surrounding West Meadow, a cleared area with an overlook at its center. Turn left and watch for a kiosk on your left, at the end of a trail of pea-sized gravel that splits

---

Directions

Take I-85 North to Exit 106 and merge onto GA 316. Drive 10.5 miles and turn left on Fence Road. Drive 5.2 miles to the park entrance, on the left.

KEY AT-A-GLANCE INFORMATION

LENGTH: 6 miles

CONFIGURATION: Multiple loops

DIFFICULTY: Easy except for the loops to the waterfalls and river valley, which are moderate

SCENERY: Waterfalls, unspoiled river valley, landscaped pond

EXPOSURE: Full sun, except on the hiking trail, which is shaded

TRAFFIC: Moderate; multiuse trail (not discussed here) permits horses

TRAIL SURFACE: Asphalt, except for the hiking trail, which is gravel

WHEELCHAIR ACCESS: Partial

HIKING TIME: 3 hours

ACCESS: Daily, year-round, sunrise–sunset; free

MAPS: At trailhead kiosk; USGS *Auburn (Georgia)*, *Hog Mountain*

MORE INFO: 770-978-5270; tinyurl.com/littlemulberry

FACILITIES: Restrooms, playground, small pond. Miller Lake can be accessed using the 0.7-mile Carriage Trail and the 2.2-mile Miller Lake Trail.

SPECIAL COMMENTS: Fishing is allowed in designated areas of the park's pond. The park has two additional entrances, at 3900 Hog Mountain Rd. and 1300 Mineral Springs Rd., both in Dacula.

DISTANCE: 25.9 miles from I-85 North/I-285 Northeast

GPS INFORMATION

N34° 2.379' W83° 52.658'

3855 Fence Rd. NE
Auburn, GA 30011

Little Mulberry Trail

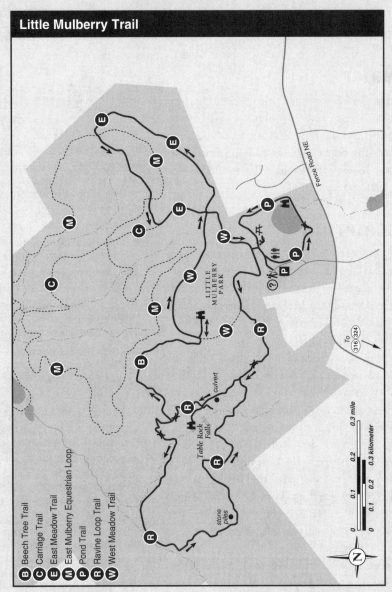

LITTLE MULBERRY PARK

Fence Road NE

To 316/324

culvert

Table Rock Falls

stone piles

B Beech Tree Trail
C Carriage Trail
E East Meadow Trail
M East Mulberry Equestrian Loop
P Pond Trail
R Ravine Loop Trail
W West Meadow Trail

0.3 mile
0.3 kilometer

N

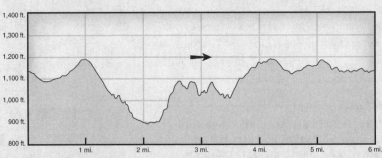

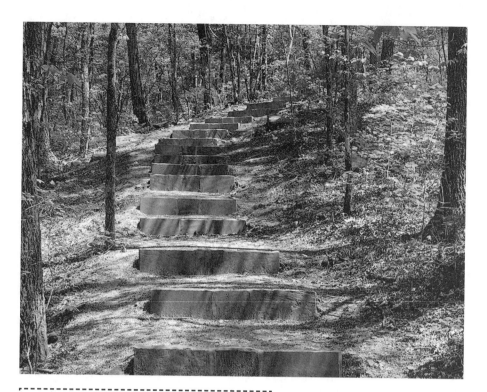

Stairs help control erosion on the climb out of the valley.

from the multiuse trail at 1.1 miles. On entering the full shade of the forest for the first time on the hike, the trail surface switches to wood chips covering compacted soil. Notice how the trees cool the air on even the hottest day. Just a few steps into the forest, the trail splits. We normally hike this section of the trail counterclockwise, so the return trail is on your left. Continue straight ahead, crossing a manmade rock-hop on a concrete culvert. The trail to the falls is on the left. After reading the interpretive sign, continue around to the left to Table Rock Falls, at 1.3 miles. Dropping 30 feet to a flat rock, the stream spreads along the rim and then free-falls another 15 feet, where it cascades, forming a small creek.

Return to the interpretive sign and continue straight, into a forest of American beeches punctuated by a red maple here and a shagbark hickory there. Return to the main trail and turn left (more of a U-turn, really). After gaining a small hill, the trail begins a moderate-to-difficult descent into the river valley, quickly passing a stone bridge and Beech Tree Trail on the right. Descending the hill, the trail switchbacks for an easy walk. Watch for a deep valley on the right as the trail descends and then crosses a stone bridge over a gently babbling brook at 1.7 miles.

In the valley the trail levels off, running alongside a couple of streams before beginning to climb back to the hilltop. On the climb, watch for rock cairns in the forest. Built by American Indians for an unknown reason (the structures hold

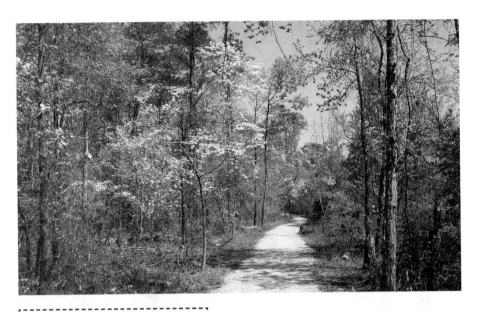

April-blooming dogwoods adorn the path.

neither bodies nor religious artifacts), many of these cairns are symmetrically stacked rocks, although some are scattered as if they had been vandalized. Protected within the park, there are hundreds of these mounds.

As you return to the top of the valley, bear left and continue to Beech Tree Trail; then turn right to exit the forest. The trail curves right as it climbs to the multiuse trail at 3.6 miles. Walk across West Meadow Trail, and make the easy climb to the overlook—one of the highest points in Gwinnett County—for some excellent scenic views into the surrounding Piedmont; then return to the West Meadow Trail and turn right. Walking downhill to a four-way intersection, head straight on East Meadow Trail and then begin climbing to another high point. The trail curves left, reaches a small hill, and then begins an extended but easy descent to the starting point. Go straight at the four-way intersection and then turn left on the connector trail. You'll see the trailhead kiosk on the right.

NEARBY ACTIVITIES

From the park, turn right on Fence Road NE, drive 0.6 mile, and make another right on Auburn Road. Drive 1.4 miles and turn left on Dacula Road. In about 0.5 mile, watch for an impressive old home on the left, at 908 Dacula Rd.—the oldest building in Gwinnett County and likely the oldest in metropolitan Atlanta. Built in 1812 and restored to its 1870s appearance, the **Elisha Winn House** is managed by the Gwinnett Historical Society. It is open for tours March–September on the second Saturday of the month and during the first weekend of October; for more information, call 770-822-5174 or 770-237-2804, or visit **gwinnetths.org**.

McDANIEL FARM PARK TRAIL 42

IN BRIEF

McDaniel Farm has been restored to depict a subsistence farm similar to many of the farms in the area in the 1930s. In addition to hiking the asphalt trail and taking a free self-guided tour of the farm, you can take the docent-led Heritage Farm tour on Friday and Saturday.

DESCRIPTION

When people think of antebellum Georgia, most picture massive cotton plantations. In the Atlanta area, however, most agriculture before the Civil War was subsistence farming— raising enough corn and wheat to meet only one family's needs. Grain from these farms had to be cracked, or ground, before being eaten; wealthier planters coined the derogatory term *cracker* to describe the poorer farmers. Atlantans, though, were proud of the term: for more than 60 years, Crackers was the name of their minor-league baseball team. Although the McDaniel family owned the farm from 1859 until it was given to the county after Archie McDaniel's death in 1999, the property is set up as a 1930s farm might have been.

From the kiosk adjacent to the restrooms, head left, following the asphalt path as it curves 180 degrees and passing a group shelter on the left before crossing a wooden bridge over a deep ravine. Watch for some larger trees here,

KEY AT-A-GLANCE INFORMATION

LENGTH: 2.5 miles

CONFIGURATION: Loop

DIFFICULTY: Easy

SCENERY: Meadowlands, Heritage Farm

EXPOSURE: Full sun

TRAFFIC: Moderate

TRAIL SURFACE: Asphalt, except at Heritage Farm

WHEELCHAIR ACCESS: Yes, but the area is hilly.

HIKING TIME: 1 hour; Heritage Farm tour adds 1 hour

ACCESS: Daily, year-round, sunrise–sunset; free to hike ($5 for Heritage Farm tour)

MAPS: Available at trailhead and Heritage Farm; USGS *Luxomni, Norcross*

MORE INFO: 770-822-8840; tinyurl.com/mcdanielfarm

FACILITIES: Restrooms at trailhead

SPECIAL COMMENTS: In spring the meadow is full of color.

DISTANCE: 10.1 miles from I-85 North/I-285 Northeast

Directions ⟶

Take I-85 North to Exit 104/Pleasant Hill Road, and turn left. Drive 0.5 mile and turn right on Satellite Boulevard. Drive 0.5 mile and turn left on Old Norcross Road. Drive 0.2 mile and turn right on McDaniel Road. Drive 0.4 mile to the parking lot, on the left.

GPS INFORMATION

N33° 58.135' W84° 7.685'

3251 McDaniel Rd.
Duluth, GA 30096

McDaniel Farm Park Trail

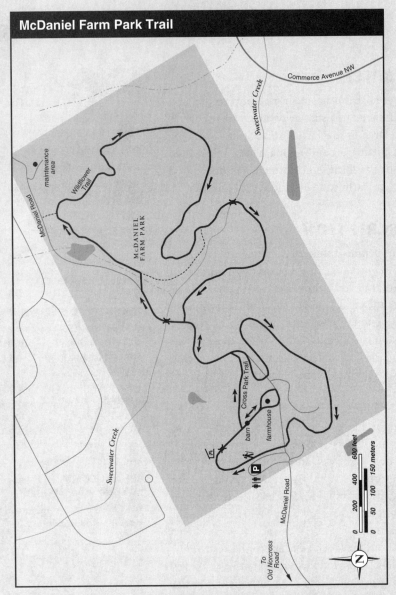

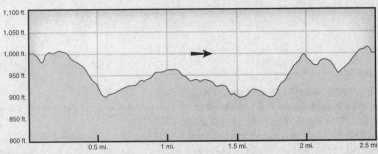

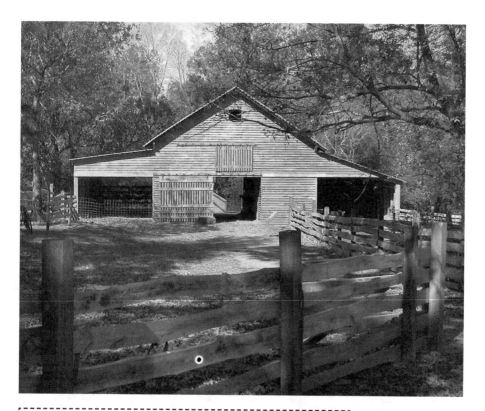

An old barn gives visitors a glimpse of life on the old McDaniel homestead.

including tulip poplars and oaks. As you cross the bridge, the farm entrance is directly ahead. Guided tours ($5 per person) are given March–November, Tuesday–Saturday, 10 a.m.–4 p.m. (call 770-814-4920 for more information). If you can't make the tour, pick up a brochure from the metal pail hanging just inside the barn on the left wall. We strongly recommend the walking tour because it gives visitors access to the farmhouse, which is the most interesting building on the farm.

The lower level of the barn was used to house animals—cows, horses, mules, and pigs. The upper floor, or loft, was used to store feed, which could be dropped down to the animals through specially built chutes. On either side are two additional covered areas where a farmer could store machinery or extra feed he couldn't get in the loft. Also notice that the barn has a lot of open spaces in the building; these allowed the air that accumulated in the mild Georgia winters to circulate through the barn all year.

Continue straight ahead to the farmhouse. A chicken coop–henhouse is to the right and a smokehouse to the left. The hens would have been kept for their eggs rather than raised for food. Smoked or salted meat cured in the smokehouse could be stored for months without refrigeration. After the Civil War, the McDaniels built the farmhouse, which is directly in front of you; it reflects the

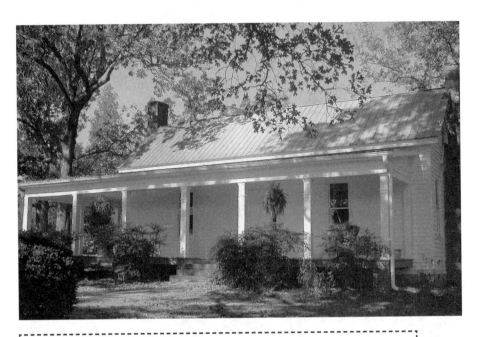

Built after the Civil War, the McDaniel farmhouse has been restored to its 1930s appearance.

family's prosperity. For the McDaniels, cotton became a cash crop after the war, adding to the farm's income.

Notice an old pear tree and pecan tree close to the house and a Chinese chestnut a bit farther back. In front and on the far side are post and white oaks. The lawn is swept—there is no grass—because tending a lawn would have taken too much time. Inside the home, photos of each family member adorn the rooms in which they slept, and letters written home by the boys during World War II are simply addressed "McDaniel, Duluth, Georgia."

Circle the farmhouse and return to the barn. Once through the barn, turn right on the asphalt path. Known as Cross Park Trail, the path begins a moderate descent to Sweetwater Creek, passing a trail to the parking lot on the right at 0.4 mile. At the bottom of the hill, just before the bridge over the creek, the return trail from the loop enters from the right.

This portion of the path was once a county roadway, but almost all evidence of this fact has been obliterated. Only in the vicinity of the farmhouse is the road evident. From the bridge the path begins to climb, bearing left at 0.65 mile at a three-way intersection. The path continues to a maintenance area, where it turns right to become Wildflower Trail. From a ridge just under a mile into the hike, you can see commercial development off to the left. At this point the trail begins an easy descent as it curves left, toward a forested area with a variety of large pines.

After the trees, a meadow where the McDaniels once planted cotton has been replanted with flowers to provide color in the spring. Cotton was grown on the

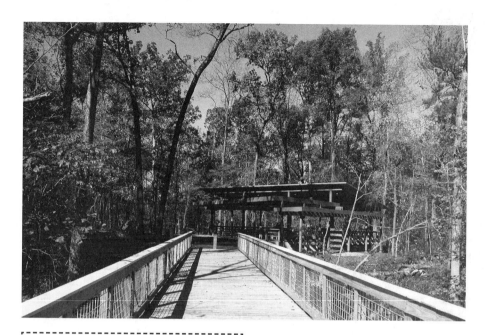

A bridge crossing comes near the start of the trail.

farm only until the 1920s, when boll weevil infestation reached Gwinnett County. After about 1925 the McDaniels planted corn, okra, and butter beans in these fields.

Where a path heads right at 1.4 miles, continue straight to another pedestrian bridge over Sweetwater Creek, less than 0.1 mile ahead. After the bridge the trail winds to the right and returns to Cross Park Trail. Turn left and climb the hill to an alternate return trail to the parking lot, at 1.9 miles. Turn left on the level path as it swings around McDaniel Farm's outer perimeter. The small house on the right, at 2.2 miles, was used by the tenant farmer who worked on the farm in exchange for food and a meager salary: $5 for all the work he did during a winter in the 1930s, according to a display inside the house. Notice the outhouse adjacent to the tenant's house. Continue on the trail to the parking lot.

NEARBY ACTIVITIES

Train and railroad buffs will enjoy the **Southeastern Railway Museum** (3595 Buford Hwy., Duluth; hours and admission info: 770-476-2013 or **srmduluth.org**). To get there, retrace your route back to Old Norcross and Pleasant Hill Roads. Turn right on Pleasant Hill Road, drive 1.6 miles, and then turn right on Buford Highway (US 23/GA 13). In 0.45 mile bear left on Peachtree Road—look carefully for a small green museum sign at the turnoff. The museum is a few yards ahead on your left, across the railroad tracks.

43 STONE MOUNTAIN LOOP

KEY AT-A-GLANCE INFORMATION

LENGTH: 5.5 miles

CONFIGURATION: Loop

DIFFICULTY: Easy

SCENERY: Views of Stone Mountain and Confederate Memorial; gristmill; covered bridge; streams; lakeshore

EXPOSURE: Full sun around carving and in some areas where trail runs on granite; mostly shaded elsewhere

TRAFFIC: Heavy between Confederate Hall and Summit Skyride, light elsewhere

TRAIL SURFACE: Compacted soil, Chattahoochee stone, granite

WHEELCHAIR ACCESS: None

HIKING TIME: 2.5 hours

ACCESS: Daily, year-round; gates open 6 a.m.–midnight; parking $10/day. General-admission tickets allow access to all attractions (see website below for pricing).

MAPS: At entrance and Confederate Hall; USGS *Stone Mountain*

FACILITIES: Restrooms at trailhead and at most attractions; playgrounds, picnic tables

MORE INFO: 770-498-5690; stonemountainpark.com

SPECIAL COMMENTS: Stone Mountain Park has a laser show, a cable-car ride, and many other attractions.

DISTANCE: 7.7 miles from US 78 East/ Stone Mountain Highway/I-285 East

GPS INFORMATION

N33° 48.639' W84° 9.714'

1000 Robert E. Lee Blvd.
Stone Mountain, GA 30083

IN BRIEF

This loop trail takes visitors to most of the major attractions at Stone Mountain.

DESCRIPTION

After parking, return to the sidewalk in front of Confederate Hall and turn left, walking Stone Mountain Loop counterclockwise. Follow the sidewalk 0.2 mile to a trestle for Stone Mountain Railroad. Walk under the trestle and turn left, entering the forest for the first time. At just under 0.4 mile, a path leads right, almost hidden in the summer months. Descend a few steps to two polished granite "bridges" across a creek. Return to the main trail and turn left.

Continue on the orange connector trail to a marked right turn at 0.6 mile. This is the entrance to the nature center, which has an interpretive display of plants native to Georgia. Among the trees are mulberries and white oaks. Plants include strawberries Christmas ferns, trumpet creepers, fragrant sumacs, and beautyberries. As you walk through the garden, keep a small building to your left and continue to the other side. Mulberry trees at 0.7 mile indicate the end of the nature center.

Directions ⟶

Take I-285 East to Exit 39B/US 78/Stone Mountain Highway (Snellville/Athens), and merge onto US 78 East. Drive 7.3 miles to the exit for Stone Mountain East Gate. The road curves right and then comes to a gate, where you pay the $10 entrance fee. After the gate, this road is known as Jefferson Davis Drive. Continue 1 mile to a fork in the road. Bear right and merge onto Robert E. Lee Boulevard. Follow it 1 mile to Confederate Hall. Turn left and park.

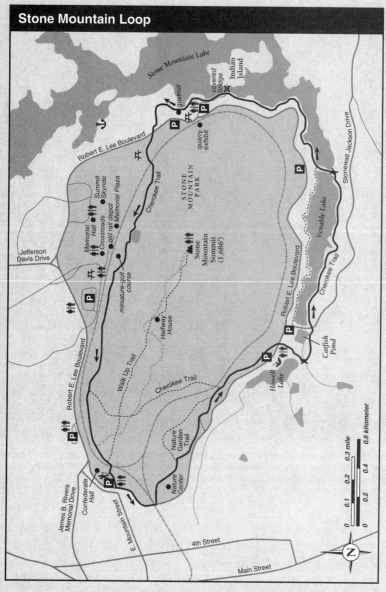

Stone Mountain Loop

Stone Mountain Lake

Indian Island

covered bridge

grist mill

quarry exhibit

Robert E. Lee Boulevard

Summit Skyride

Memorial Hall

Memorial Plaza

Crossroads

old rail depot

STONE MOUNTAIN PARK

Stonewall Jackson Drive

Venable Lake

Cherokee Trail

Jefferson Davis Drive

Stone Mountain Summit (1,686')

miniature-golf course

Robert E. Lee Boulevard

Cherokee Trail

Catfish Pond

Halfway House

Walk-Up Trail

Cherokee Trail

Howell Lake

Robert E. Lee Boulevard

Nature Garden Trail

James B. Rivers Memorial Drive

Confederate Hall

Nature Center

0.6 kilometer

0.3 mile

0.4

0.2

0.2

0.1

0

0

E. Mountain Street

4th Street

Main Street

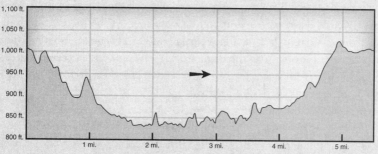

1,100 ft.
1,050 ft.
1,000 ft.
950 ft.
900 ft.
850 ft.
800 ft.

1 mi.   2 mi.   3 mi.   4 mi.   5 mi.

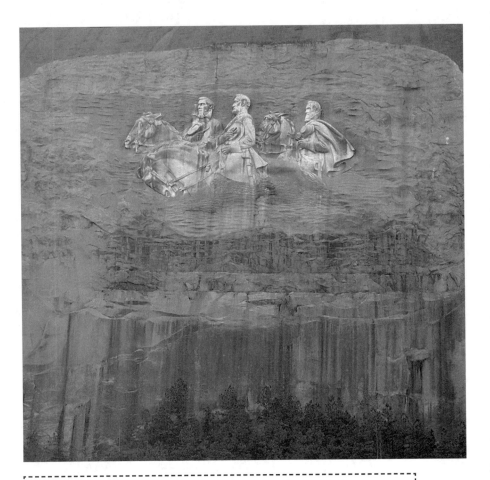

Jefferson Davis, Robert E. Lee, and Stonewall Jackson forever ride on their favorite mounts in the famous carving on the face of Stone Mountain.

The footpath bears right, coming to an intersection with Cherokee (Red) Trail. Turn right and continue to the remains of a house at 1 mile. You can see the roofline cut in the chimney about two-thirds of the way to the top. There are wire cuts in a tree on the opposite site of the house as well. The path bears right at 1.3 miles, climbs a set of railroad-tie steps, and crosses Robert E. Lee Boulevard. Keep a green-fenced playground to your right as you reenter the forest. The trail circles the playground, turning left on a gravel road and then crossing the dam that forms Howell Lake. Step down into the cement overflow and climb a similar step on the other side. As the path bears left, a railed bridge crosses a creek at 1.5 miles. Just 0.1 mile later, the path crosses Stonewall Jackson Drive.

Venable Lake, on your left, is named for Sam Venable, who ran the quarry here in the early 20th century. About halfway around the lake, the trail bears right, crosses a beautiful stream with cascades flowing over a series of large rocks, and then bears left to return to the lakeshore. At 2.5 miles the footpath makes a hard left, crossing an earthen dam and turning right on the far side of the lake. On your right is the largest body of water in the park, Stone Mountain Lake.

Just before 2.8 miles, Stone Mountain Loop rises around a rock outcrop, turning inland before turning right just before the road, and then falling to a creek. The trail becomes undefined as it crosses granite outcrops, but watch for white blazes on the rock. The number of trails to the lakeshore increases, and the covered bridge comes into view at 3.2 miles. African American bridge builder W. W. King constructed the lattice bridge in 1891. Originally, the bridge spanned the Oconee River in Athens, but when the Georgia Department of Transportation replaced the bridge in 1965, they offered it to Stone Mountain Park for $1. The park accepted and moved the bridge to its present site at a cost of $18,000.

The footpath falls to the lakeshore and crosses an outflow on two granite tablets. The path runs along the lake, inches above the water level and with a granite wall to your left. Watch for two sets of two granite hearts put in the pathway by an energetic stonemason. As the path curves left and away from the lake, concrete walkways replace the trail at 3.6 miles. The network of walkways offers views of the Stone Mountain gristmill, but head for the mill wheel and a boardwalk that runs next to the mill for a close-up look at the structure. At the far end of the boardwalk, turn right and continue uphill to a granite sluice and springhouse. Keeping the sluice on your right, cross a field and a small stream, turn left, and climb to Robert E. Lee Boulevard.

After you cross the road, the trail winds through second-growth forest, mostly oaks and beeches, and then climbs railroad-tie steps to cross the tracks at 4 miles. A nature garden, established by the Atlanta branch of the National League of American Pen Women in 1961, is on the left. After you pass under the alpine-style Summit Skyride cable cars, keep a small garage at 4.4 miles to your right as you circle right and climb to Memorial Plaza. As the path curves left, it turns to Chattahoochee stone, and the carving comes into view for the first time.

The massive bas-relief sculpture of Jefferson Davis, Robert E. Lee, and Stonewall Jackson was carved out of the world's largest piece of solid rock and represents the work of three sculptors over a period of 56 years. Gutzon Borglum began working on a concept for the sculpture in 1916, although actual carving did not begin until 1923. Borglum quickly ran into problems—not only with the creative process, which proved tedious and frustrating, but also with the other people involved in the project, whom he alienated with his explosive temper and domineering ways. Ultimately, he fled Georgia just ahead of a police car. Sculptor Augustus Lukeman took over in 1925, blasting Borglum's work off the face of the mountain. (Two years later, Borglum began work on another project, Mt. Rushmore.) Lukeman had made significant progress on the current carving when the project failed to meet its deadline in 1928. The carving sat unfinished for 30 years at the intersection of two rural highways.

When the state of Georgia purchased the land in 1958, plans were immediately set in motion to complete the project. Sculptor Walker Hancock was picked

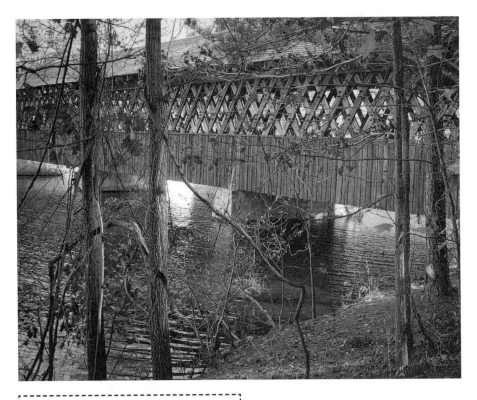

A historic covered bridge crosses to Indian Island.

for the task, although Roy Faulkner, a former Marine with no prior experience carving stone, did most of the work under Hancock's supervision. Dedicated in 1970, the project was finally declared complete in 1972. On the right, across an open field, is Memorial Hall, which contains an excellent museum that highlights the mountain, the sculptors, and some local history.

Stone Mountain Loop reenters the forest as it leaves Memorial Plaza. On your right at 4.5 miles, on the far side of the miniature golf course and the tracks, is a re-creation of the Atlanta rail depot that General William Tecumseh Sherman destroyed in his 1864 March to the Sea. Behind the depot is the recently added Crossroads, an area of shops designed to resemble a frontier village, with areas called the Treehouses and the Great Barn, and a 4-D theater with a film about the Southern art of storytelling.

Past the miniature golf course, the trail runs between the mountain and the railroad and continues in a shortleaf-and-loblolly-pine forest on a frequently rocky path, occasionally moving into full sun when it climbs solid-granite outcrops of the mountain. The red-blazed Cherokee Trail heads left at the marked intersection at 5.2 miles; then Stone Mountain Loop runs adjacent to the tracks as it crosses a paved road and enters the Confederate Hall complex.

STONE MOUNTAIN WALK UP TRAIL

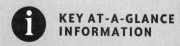

44

IN BRIEF

This trail climbs on solid granite and through boulder fields to the top of Stone Mountain, some 780 feet above the surrounding Georgia Piedmont.

DESCRIPTION

Climb the Walk Up Trail to the top of Stone Mountain, and you walk through 200 years of American history, 400 years of European history, thousands of years of American Indian history, and millions of years in geological history. To call this trail historic is an understatement.

Formed 7 miles beneath the Earth's surface more than 350 million years ago, Stone Mountain is what geologists call a pluton. Molten lava, created by the massive collision of tectonic plates during the formation of the Blue Ridge Mountains, forced its way into an underlying fold over many millions of years. The east side of the mountain was the first side to be formed. Stone Mountain granite is significantly different from the underlying Lithonia granite belt that runs east and south of the mountain. Archaic American Indian sites dating back 8,000 years have been found

KEY AT-A-GLANCE INFORMATION

LENGTH: 2.4 miles round-trip

CONFIGURATION: Out-and-back, with a small loop on the mountaintop

DIFFICULTY: Hard

SCENERY: 360-degree vista of the Georgia Piedmont, including long-distance views of central Atlanta, Buckhead, and Decatur

EXPOSURE: Full sun for entire hike

TRAFFIC: Heavy

TRAIL SURFACE: Granite rock and boulders

WHEELCHAIR ACCESS: None

HIKING TIME: 2 hours, including time to browse a small museum at the top

ACCESS: Daily, year-round; gates open 6 a.m.–midnight; parking $10/day. General-admission tickets allow access to all attractions (see website below for pricing information).

MAPS: At entrance and Confederate Hall; USGS *Stone Mountain*

MORE INFO: 770-498-5690; stonemountainpark.com

FACILITIES: Restrooms, vending machines

SPECIAL COMMENTS: Stone Mountain Park has a laser show, a cable-car ride, and many other attractions.

DISTANCE: 7.7 miles from US 78 East/Stone Mountain Highway/I-285 East

GPS INFORMATION

N33° 48.639' W84° 9.714'

1000 Robert E. Lee Blvd.
Stone Mountain, GA 30083

Directions

Take I-285 East to Exit 39B/US 78/Stone Mountain Highway (Snellville/Athens), and merge onto US 78 East. Drive 7.3 miles to the exit for Stone Mountain East Gate. The road curves right and then comes to a gate, where you pay the $10 entrance fee. After the gate, this road is known as Jefferson Davis Drive. Continue 1 mile to a fork in the road. Bear left and merge onto Robert E. Lee Boulevard. Follow it 1 mile to Confederate Hall. Turn left and park.

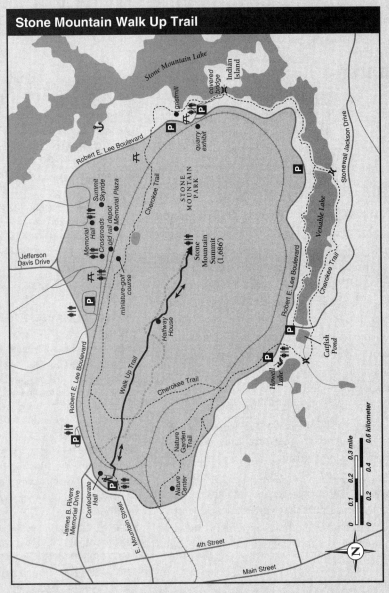

Stone Mountain Walk Up Trail

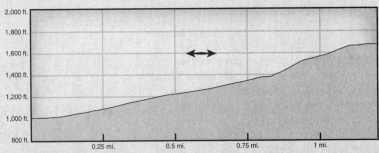

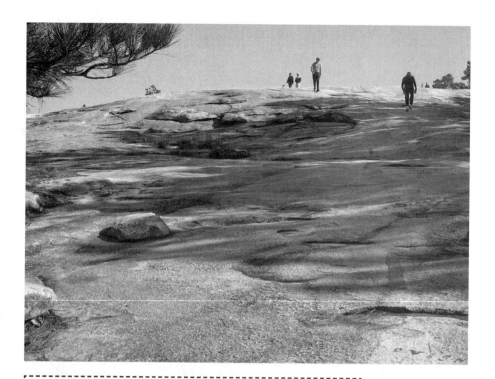

The trail to the mountaintop is marked with yellow lines painted on the rocks. *Note:* The trail surface is very slippery when wet.

near the mountain, along with Woodland Indian sites, Mound Builder settlements, and Creek villages.

When Spanish explorers first visited the mountain (in about 1560), they called the monadnock Crystal Mountain because of the quartz that they found around the base and embedded in the rock. The Creeks regularly climbed the trail to the mountaintop, frequently using the site to meet with nearby Cherokees. In 1790 Colonel Marinus Willet met Creek chiefs at the top of the mountain and escorted them to New York City to meet with President George Washington.

Settlers moving west along Hightower Trail called the peak Rock Fort Mountain because of the wall that Woodland Indians had built around the top. Over time the name was shortened to Rock Mountain. Baptist minister Adiel Sherwood, one of the founders of Mercer College (now Mercer University) in Macon, renamed the peak Stone Mountain. Large-scale granite quarrying began about 1847, the same year that the nearby town changed its name from New Gibraltar to Stone Mountain. Civil War battles briefly raged near the mountain in July 1864, and the left wing of General William Tecumseh Sherman's army passed just north of the mountain in November 1864 on its March to the Sea. In 1958 the state purchased the mountain and surrounding land and turned it into a state park. One of the first buildings in the park was Confederate Hall, on your left as you approach the railroad crossing that marks the start of the trail.

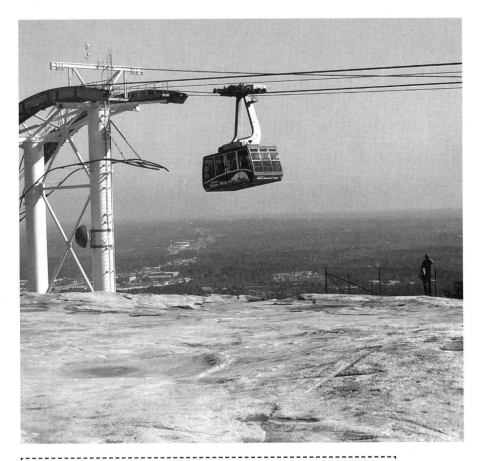

The appropriately named Summit Skyride carries visitors to the top of Stone Mountain.

Once across the tracks, the trail begins its climb—easy at first but quickly increasing in grade. You'll find no level or downhill sections until the return trip. At 0.3 mile into the hike, power lines come in from the left and follow near the rock path to the mountaintop. During this part of the ascent, boulders straddle the path; climbing them can take a while.

Just over 0.6 mile into the hike is a picnic shelter. Look closely on the right to see a barbecue grill, marking the start of the steepest portion of the climb. Keep your eyes on the trail: embedded in the granite a short distance past the shelter, an engraved plaque marks Cherokee Trail, a historic pathway that crosses Walk Up Trail at this point. Just a few steps up from the plaque, parallel metal railings help unsteady visitors up a particularly steep section of the footpath, but experienced hikers can easily bypass these structures by bearing left at a split in the trail before the railings. Follow this trail through a large boulder field, watching for Bubble Gum Rock, where visitors have left their chewing gum for many years.

Now the trail has climbed far enough to allow stunning views of the relatively level Piedmont surrounding Stone Mountain. Moving left, closer to the sheer northern face where the carving is, the trail passes a series of metal structures attached to the mountain. These are remnants of the scaffolding that supported the sculptors as they worked. Rising toward the peak, the trail passes near a vernal (spring) pool with red moss. These pools fill with rainwater in the spring and literally come to life. Tiny fairy shrimp, whose lifespan is measured in days, not years, are born, reproduce, and die. When the pools dry up during the winter or in heavy drought years, animals and wind spread the eggs to other vernal pools.

On one visit, tour guide Matt Wood met us at the summit to show us some of the highlights. Walking near the steep north face of the mountain, where we enjoyed an incredible long-distance view, we listened as Matt told us of Elias Nour, who was frequently called to rescue people from the cliff face. His legendary exploits, some of which are discussed in David B. Freeman's book *Carved in Stone,* include pushing a burning car off the face of the mountain as a stunt to attract visitors.

At the top of the mountain is a dual-purpose structure: it serves as both a dock for the Summit Skyride and a small museum with interesting information on the natural history of Stone Mountain. As we walked toward the building, we passed the highest point on the mountain. Yellow paint on the northeast side of some rock was the next point of interest. In the early 1920s, before airplanes had directional systems, the rock was painted with the word ATLANTA and a huge arrow pointing toward the city. Stone Mountain, visible for 50 miles on a clear day, was the guiding point for pilots from the Northeast. At the museum–cable car dock, Matt told us that the alpine-style lift was one of the park's first attractions. As we began to circle back to our starting point, we saw a white line designating a drivable road down the mountain. A large, fenced-off area protects the fragile habitat of the fairy shrimp and other species.

At the end of the loop, turn left to retrace your steps to your car.

NEARBY ACTIVITIES

Confederate Hall (770-498-5658), at the base of the mountain, contains extensive information on the geology and environment of Stone Mountain, plus an excellent display on the Civil War in Georgia, narrated by Hal Holbrook. **Stone Mountain Village** (770-413-0607; **stonemountainvillage.com**) is home to eclectic shops, art galleries, and restaurants.

45   SUWANEE GREENWAY

KEY AT-A-GLANCE INFORMATION

LENGTH: 9.5 miles round-trip

CONFIGURATION: Out-and-back

DIFFICULTY: Moderate

SCENERY: Multiple creekside views and forested wetlands

EXPOSURE: Full sun, except for either end of the trail and in the vicinity of McGinnis Ferry Road, where the trail is mostly shaded

TRAFFIC: Moderate; multiuse trail

TRAIL SURFACE: Paved except for compacted soil at the beginning, at George F. Pierce Park

WHEELCHAIR ACCESS: None

HIKING TIME: 4.5 hours

ACCESS: Daily, year-round, sunrise–sunset; free

MAPS: USGS *Suwanee*

MORE INFO: 770-945-8996; suwanee .com/cityservices.recreationparks.php

FACILITIES: Restrooms and picnic areas at both ends; picnic area at Martin Farm Road parking area. More facilities are planned.

SPECIAL COMMENTS: This river environment has abundant wildlife, especially in the wetland areas. The area is popular with birders.

DISTANCE: 19.6 miles from I-85 North/I-285 Northeast

GPS INFORMATION

N34° 3.571' W84° 3.501'

IN BRIEF

This hike follows the floodplain of Suwanee Creek from George F. Pierce Park to Suwanee Creek Park.

DESCRIPTION

It's no exaggeration to call Suwanee Greenway the environmental success story of the Atlanta area. Suwanee Creek was all but destroyed by source-point pollution. The Bona Allen Tannery, founded in 1873, operated for a century on the creek in Buford. For decades, untreated chemicals used in the leather-tanning process—acid, lime, and dyes—were pumped into the waterway, killing virtually all living creatures and creating a 15-mile environmental disaster area. By the time the tannery shut down in the late 1970s, scientists estimated that the creek could take 100 years to return to normal.

Today Suwanee Creek has risen from the dead, more than 30 years after the factory closed. Stretching from George F. Pierce Park (a 300-acre Gwinnett County park) to Suwanee Creek Park (an 85-acre park developed by the city of Suwanee), the Suwanee Greenway offers visitors the chance to hike, bike, walk, run, or skate along a level 4-mile paved trail; additional paved and gravel hiking is available in the parks at either end. Between the two

----

Directions ─────────────────➤

Take I-85 North to Exit 111/Lawrenceville–Suwanee Road/GA 317. Turn left on GA 317 and drive 2.3 miles to Buford Highway/US 23. Turn right, drive 0.3 mile to the first traffic light, and make a right into George F. Pierce Park. Drive 1 mile to the parking area and turn left down the first aisle. Park at the far end of this aisle, near an embankment.

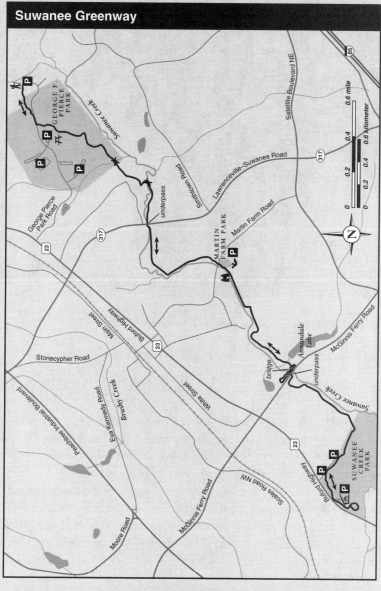

Suwanee Greenway

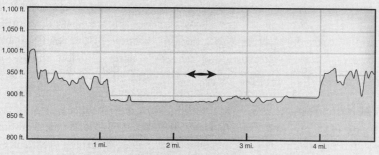

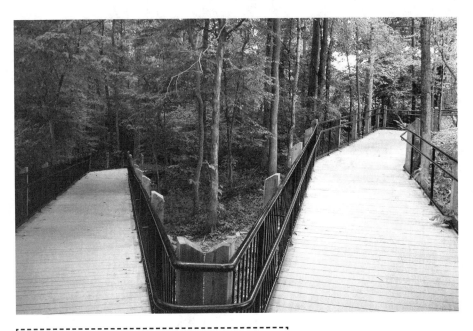

This wooden walkway snakes its way to McGinnis Ferry Road.

parks, the renewed creek shelters a wide range of native and nonnative trees and shrubs, waterfowl, and wildlife.

Our hike begins at the south end of Pierce Park. Although we love the greenway, starting here rather than at Suwanee Creek Park gives us at least a little time away from the cyclists and in-line skaters who dominate the paved portion of the hike. Climb the embankment and turn left after entering the mostly oak forest. (We once ran into a rooster not very far along the trail.) The unblazed-but-easy-to-follow footpath descends into the watershed of a tributary of Suwanee Creek, winding as it climbs to a paved road at 0.3 mile. Turn right, follow the road 200 feet to the NATURE TRAIL sign, and turn left. A short way down this compacted-soil trail, a RULES OF THE ROAD sign indicates the start of the multiuse trail.

The forest is replaced by manicured grass as you enter full sun, but it returns at 0.5 mile. The trail becomes a gravel road and continues an easy descent. On the left, a wetland stretches across a low floodplain between the road embankment and Suwanee Creek. Waterfowl and larger predators inhabit this floodplain throughout the year. Just past a bench on the right, the road makes a sharp right turn and continues skirting the creek until it makes another right, onto a long bridge with wooden slats and a metal railing. For the first time, the trail enters the wetland and excellent long-distance views open up. At 1.2 miles the trail turns left on a wooden bridge and crosses Suwanee Creek, again affording great river views. About midway across the bridge, the trail turns right and then comes to an asphalt path. Bear left and continue across another wooden bridge. At the end of the bridge the trail bears left, quickly coming to an underpass at 1.5 miles, where the trail narrows.

Emerging from the underpass, Suwanee Greenway turns left and begins to meander through the manicured grass of the wide floodplain of Suwanee Creek, heading west and following the river as it curves left and begins to flow southward. At 2.2 miles the pathway crosses Martin Farm Road, and a side trail on the left takes you to a parking area with some playground equipment. The greenway changes noticeably, with wetlands frequently engulfing the path, which has almost imperceptibly turned west again. This habitat, which also serves as a breeding ground and rest stop for migratory birds, shows how dramatically the creek and the nearby wetlands have recovered. Among the species that make use of this once-polluted ecosystem are great blue herons, black vultures, red-tailed and red-shouldered hawks, ospreys, and American bald eagles. Watch for typical water-loving grasses, such as goldenrods and cattails, and trees including river birch and white ash.

The Suwanee Greenway then enters a swamp created by an active beaver dam. As the paved road rises, Annandale Lane, a residential street, dead-ends into the greenway at 2.7 miles. Following the road the trail runs above an area of immense trees. Among the varieties of oaks grow loblolly and shortleaf pines, tulip poplars, sweet gums, and red maples. A ramped, switchbacking wooden walkway takes you up to McGinnis Ferry Road. At the road the trail turns right, using the curbed sidewalk on the bridge to cross Suwanee Creek, and then it turns right again, easily curving right, descending to the creek, and passing under the bridge. As the path comes out the other side, it curves right again and rises to the Burnette Road parking lot, where it makes a 90-degree left turn.

From McGinnis Ferry Road to Suwanee Creek Park, the paved trail repeatedly rises on low wooden bridges to cross thriving, sensitive wetlands. Once again, be ready to see a good deal of wildlife, although we've typically spotted only smaller mammals such as raccoons and rabbits. At 4 miles, the last bridge ends and the trail splits in a garden of native plantings. The trail on the right is a quick, refreshing thigh-stretch to Suwanee Creek Park, while the trail straight ahead is more gradual, intended for cyclists.

The city of Suwanee has created a wonderful environment in the park. The paved trail explores a small knoll that is vastly different from the greenway. At a four-way intersection with a parking lot immediately on the right, go straight to explore the park. Pavilions and picnic tables dot the landscape as the trail crosses the entrance road at 4.3 miles. As the pathway approaches Buford Highway, it makes a U-turn deep in a forested cove on a wooden bridge across a gully; then it rises and parallels the roadway to a parking lot. Walk past the pavilion on the far end of the parking lot and turn right.

An overlook allows hikers to view Suwanee Creek from above. Then the footpath continues, curving to the right to an unobstructed (although decidedly

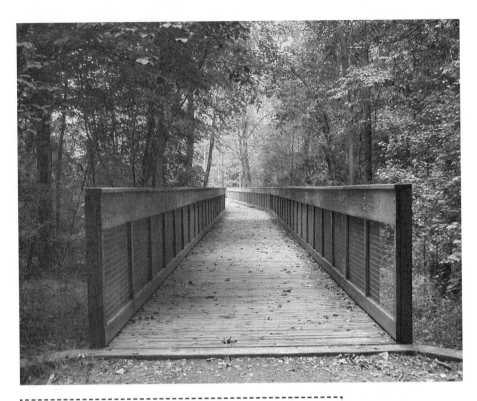

Numerous bridges and boardwalks span environmentally sensitive areas.

suburban) view at 4.7 miles. The trail loops right, returning to the inbound trail. Turn left and retrace your steps to your car.

NEARBY ACTIVITIES

At Lawrenceville–Suwanee Road, the Suwanee Creek Greenway connects to **Suwanee Town Center,** a mixed-use public–private development with a 10-acre urban park at its heart (770-945-8996; **suwanee.com/economicdevelopment.towncenter .php**). Nearby are restaurants and a kid-friendly fountain.

TRIBBLE MILL TRAIL 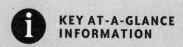 46

IN BRIEF

This multiuse trail explores a portion of 800-acre Tribble Mill Park and one of its two artificial lakes.

DESCRIPTION

The town of Grayson and its environs lie within the first part of Gwinnett County that was settled by farmers from the east. The land was originally part of Franklin County, incorporated in 1784, but was later ceded to Gwinnett County, established in 1818. Founded in 1881, Grayson was originally called Trip. The name was changed to Berkeley in 1901, and finally to its present name in 1902 since there was already a Berkeley elsewhere in Georgia.

Two artificial lakes—Ozora (109 acres) and Chandler (40 acres)—form the centerpiece of Tribble Mill Park, and the paved, multiuse trail circles most of Ozora Lake. From the parking lot you have a good long-distance view up the lake. At the road, turn right on the trail, which begins to rise as it parallels Tribble Mill Parkway. It dips into a

- -

Directions ⟶

Take I-285 East to Exit 39B/Stone Mountain Highway/US 78 East (Snellville/Athens), and merge onto US 78 East. Drive 16.2 miles to Grayson Parkway/GA 84—begin watching for this road after you cross Scenic Highway/GA 124 in downtown Snellville—and turn left. *Note:* At 3.6 miles, Grayson Parkway/GA 84 becomes Grayson–New Hope Road. Drive a total of 6.8 miles on this combined road to a four-way stop at New Hope Road. Turn right and drive 0.5 mile; then turn right on Tribble Mill Parkway SE. Drive 0.7 mile and turn left into the parking lot.

KEY AT-A-GLANCE INFORMATION

LENGTH: 3 miles

CONFIGURATION: Loop

DIFFICULTY: Easy

SCENERY: 2 lakes, forested wetlands

EXPOSURE: Full sun

TRAFFIC: Moderate; multiuse trail

TRAIL SURFACE: Paved asphalt

WHEELCHAIR ACCESS: Yes

HIKING TIME: 1.5 hours

ACCESS: Daily, year-round, sunrise–sunset; free

MAPS: At both entrances; USGS *Lawrenceville*

MORE INFO: 770-822-5414 (general); 770-978-5270 (trail hotline); tinyurl.com/tribblemill

FACILITIES: Restrooms, picnic tables with grills and pavilions, playground, meadow area with wildflowers, amphitheater

SPECIAL COMMENTS: Within the park are an additional 18 miles of equestrian and mountain bike trails, along with a fishing lake (nonmotorized and electric boats allowed).

DISTANCE: 24 miles from US 78 East/Stone Mountain Highway/I-285 East

GPS INFORMATION

N33° 54.724' W83° 54.709'

2125 Tribble Mill Pkwy. SE
Lawrenceville, GA 30045

Tribble Mill Trail

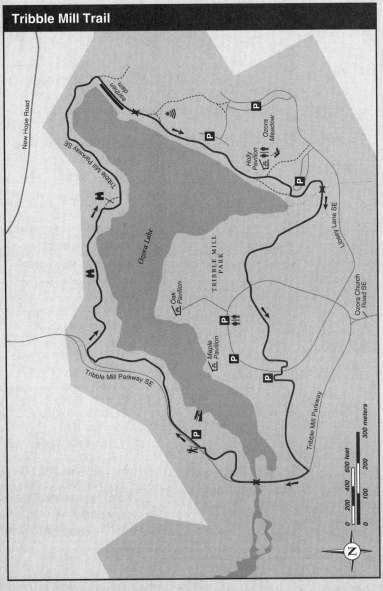

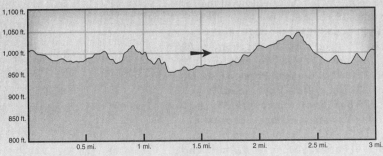

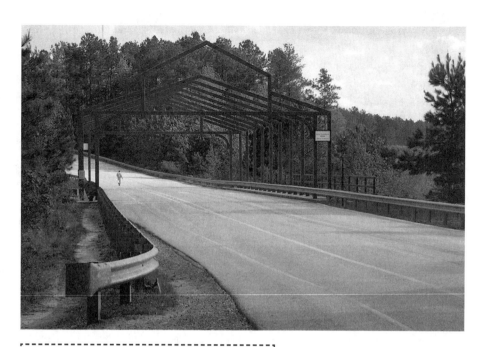

The striking Julian W. Archer Sr. Bridge spans Ozora Lake.

forest of pines and dogwoods, quickly returning to the parkway. The second time the trail descends, it begins to drop steeply past a post designed to prevent vehicular traffic from entering the multiuse trail.

The trail parallels the lakeshore, running above it to offer good long-distance views, and the forest diversifies. By the time the trail makes a hard left at 0.4 mile, white and post oaks, American beeches, maples, and elms have all joined the loblolly–shortleaf pine forest. An overlook made from granite, with steel seats, yields a somewhat blocked view of the lake and Ozora Meadow in the distance. Turn left at 0.8 mile, where the trail splits, and you'll come to a much better overlook, on the right. Where the trails rejoin, turn left; the pathway continues to bear left, following the curve of the lake. As the lakeshore begins to curve to the right, the trail makes a corresponding curve, crossing an earthen dam with a spillway at 1.3 miles.

After the dam, take the trail to the right as it continues to follow the lakeshore. On your left, past the amphitheater, is Ozora Meadow, an open field where kids can play. After the field and the playground, turn left and climb to the restrooms. To return to the main trail, take the next right and then another right at the parking lot. When you reach the lakeshore, turn left to enter full shade for the first time on the hike. The trail curves left and follows a stream on the right to a boardwalk bridge. Trails that allow you to explore the area below the boardwalk can be accessed before the boardwalk or from a sitting area on the left, after the bridge.

Following the bridge, the trail begins a good thigh-burning climb to the top of a small ridge. Multiple mountain bike paths cross the trail here; you can take any of these to further explore the area. The trail begins to curve more, falling to a roadbed at 2.1 miles and then continuing an easy climb. Just 0.2 mile later the trail crosses a second road, curves right, and then makes a U-turn as it begins to descend. After crossing a wooden bridge with metal railings, the path turns right as it runs adjacent to Tribble Mill Parkway, under the Julian W. Archer Sr. Bridge, on its way back to the parking lot.

NEARBY ACTIVITIES

Once you're done hiking Tribble Mill, retrace your route back to the intersection of US 78 West and GA 124 in downtown Snellville, and turn left on GA 124, signed as Scenic Highway and then Centerville Highway. Drive 4.2 miles and turn right on Annistown Road. Drive 2 miles and, just after you cross the Yellow River, turn left on Juhan Road SW. Turn into the first parking lot on the left, which is the starting point for a paved 1-mile **multiuse trail**—a good place to let the kids pedal off some steam. If you want to try the 5.7-mile **mountain bike trail** (which can also be hiked) or the **equestrian trail,** use the second parking lot, also on the left.

On the north end of the multiuse trail, a meadow and "council area" are planted with native grasses and wildflowers, and an observation deck yields lovely views of the Yellow River. Continuing past the end of the pavement, a pedestrian trail climbs a hill with a creek on the left, loops back to the equestrian trail, and drops with the same creek on the right, returning to the paved multiuse trail.

The bike paths form a double loop, one south and one north of the mountain bike parking area. The southern loop has less elevation change and is slightly shorter; the northern loop climbs out of the river valley to nearby knolls.

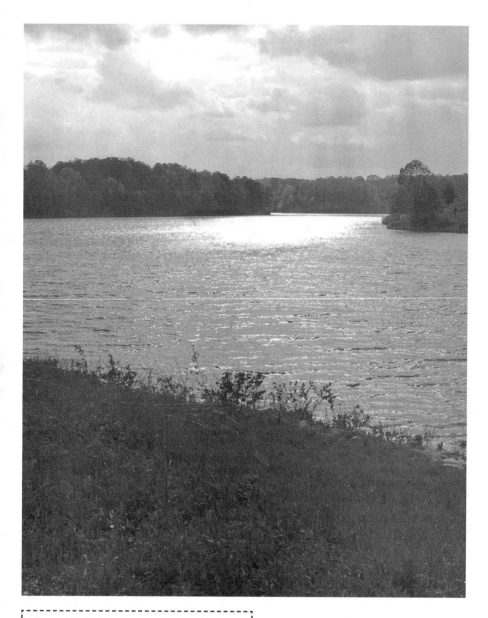

The sun breaks through the clouds over Ozora Lake.

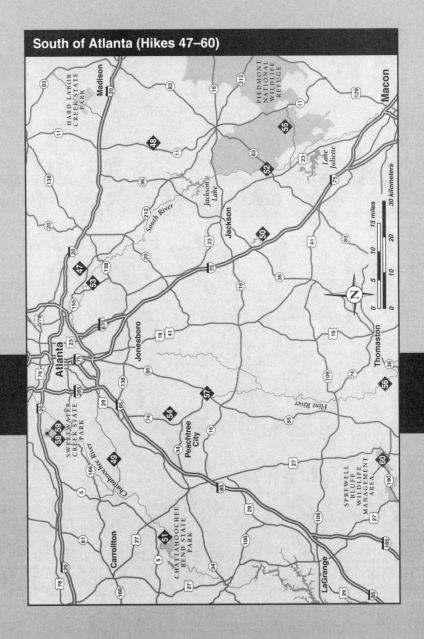

SOUTH OF
ATLANTA

47 ARABIA MOUNTAIN TRAIL

KEY AT-A-GLANCE INFORMATION

LENGTH: 5.1 miles

CONFIGURATION: Double loop with connecting trail

DIFFICULTY: Moderate

SCENERY: Long-distance mountaintop views, 2 lakes, forested wetlands, small streams

EXPOSURE: Full sun with some areas of partial shade, including the area around Arabia Lake

TRAFFIC: Moderate

TRAIL SURFACE: Stone, compacted dirt, some pavement

WHEELCHAIR ACCESS: None

HIKING TIME: 3 hours

ACCESS: Daily, year-round, sunrise–sunset; free to hike (some special programs charge fees)

MAPS: Available at nature center and both trailhead kiosks; USGS *Conyers, Redan*

MORE INFO: 770-492-5231; arabiaalliance.org

FACILITIES: Restrooms, nature center

SPECIAL COMMENTS: Formed by metamorphosed granite, Arabia Mountain is much older than nearby Stone Mountain.

DISTANCE: 10.1 miles from I-20 East/I-285 East

GPS INFORMATION

N33° 39.562' W84° 7.402'

3787 Klondike Rd.
Lithonia, GA 30038

IN BRIEF

This hike explores the Davidson–Arabia Mountain Nature Preserve area, composed of three distinct "mountains"—Bradley, Arabia, and Little Arabia—made of Lithonia gneiss. From the top of Bradley Mountain the trail is unmarked, but it's easy to pick up near the bottom.

DESCRIPTION

On first sight Arabia Mountain looks a lot like Stone Mountain, because both are rock outcrops. The difference lies in the type and age of the stone, and in the size of the two formations. Arabia Mountain is made of Lithonia gneiss—metamorphosed granite that is 700 million years old—whereas Stone Mountain is made of granite half that age. Aside from that, the barren landscape is surprisingly similar. Both formations have vernal pools and Georgia oaks, and both supported quarrying operations from the mid-1800s on. Like Stone Mountain, Arabia Mountain is near a crossroads. In fact, the nearby city of Lithonia ("stone place" in Latin) was originally called Crossroads.

From the parking lot, walk toward the elongated wooden trailhead kiosk and a

----

Directions ────────────────────→

Take I-20 East to Exit 74/Evans Mill Road. At the end of the ramp, turn right on Evans Mill Road. At 0.1 mile continue straight through a traffic light on Woodrow Drive (Evans Mill turns right). Continue 0.8 mile on Woodrow Drive to Klondike Road. Turn right and watch for Davidson–Arabia Mountain Nature Preserve, on the right at 1.2 miles, but continue on to the Arabia Mountain parking area, on the left at 2 miles. If this lot is full, use the parking area at the nature preserve.

Arabia Mountain Trail

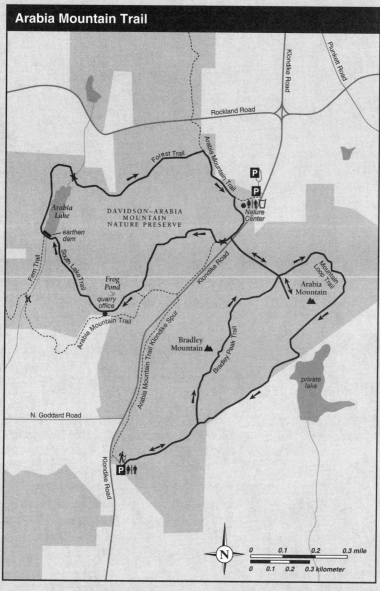

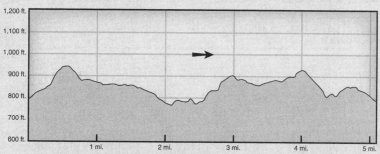

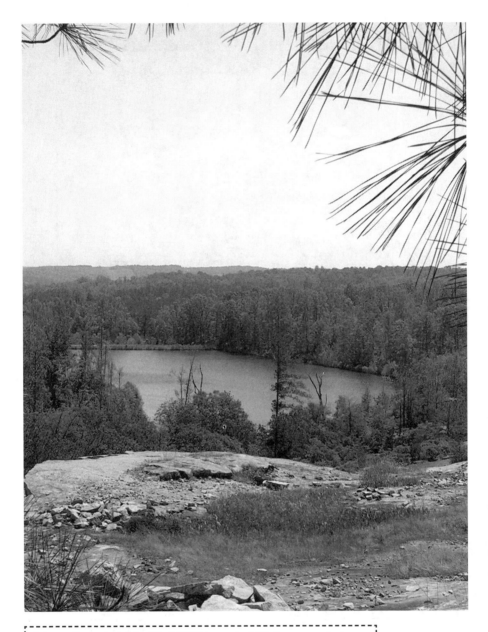

Enhanced by a private lake, this delightful scene is visible from an overlook on the trail to Arabia Mountain.

split rail fence. After traversing a stunted-pine forest, the path curves left, dipping through a low area with more pine trees; then the path begins the easy climb to the top of the first hill, Bradley Mountain. Knee-high cairns guide hikers to the top of the mountain, and not very far into the hike visitors are rewarded with an astounding view of the rolling hills of the Georgia Piedmont. Atop Bradley Mountain, 0.6 mile into the hike, you have a 360-degree view, with Arabia Mountain ahead on the right.

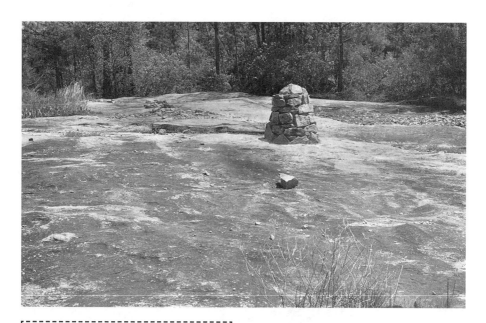

One of numerous rock cairns marking the trail

As you face Arabia Mountain at the top of Bradley Mountain, look down to your left at about 10 o'clock. An unmarked stone path with trees on either side will lead you down to an opening in the trees, where a glass-covered box explains the flora of Arabia Mountain. If you can't find the correct path, don't worry: simply walk to the treeline at the bottom of the mountain and follow it until you come to the opening. When you pass through the opening, turn left at 1 mile on an old roadbed and walk to Klondike Road. After crossing the road, turn left on the asphalt-paved multiuse trail connecting Arabia Mountain to The Mall at Stonecrest in Lithonia. Follow the paved trail across a bridge, and turn right on a wide, sandy road covered with pine leaves that leads to a three-way intersection at 1.2 miles. Turn left and continue on this path until it turns to solid rock; you'll immediately see the first cairn.

As the trail meanders over the rock, watch for areas that have been quarried, as well as for indigenous plant life such as red moss. At 1.4 miles, a large indentation that is normally wet has an interpretive sign about the frogs living there. From here the trail turns left, then right, and comes to a one-story building made of Lithonia gneiss. This is the remains of the old quarry office and weigh station, just over 1.7 miles into the hike. The paved-asphalt trail is directly in front of you—turn right, keeping the stone building to your left, and take the wide, partially shaded, pine leaf–covered road that turns into South Lake Trail. As the trail returns to full sun, the cairns guide you to the top of an unnamed stone knoll. From your vantage point here, look for more cairns to the left as you face north. This is where the trail enters a pine forest adjacent to Arabia Lake.

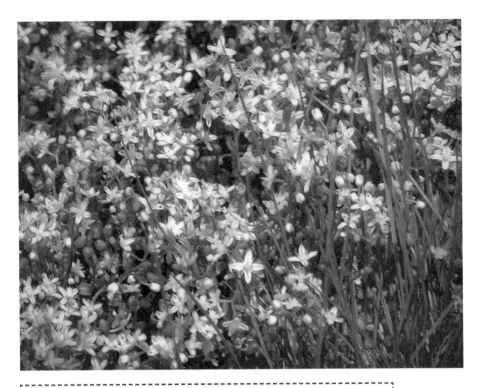

Crevices in Arabia Mountain come to life in the spring when colorful red moss blooms.

Quickly reach the lake at a stone ramp and take a couple of minutes to walk down to the shore. Metallic structures at the far end make for an intriguing photo, especially in the midafternoon sun. Return up the stone path, turning into a small opening on a well-worn trail. A few steps in, the fully shaded forest opens up, with a creek to your right. Up the creek are a rock dam and wall. Just past the wall is the earthen dam that forms the lake. Turn off the roadlike trail, rock-hop across the stream, and look for a large loblolly pine. Behind the tree are a step up to the wall and a path that leads to the top of the earthen dam. After crossing the dam, turn left for additional lakeside views.

Leaving the dam, the path curves right at 2.1 miles, following the shore of Arabia Lake, where it occasionally breaks into full sun. The metallic structures, which appear to be pumps of some kind, come into close range. Passing them on the right, the lake returns to a creek with extensive wetlands. At the north end of the wetlands, the narrow path curves right, crossing the wetlands in two places. This area may be impassable after a heavy rain. After the second muddy area, the path climbs a small knoll to a wooden bridge, still in full shade. At a three-way intersection at 2.5 miles, turn right on the Arabia Mountain Trail and watch for a path on the left with a NATURE CENTER sign and arrow.

Turn right to stay on the Arabia Mountain Trail, a paved multiuse trail, and follow it as it veers right. Turn left at a three-way intersection, crossing Klondike

Road at 3.4 miles. Follow the path until it turns to stone. You're standing between Bradley Mountain and Arabia Mountain. Directly in front of you and off to the right are two quarried ledges. The roads within the complex were used to haul stone back to the office, where it was weighed. Men were paid based on the amount of material quarried and the price of the rock on the open market.

Turn around and return to the four-way intersection; then turn right. The road curves right, and the path returns to full sun as you walk out on the mountain. There are no cairns, but the path is easy to follow—it's about 20–30 feet to the right of the treeline at the bottom of Arabia Mountain. When you approach the treeline, you'll easily spot the path through the trees. A large private lake on the left can be used to judge your location on the map. You'll see cairns as you descend Bradley Mountain; follow them to the trail into the trees, where you join the marked trail. Return along this path to your car.

NEARBY ACTIVITIES

Both **Stone Mountain Park** (see Hike 43, page 204, and Hike 44, page 209) and **Panola Mountain State Park** (see Hike 53, page 254) feature trails that climb to the top of similar rock structures. Site of the 1996 Olympic equestrian events, **Georgia International Horse Park** (1996 Centennial Olympic Pkwy., Conyers; 770-860-4190; **georgiahorsepark.com**) is also the scene of many events and festivals throughout the year.

48 CHARLIE ELLIOTT WILDLIFE CENTER TRAILS

KEY AT-A-GLANCE INFORMATION

LENGTH: 3 miles

CONFIGURATION: Extended loop

DIFFICULTY: Moderate

SCENERY: 3 lakes, each with abundant wildlife; cascades on Murder Creek

EXPOSURE: Areas of full sun, especially during the first mile, then partial sun–full shade

TRAFFIC: Light

TRAIL SURFACE: Rocky dirt; gravel and old roadbed; manicured grass

WHEELCHAIR ACCESS: None

HIKING TIME: 1.7 hours

ACCESS: Trails: daily, year-round, sunrise–sunset; free. Visitor center: Tuesday–Saturday, 9 a.m.–4:30 p.m.; closed state holidays.

MAPS: Available at visitor center, and at a station near the entrance; USGS *Farrar*

MORE INFO: 770-784-3059; georgiawildlife.org/charlieelliott

FACILITIES: Restrooms, picnic tables

SPECIAL COMMENTS: The Visitor Center and Museum offers a variety of activities and programs. The wildlife center features fishing, bird-watching, horseback riding, and primitive camping, among other activities. Dogs must be leashed.

DISTANCE: 41.7 miles from I-20 East/I-285 East

GPS INFORMATION

N33° 27.756' W83° 44.031'

543 Elliott Trail
Mansfield, GA 30055

IN BRIEF

You can see a wide range of wildlife—including wild hogs, otters, beavers, deer, American bald eagles, and waterfowl—on this relatively short hike.

DESCRIPTION

One of two parks under the management of Georgia's Wildlife Resources Division, the Charlie Elliott Wildlife Center is named for a conservationist and educator who developed Georgia's state-park system and the Department of Natural Resources. Inside, a museum tells Elliott's life story along an indoor hiking trail. After Elliott died in 2000 at age 93, his ashes were buried under a white pine that grows near the center.

This well-marked, well-maintained trail system is composed of four trails designated by the colors red (Clubhouse Trail), white (Pigeonhouse Trail), yellow (Murder Creek Trail), and blue (Granite Outcrop Trail). Hunting is prohibited near these footpaths but is

----

Directions

Take I-20 East to Exit 98/Monticello/Mansfield, and turn right on GA 11 South. At 0.8 mile the road crosses US 278 at a four-way stop—continue straight. At 4.3 miles you come to a second four-way stop—again, continue straight. At 9.5 miles turn left at the signed entrance to Charlie Elliott Wildlife Center, on Marben Farm Road. Drive 1.2 miles, turn right on Elliott Trail, and proceed to the visitor center at 0.8 mile. Park and walk toward the front entrance of the green-roofed visitor center. As you approach the museum, a path marked by a brown hiker sign heads right. Follow the path 250 feet to a bulletin board. Look to the left for a red blaze to begin the hike.

Charlie Elliott Wildlife Center Trails

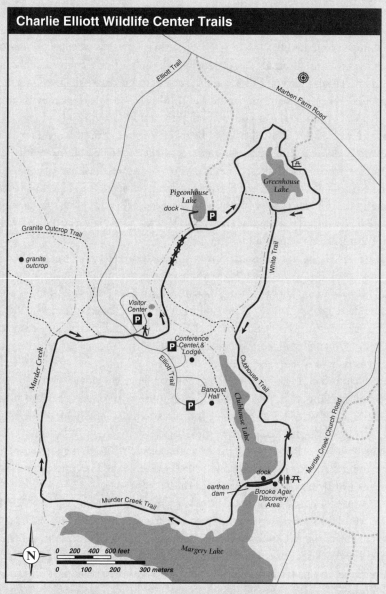

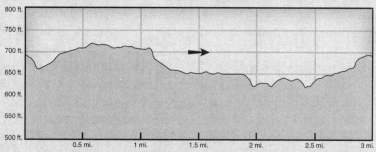

permitted outside the safe zone, so stay on designated trails at all times. The hike begins in a heavily shaded forest and makes an easy, steady climb to the trail's high point almost immediately. Toward the back of the visitor center, a man-made stream flows to a small pond. Passing the pond, the pathway curves left. Notice as you turn and climb that you can always see the next blaze. Near the top of the hill, a steep-sided valley spreads out on the right. In the center of the valley is an island of large granite boulders. On your left, slightly uphill, are more boulders.

At 0.2 mile, after a small bridge, bear left on the white-blazed Pigeonhouse Trail, which begins a long, sweeping curve to the right, leading to both Pigeonhouse and Greenhouse Lakes. The footpath continues a slow, easy-paced rise between two ravines that run after a rain. As the trail nears the ridgetop, you come to a small area for interpretive meetings to the left. Shortly after the benches, an old road leads left. Three wooden walk-overs in quick succession come at 0.3 mile; a fourth bridge comes a bit later.

Less than 50 feet past this last bridge, the trail suddenly emerges onto a manicured grass trail in full sun, with Pigeonhouse Lake to your left. A dock slightly off the trail affords an excellent viewing platform for bird-watchers (fishing is allowed for designated groups only). When approaching the lake during one hike, we flushed a blue heron, which flew off and circled some tall pines on the north side of the lake. Once convinced that we meant no harm, the heron returned, busily looking for fish. You may also see otters and beavers at the preserve's lakes.

Turn around and walk straight ahead as you leave the dock. On the other side of the small parking area, pick up the Pigeonhouse Trail once again and turn left. At 0.6 mile a pathway heads right—continue straight. Shortly after the intersection, the trail dips, and Greenhouse Lake comes into view. When the area was known as Preacher's Rock, this artificial lake was called Boyle Lake Number One. You may hear frequent loud firecracker-like pops of handguns and the rat-a-tat of small-arms fire from a shooting range in the vicinity.

A century oak towers on the left side of the path, which begins to circle the lake. On the lake's north end, you enter the forest; the pathway makes a quick ascent and turns right. Quickly leaving the forest, the trail returns to full sun and manicured grass. After passing under power lines, the Pigeonhouse Trail bears right.

Continue on this trail to a gazebo near the lakeshore. Walk past the gazebo on the lakeshore side, and bear slightly left. Normally the trail is well blazed, but you'll encounter a short stretch where no white blazes are apparent. At the next intersection, bear right as the trail follows the water's edge. At 1.1 miles the pathway returns to shaded forest, and a few steps later you come to a three-way intersection where all the trails bear a white blaze. Take the path that runs by the lakeshore for a few feet to another dock, for another opportunity to see waterfowl. As you leave the dock, turn left, return to the intersection, and then turn right.

Over the next 1.5 miles, the trail is a mostly downhill affair in shaded forest, first following a creek to Clubhouse Lake and then the lakeshore to Margery Lake. Step across a creek at 1.3 miles; the trees are larger here, indicative

Charlie Elliot Wildlife Center encompasses 6,400 acres and a wide range of woodland and lake habitats. More than 200 bird species use these diverse habitats, and the center was designated an Important Bird Area in 2002 by the Atlanta Audubon Society.

of older growth. Look across the small gully ahead and to the right to see a wooden-slat ladder climbing to a hunter's stand. A tenth of a mile later, the white trail ends at the red-blazed Clubhouse Trail. Turn left and continue on the red trail, which quickly curves right. Clubhouse Lake is on your right, shortly after the intersection.

From a distance, the sound of croaking frogs fills the air. Side trails allow fisherfolk access from a low ridge, which the red trail follows. A bridge with stairs on each end marks the hike's halfway point. After the bridge, the trail moves away from the lake along an old roadbed, returning to Clubhouse Lake at the Brooke Ager Discovery Area. In addition to having an educational area, the center has picnic tables, restrooms, a small clubhouse, and a dock. On one visit we spied a large number of crows—technically, a murder of crows—in the area when we hiked this trail, perhaps giving Murder Creek its name. Turn right, walk down a set of stairs, and walk out on the dock.

Returning to the shore, turn right and cross an earthen embankment that impounds Clubhouse Lake. On the dam, the trail becomes the yellow-blazed

Murder Creek Trail. Note the significant difference in the levels of Clubhouse Lake (right) and Margery Lake (left). At the end of the embankment, the trail begins to zigzag, ending with a short climb as it becomes rocky and heavily rooted. The pathway may be loaded with spiderwebs, so duck under and around them when possible, or go with a group and volunteer to bring up the rear. Just shy of 2.5 miles, the trail turns right and begins an easy climb alongside Murder Creek. The cascading creek creates opportunities for photographers who aren't afraid to get their feet wet. At 2.8 miles the Murder Creek Trail reaches a T-intersection with the blue-blazed Granite Outcrop Trail. Turn right on the Granite Outcrop Trail, which begins as a narrow path on a level, grassy plain and then climbs toward the visitor center and the trailhead.

COCHRAN MILL TRAIL 49

IN BRIEF

After crossing Little Bear Creek, the trail follows an old road to Bear Creek, where it climbs along the riverbank to two falls. From the second falls, it rises to an old road and explores the Bear Creek watershed.

DESCRIPTION

Cochran Mill is one of those great hikes full of unexpected bonuses. Owen Henry Cochran inherited his father's land near Bear Creek and for many years ran a water-powered gristmill that his father had built. His brothers expanded the operation around the start of the 20th century. With the coming of electricity to rural Georgia, water power was no longer desirable, and the mill was abandoned. In the 1940s the land was used by the Ku Klux Klan for undisclosed purposes. Unfortunately, both mills were burned, and the dam that created the millrace was partially destroyed by vandals. A 48-foot-wide fieldstone dam built by one of Owen's brothers remains. Fulton County built facilities on the 800-acre site, and in 1985 the private Cochran Mill Nature Center was built beside the public Cochran Mill Park.

From the parking lot, cross Cochran Mill Road and then follow the gravel road as it curves left and begins a moderate descent to Little Bear Creek. A concrete bridge has been sealed off to prevent people from using

KEY AT-A-GLANCE INFORMATION

LENGTH: 3 miles

CONFIGURATION: Loop

DIFFICULTY: Easy

SCENERY: 3 separate falls, large rock outcrops and boulders

EXPOSURE: Full sun until you cross Bear Creek, then mostly shaded

TRAFFIC: Heavy to Bear Creek, moderate to the falls, then light

TRAIL SURFACE: Compacted dirt; portions traverse rock outcrops

WHEELCHAIR ACCESS: None

HIKING TIME: 2 hours

ACCESS: Monday–Saturday, 9 a.m.–3 p.m.; $3 adults, $2 kids ages 3–12, free for kids age 2 and younger and Cochran Mill Nature Center members

MAPS: At the nature center; USGS *Palmetto*

MORE INFO: 770-306-0914; cochranmillnaturecenter.org

FACILITIES: Restrooms at the nature center; picnic tables and restrooms ($20 key deposit) next door at Cochran Mill Park

SPECIAL COMMENTS: Neighboring Cochran Mill Park (770-463-8881; chatthillsga.us/cochranmillpark.aspx) has separate trails for mountain bike enthusiasts and equestrians.

DISTANCE: 14 miles from I-85 South/I-285 Southwest

Directions ⟶

From the I-85/I-285 junction, follow the signs to GA 14 West, which becomes South Fulton Parkway. Drive 12.7 miles to Cochran Mill Road and turn right. Drive 0.5 mile to the parking area on the left. Cochran Mill Nature Center is ahead on the right.

GPS INFORMATION

N33° 34.276' W84° 42.770'

6300 Cochran Mill Rd.
Palmetto, GA 30268

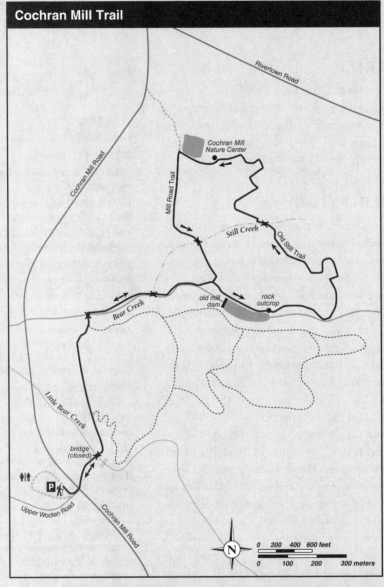

Cochran Mill Trail

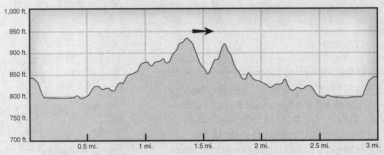

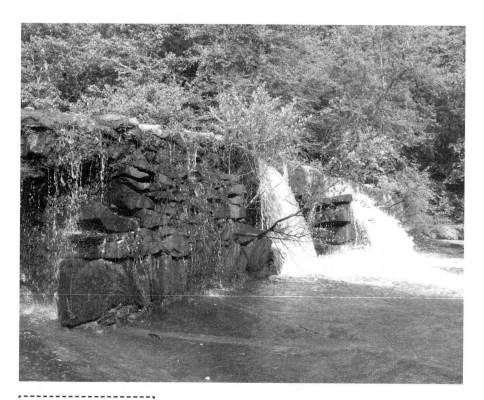

Old Mill Dam at Cochran Mill

it—carefully step down to the creek, on the left side of the bridge. This is one crossing we do barefoot because the creek is deep and wide.

As you cross the creek, watch on the right for the first of three falls. (Don't forget to put your shoes back on after you cross.) At the top of the hill near the bridge, you'll have additional scenic views of the falls. From the bridge, travel straight ahead and down a level gravel road that takes you into a diverse hardwood forest. At 0.3 mile you'll find wild strawberries at the base of a large rock outcrop on the right. When the road forks 0.1 mile ahead, take the path on the right and continue to a second bridge, this one over Bear Creek. A cleverly arranged entrance is designed to be wide enough for a human but too narrow for bikes and horses. After crossing the bridge, turn right and begin to climb in full shade at an easy-to-moderate grade along the bank of Bear Creek.

If you watch closely, you'll see an old yellow blaze every once in a while, but don't worry if you don't see it. Except in a couple of places on rock outcrops, the trail is well worn and easy to follow. One of these outcrops comes quickly, at 0.7 mile into the hike. Keep the river and falls to your right and climb until the trail enters the woods, still near the stream's bank. As you reenter the full shade of the forest, you encounter an area of perma-mud. At 0.8 mile the trail splits; bear right—the other path is the return from the loop. Following the split, the footpath begins to make a significant moderate climb.

Watch for the destroyed dam on the right; water emerges on the left, falls a few feet, and slides back to the right. Not much else remains of Owen Cochran's mill. As you climb the outcrop, you'll see a large stone with a square center cutout. The rock marks the path, which rises to a level road with an embankment on the left. Still following the creek, the trail begins to curve left at 1.2 miles. At the curve, watch for an excellent view of wetlands in the distance.

Climbing into the watershed of Bear Creek on a moderate grade, you'll reach the top of an unnamed knoll. The trail then falls to a small creek, which it crosses on a wooden plank bridge with no railings. After the bridge, the trail bears right and begins to climb the next knoll. Just before the top, the path turns left and then descends to Cochran Mill Nature Center. Entering from the back, you'll pass a large iguana and other animals before coming to the wooden building.

With the pond to your right, walk along a gravel road to a trailhead kiosk, off the road on the left. Follow the path as it descends to a left turn at 2.1 miles. About 0.2 mile later bear right at a three-way intersection, and continue right where the trail crosses a stone outcrop to return you to the middle falls of Bear Creek, on your left. Continue along this trail back to your car.

NEARBY ACTIVITIES

From mid-April to the first week in June, the **Georgia Renaissance Festival** in Fairburn takes visitors back to 16th-century Europe. Performers such as the Tortuga Twins and Friar Finnias Finnegan entertain the masses until it's time for jousting. The festival is held weekends, including Memorial Day, 10:30 a.m.–6 p.m. For more information, call 770-964-8575; buy tickets and view event schedules at **garenfest.com**.

HIGH FALLS TRAIL 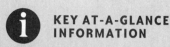 50

IN BRIEF

This trail explores High Falls State Park, including the waterfalls on the Towaliga River and a mill and sluice.

DESCRIPTION

From the overlook, look just right of the modern road to the remains of a gristmill. Built before the Civil War on the Old Alabama Road, the mill had attracted a small community by 1860. Confederate troops burned the mill as Union troops advanced toward it during General William T. Sherman's March to the Sea. Following the Civil War, the mill was rebuilt and the town once again began to grow. In addition to the gristmill there was a post office, cotton mill, factories, and a blacksmith shop. A major east–west connector, the Old Alabama Road gave the settlers the means to transport their goods.

Once known as Unionville, the city was renamed High Falls after the Civil War. Construction on the dam to the right was begun in 1890 by the Towaliga Falls Power Company. (According to local legend, *Towaliga* means "roasted scalp" in Creek, but the most probable translation is "sumac place.") Shortly thereafter, the city found out that the railroad was passing them by. Many residents decided to

KEY AT-A-GLANCE INFORMATION

LENGTH: 1.5 miles

CONFIGURATION: Loop

DIFFICULTY: Moderate

SCENERY: Cascades and waterfalls along the Towaliga River

EXPOSURE: Full sun near the dam, partial sun–full shade elsewhere

TRAFFIC: Heavy on the Falls Trail, light elsewhere

TRAIL SURFACE: Packed dirt

WHEELCHAIR ACCESS: None

HIKING TIME: 1.5 hours

ACCESS: Daily, year-round, 7 a.m.– sunset; $5 state-park fee

MAPS: Handout at kiosk; USGS *High Falls*

MORE INFO: 478-993-3053; gastateparks.org/highfalls

FACILITIES: Swimming area, picnic tables, restrooms

SPECIAL COMMENTS: Close to I-75, this state park has 4.5 miles of hiking trails along with many additional outdoor activities, including boating, geocaching, swimming, fishing, and miniature golf. Be aware that during drought conditions you may not see water spilling over the dam and/or the falls.

DISTANCE: 42 miles from I-75 South/I-285 South

Directions ———→

Take I-75 South to Exit 198/High Falls Road. At the end of the ramp, turn left—there is no traffic light. At 1.7 miles, cross the bridge and turn left on High Falls Pool Drive. After paying the $5 day-use fee at the entrance kiosk, find a parking spot on the left side of the road and walk to the overlook. The hike begins to the right of the kiosk.

GPS INFORMATION

N33° 10.775' W84° 1.090'

High Falls Pool Dr.
Jackson, GA 30233

High Falls Trail

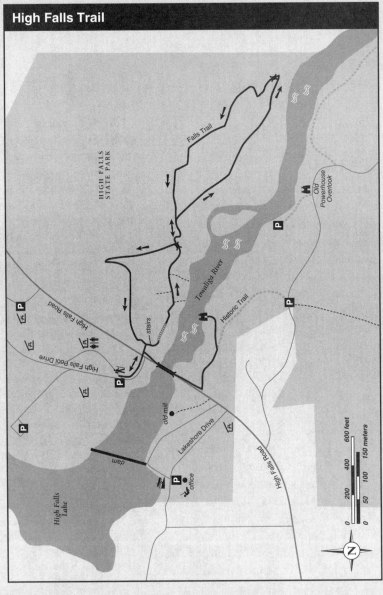

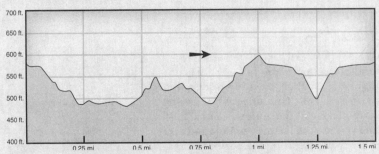

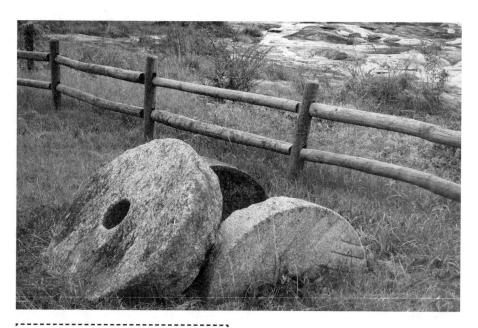

Historical millstones rest casually near the trail.

follow the railroad to Jackson, and work on the dam came to a halt. In 1905 the property was sold to the Georgia Hydro-Electric Company, which finally completed the dam.

In 1902 a steel bridge was completed, spanning the Towaliga River above the falls. The remains of the bridge are still visible. Flooding that followed Hurricane Alberto in 1994 brought so much debris down the river that the supports for a portion of the bridge were destroyed, and the bridge collapsed. From the overlook, follow the road past the kiosk and cross the street, stepping up to a decklike structure on the far side of the road. This is the trailhead for both High Falls Nature Trail and Falls Trail. Walk past the nature trail on the left, down to the signed entrance to Falls Trail on the right. Descend a set of alternating wooden steps and boardwalk until the trail turns left at the end of the boardwalk and runs near the bank of the river. The compacted-soil trail is covered with gravel to help with footing in this moist environment. Finally, at 0.2 mile, the view opens and the Towaliga River becomes a series of cascades and falls on the right, the water playfully darting between and over large boulders in the river. In the center, the 20- to 30-foot drop is the falls' largest.

The red-blazed trail parallels the river but does not run adjacent to it at all times. Trails to the right provide access for fishing or for better views of the falls; trails to the left allow hikers to explore the river's small floodplain. The mixed second-growth Piedmont forest is composed of American beeches, shortleaf pines, and hemlocks. At just under 0.3 mile the trail approaches a confusing intersection at a bridge, where you turn right and cross the bridge; then turn

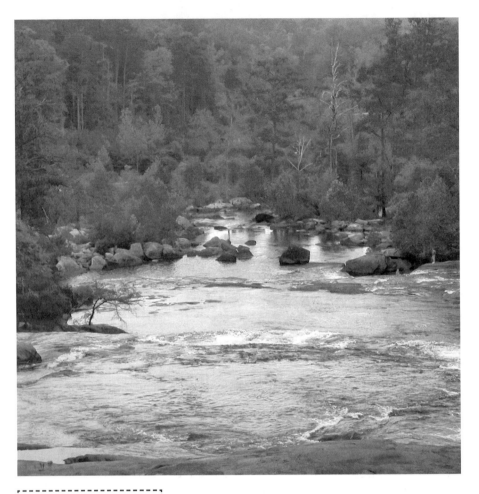

The enchanting Towaliga River

right again. Ignore the red blazes straight ahead at the bridge—these are for the return trail, which also uses this bridge.

Running some 20 feet above the river, the trail now offers occasional long-distance scenic views, especially in winter and early spring. Boulders are scattered about here, with some impressive rock outcrops that combine to create something of a maze, which the kids should love. Watch for the blazes, and follow the well-worn trail where there are none. Don't get discouraged by the lack of blazes; one time we were about to turn around when a red blaze suddenly appeared high on a tree.

As the path climbs away from the river, a switchback eases the rise. Near the top of the hill, turn right where the trail reaches a three-way intersection. Now the trail begins to undulate, becomes rockier, and follows the curves of the hills as it runs some 60 feet above the Towaliga River. A boulder-strewn tributary at 0.5 mile makes for a good photo opportunity. The trail soon makes a hard left. A few feet ahead, a wooden bridge spans another scenic creek. After crossing the bridge, the trail turns right and begins a rapid ascent, curving back around to the left. The wooden bridge is now down a steep embankment on your left as the trail slowly comes around to the right. Crossing the outgoing trail, the path comes to the confusing bridge, and the markings are now easy to understand. Cross the bridge and turn right, following the path as it climbs a ridge.

A few feet past a double blaze, the footpath makes a hard left and joins High Falls Nature Trail. According to the High Falls map, the blaze on the nature trail is white, but it seems to have a yellowish tint; there are red blazes as well. On returning to the deck, turn right and then left to cross the bridge. Turn left at the HISTORIC TRAIL sign. Almost immediately on the right is a sluice that powered an electric plant farther down the river. This plant supplied power to area businesses from 1905 until 1958. Georgia Power transferred the plant and some adjoining land to the Hiawassee Timber Company, which gave it to the state of Georgia in 1966.

On the left, 1.2 miles into the hike, a trail departs at a 45-degree angle. Follow this down to an overlook that affords an excellent view of High Falls. Retrace your route to the parking area.

NEARBY ACTIVITIES

Fresh Air Bar-B-Que (1164 GA 42 South, Jackson; 770-775-3182; **freshairbarbecue .com**) has been serving Georgia-style 'cue since 1929 and has been honored as the best in the state.

Other attractions nearby include the following: **Indian Springs State Park** (770-504-2277; **gastateparks.org/indiansprings**; $5 state-park fee), with a 3.25-mile multiuse trail that links to **Dauset Trails Nature Center** (770-775-6798; **dausettrails.com**; free); **Jarrell Plantation State Historic Site** (open Thursday–Saturday only; 478-986-5172; **gastateparks.org/jarrellplantation**; $4–$6.50); **Chattahoochee-Oconee National Forest** (770-297-3000; **fs.usda.gov/main/conf**); and **Piedmont National Wildlife Refuge** (478-986-5441; **fws.gov/piedmont**), with 7 miles of walking trails.

51 McINTOSH RESERVE TRAIL

KEY AT-A-GLANCE INFORMATION

LENGTH: 5.2 miles

CONFIGURATION: Loop

DIFFICULTY: Moderate

SCENERY: River views, extensive forested wetlands, beaver pond, historic building

EXPOSURE: Full sun in the Chattahoochee floodplain, mostly shaded as the trail climbs into the watershed

TRAFFIC: Light; multiuse trails allow horses.

TRAIL SURFACE: Compacted dirt, some gravel roads

WHEELCHAIR ACCESS: None

HIKING TIME: 2.5 hours

ACCESS: Daily, year-round, 8 a.m.–sunset; closed January 1, Thanksgiving, and December 25; $3 day-use fee for non–Carroll County residents

MAPS: Available at park office; USGS *Whitesburg*

MORE INFO: 770-830-5879; tinyurl.com/mcintoshreservepark

FACILITIES: Restrooms, picnic tables, playground

SPECIAL COMMENTS: On the road to the trailhead are the homestead and grave of chief William McIntosh. The original homestead was burned by Red Sticks on the night they murdered McIntosh.

DISTANCE: 39.2 miles from I-85 South/I-285 Southwest

GPS INFORMATION

N33° 26.535' W84° 57.153'

1046 W. McIntosh Cir.
Whitesburg, GA 30185

IN BRIEF

The trail explores the banks of the Chattahoochee River, then turns inland and climbs to check out the adjacent watershed.

DESCRIPTION

Creek chief William McIntosh was the son of Captain William McIntosh of the Georgia militia and a Creek woman. When the United States declared war in 1813 on a breakaway band of Creek Indians known as the Red Sticks, McIntosh joined Andrew Jackson and led Creek warriors against this violent faction. But in spite of McIntosh's service, Jackson demanded millions of acres of land from the larger Creek Confederacy.

McIntosh's cousin, George Troup, advanced a political platform that espoused removal of the Creeks during his successful bid for governor of Georgia in 1823. In 1825 McIntosh signed the Treaty of Indian Springs, which relinquished control of much of the remaining Creek land in Georgia; as a reward for his cooperation, McIntosh received a

----

Directions

Take I-85 South to Exit 47/GA 34 (Newnan/Shenandoah). At the end of the ramp, turn right on Bullsboro Drive/GA 34. Drive 1 mile and, at the KFC, turn right on Millard Farmer Industrial Boulevard/GA 34 Bypass. At 4 miles turn right on GA 16 North/US 27 Alternate. At 8.4 miles turn left at the Citgo station on GA 5 North in downtown Whitesburg. Drive 2.3 miles and turn left on Burnett Road/West McIntosh Circle at the sign for McIntosh Reserve. At 1.6 miles register at the ranger station and pay the $3 day-use fee. The road passes the McIntosh homestead, which is also the site of the Creek chief's grave. A parking lot is on the left, at the end of the road.

McIntosh Reserve Trail

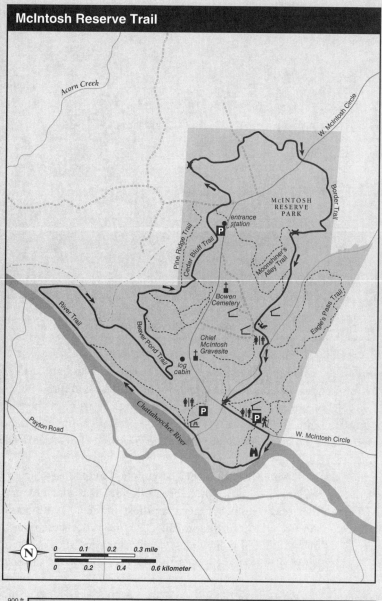

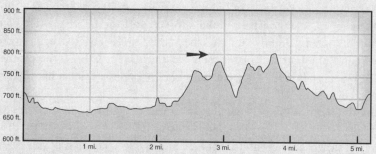

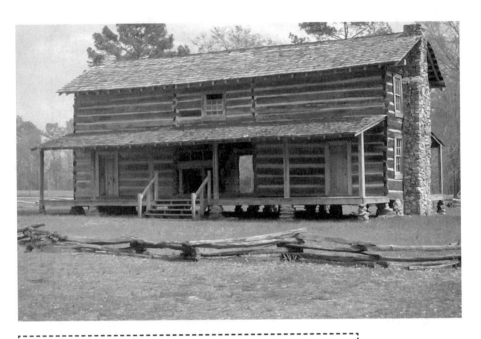

This 1840s-style log cabin is similar to the one that William McIntosh lived in.

plantation on the Chattahoochee River. When the Creeks heard about this, a supporter of the Red Sticks led a raid in which McIntosh was murdered.

Beginning as a gravel roadbed to the right of the restrooms, the trail turns right at a brown gate and falls quickly to a 90-degree turn in the Chattahoochee River. Here, you'll enjoy an excellent view of the river as it flows south. The footpath turns right and follows the river past an overlook in the picnic area atop a rock bluff. The fast-flowing Chattahoochee has ample floodplains, which this hike explores during the first 1.3 miles. These broad floodplains, which extend up to 0.5 mile wide in the area, are much larger than those in the Chattahoochee River National Recreation Area parks farther north. Their size reflects the river's growing power as it flows south. For many miles, small tributaries, such as the one you cross on a bridge at 0.4 mile, have joined the river as it flows to the southwest corner of Georgia.

A series of rock outcrops at 0.6 mile extends into the riverbed as a shoal. Just past the outcrop, a sign instructs hikers to keep off the riverbank just before the footpath juts inland slightly. Stately oaks, elms, and beeches struggle to stabilize the riverbank in an area of picnic tables and grills. At 0.9 mile the picnic area is replaced by an open field designed for a variety of sports, including flying radio-controlled airplanes.

Continuing in full sun, the footpath turns left at 1.6 miles and follows the shore of an extensive forested wetland—identified as a beaver pond on the map— as it curves slowly to the right. Coming off to the left, a side trail briefly explores the low pond. The footpath makes a U-turn at the end of the pond as it continues to follow the edge; then it quickly makes a second U-turn before it begins to climb into the watershed of the Chattahoochee River. The trail turns left at a cut in the rocks and descends to an old railroad bed, which it leaves at 2.4 miles to enter a forest of oaks, beeches, and pines.

McIntosh Reserve Trail now begins a steady climb as it sweeps right around a tall knoll. At 2.7 miles the trail splits. Take the trail that bears left; it comes to a boundary marker that runs along a dirt road marking the edge of the park. The trail soon turns right, back into the park. When you come to a yellow-blazed trail, turn left. Note the trees on the right with embedded barbwire.

Crossing a bridge over a stream at 3.5 miles, the trail climbs to an old road-bed, which it follows to a DETOUR sign before leading to a trail that climbs into the woods. After crossing a gravel road, the trail levels and then begins a moderate climb to its high point at 3.8 miles, where it crosses the paved road into the park. From this point the trail falls at an easy-to-moderate grade, reaching a wet-footed stream crossing at 4.1 miles; then it turns right and climbs a hill as the trail curves left. Less than 0.1 mile later, a trail branches off to the right—continue straight. Numerous wooden platforms in the area indicate that this was once a developed campsite. A second trail, to the right at 4.4 miles, leads to a trash dump.

From this point the trail enters full sun in an open field. As you enter an area with a playground and restrooms, watch the bushes on the left side of the field for an opening that leads to a wide stream crossing. Take a few steps to the right, where the river is easier to cross. After crossing, turn right and follow the trail as it winds through the floodplain. Occasionally the trail splits, almost always to avoid a wet area. At 5 miles the trail crosses the stream on a wooden bridge before turning left on the paved park road.

NEARBY ACTIVITIES

The **Coweta County Courthouse** in downtown Newnan, which also houses the Coweta County Visitors Center, was built in 1904 (200 Court Square; 770-254-2627; **explorecoweta.com/attractions2.htm**). The tower reaches 100 feet and dominates the county seat, which is also country-music star Alan Jackson's hometown. Newnan also sports Georgia's newest state park, **Chattahoochee Bend,** with 6 miles of hiking trails (770-254-7271; **gastateparks.org/chattahoocheebend**).

52 OCMULGEE RIVER TRAIL

KEY AT-A-GLANCE INFORMATION

LENGTH: 5.2 miles round-trip

CONFIGURATION: Out-and-back

DIFFICULTY: Easy

SCENERY: View of the Ocmulgee River and its floodplain

EXPOSURE: Some sun

TRAFFIC: Light; horseback riding allowed

TRAIL SURFACE: Packed dirt

WHEELCHAIR ACCESS: None

HIKING TIME: 2 hours

ACCESS: Daily, year-round, sunrise–sunset; $5 use fee

MAPS: USGS *Berner*

MORE INFO: 706 485-7110; tinyurl.com/ocmulgee

FACILITIES: None

SPECIAL COMMENTS: The footpath continues to the Ocmulgee River bluffs, about 16 miles from the trailhead.

DISTANCE: 63.1 miles from I-75 South/I-285 South

GPS INFORMATION

N33° 9.926' W83° 48.936'

IN BRIEF

The trail parallels the Ocmulgee River along its floodplain, occasionally moving inland to circumvent a tributary or marshy area.

DESCRIPTION

Ocmulgee, meaning "bubbling (or boiling) water," is the name given to this strong, wide river by the Hitchiti tribe. Early British explorers knew it as Ocheese Creek and referred to the native people living along the river (near present-day Macon) as the Creek Indians. The Hitchiti were one nation within the Creek Confederacy. It is believed, but cannot be proven, that the Creek were the descendants of Mound Builders who built cities near the confluence of two or more rivers throughout Georgia. Ocmulgee, Etowah, and Kolomoki mounds are all examples of the work of America's first tribal civilization in Georgia.

On one visit, as we pulled into the Oconee National Forest parking area, a family of wild turkeys hurried away from the rear of the parking area, so watch for wildlife throughout the hike. Ocmulgee River Trail begins by rising through the forest and quickly beginning an easy, even descent toward the river on a wide,

----

Directions ———————————→

Take I-75 South from Atlanta to Exit 187/GA 83 (Forsyth/Monticello). Turn left on GA 83, known locally as North Lee Street and Cabaniss Road, and drive a total of 11.9 miles, noting the following: the highway crosses US 23 and descends to the Ocmulgee River. After you cross the river on a double bridge, the road begins to rise. Watch on the left for an unmarked pull-off area big enough for five or six cars. The trailhead is on the river side of the parking area, near the highway atop a small mound.

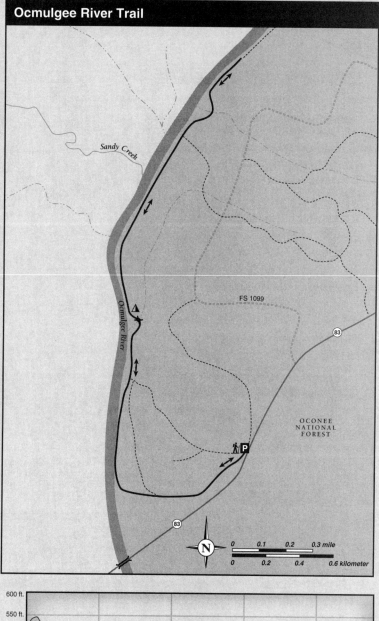

Ocmulgee River Trail

Sandy Creek

Ocmulgee River

FS 1099

83

OCONEE
NATIONAL
FOREST

83

N

| 0 | 0.1 | 0.2 | 0.3 mile |

| 0 | 0.2 | 0.4 | 0.6 kilometer |

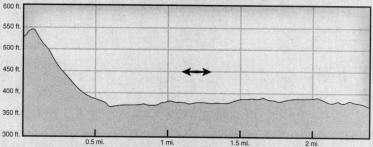

600 ft.
550 ft.
500 ft.
450 ft.
400 ft.
350 ft.
300 ft.

0.5 mi.   1 mi.   1.5 mi.   2 mi.

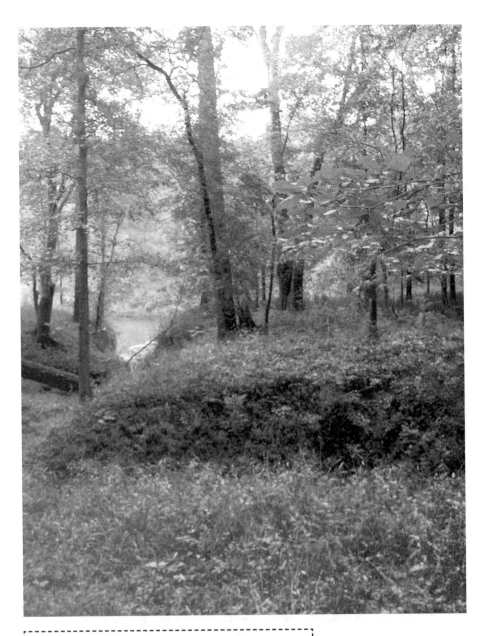

A lush green carpet enshrouds this bank on the Ocmulgee River.

roadlike path. Throughout most of the hike, the trail is wide, narrowing occasionally to cross a stream or swampy area, making this a good family hike. After dropping 200 feet in 0.6 mile, the trail reaches the Ocmulgee River and gently curves right to parallel the wide, fast-flowing watercourse. Throughout the hike, the Ocmulgee will be to your left on the way out and to your right on the way back.

Car noise quickly disappears as you walk away from GA 83 along the riverbank. From here on, watch carefully for poison ivy.

You'll get occasional long-distance views from the trail, and oaks and elms line the path. Many of the elms are large and deeply furrowed, with ashen-gray bark, indicating that they're fairly old. These elm trees, along with substantial oaks, anchor the healthy riparian zones on either side of the river. The US Forest Service, which manages the area, permits horseback riding on the trail. You may notice evidence of horses and spot a number of fairly common birds and wildlife, including wood ducks, vireos, squirrels, deer, and raccoons. Because the river flows along a migration path, large numbers of waterfowl can be spotted during the spring and fall.

As the trail comes to the first tributary of the Ocmulgee, it bears right (inland), making a wet-footed crossing of a stream at just under 1 mile. The trail climbs away from the river again at 1.2 miles, crossing a wooden bridge without rails, and climbs again to a primitive-camping area, at 1.3 miles. You can walk through the campground to a small US Forest Service parking area or simply make a hard left where the campsites start. On the trail's return to the Ocmulgee, the river traverses a swampy area before climbing to the riverbank 0.1 mile later. From here the trail follows the bank closely, dropping only occasionally into the lightly forested floodplain. At 2.6 miles the trail turns inland to cross another stream. Turn around to head back to your car.

NEARBY ACTIVITIES

The Ocmulgee River flows south to Macon, where it passes through **Ocmulgee National Monument,** an early Mississippian Mound Builder site that flourished between 900 and 1150 AD (478-752-8257; **nps.gov/ocmu**; free). On the park grounds are a museum and several large mounds that are fun to climb. To get there, return to I-75 South, take Exit 165, and follow the signs to I-16. Take Exit 2 and turn left on Coliseum Drive. In 0.6 mile turn right on Emery Highway and drive 0.8 mile. The entrance is on the right.

For more hiking, the **Ocmulgee Heritage Trail,** on 1,413 acres in Macon (478-722-9909, ext. 107; **ocmulgeeheritagetrail.com**), has 9 miles of completed trail and a projected finished length of 22 miles.

53 PANOLA MOUNTAIN TRAIL

KEY AT-A-GLANCE INFORMATION

LENGTH: 1.75 miles

CONFIGURATION: Double loop

DIFFICULTY: Easy

SCENERY: Long-distance views from rock outcrop

EXPOSURE: Much of the trail lies in full sun.

TRAFFIC: Moderate, especially on weekends

TRAIL SURFACE: Mostly dirt, some stone

WHEELCHAIR ACCESS: None

HIKING TIME: 1.5 hours

ACCESS: Daily, year-round, 7 a.m.– sunset; $5 state-park fee

MAPS: Interpretive maps at trailhead kiosk; USGS *Redan, Stockbridge*

MORE INFO: 770-389-7801; gastateparks.org/panolamountain

FACILITIES: Natural-history exhibits; interpretive trails; restrooms

SPECIAL COMMENTS: Panola Mountain Nature Center is open daily, 8:30 a.m.–5 p.m., except Wednesdays. The park also has a 1-mile Fitness Trail. For those who enjoy bicycling and jogging, there is access to the paved 12-mile Rockdale County–South River– Arabia Mountain PATH Trail.

DISTANCE: 8 miles from I-20 East/I-285 East

GPS INFORMATION

N33° 37.494' W84° 10.263'

2600 GA 155
Stockbridge, GA 30281

IN BRIEF

Two interpretive loop trails take hikers through two very different environments. The first trail drops to a creek that is occasionally dry, while the second climbs one of Panola Mountain's many outcrops.

DESCRIPTION

Georgia's first state conservation park, Panola Mountain was established in 1971. Perched on a massive granite rock outcrop, its purpose is to protect the environmentally sensitive areas, both biologic and geologic, on this 100-acre monadnock, or rock hill, that stands isolated in an otherwise-level area. The trails within the park are individual loops, and the only developed side trails take visitors to interpretive areas. Elevation change on the trails is minimal—less than 150 feet—with the greatest part of that on the Watershed Trail.

Exiting the nature center, continue to a large trailhead sign and turn right. After passing through a fire area, the Watershed Trail descends gently to a fertile Piedmont lowlands filled with hickory, oak, and sumac trees. The trail is wide and strewn with wood chips, but the surface changes to dirt as the path drops at an easy grade to a three-way intersection. Continue straight, as directed in the nature-center pamphlet, to reach a creek. Watch for

Directions

Take I-20 East to Exit 68/Wesley Chapel Road. Turn right and, at 0.3 mile, turn left at the light onto Snapfinger Road/GA 155. The entrance to the park is 7 miles ahead, on the left. Continue to the end of the road, enter the nature center, and pick up two pamphlets, one for Watershed Trail and another for Rock Outcrop Trail.

Panola Mountain Trail

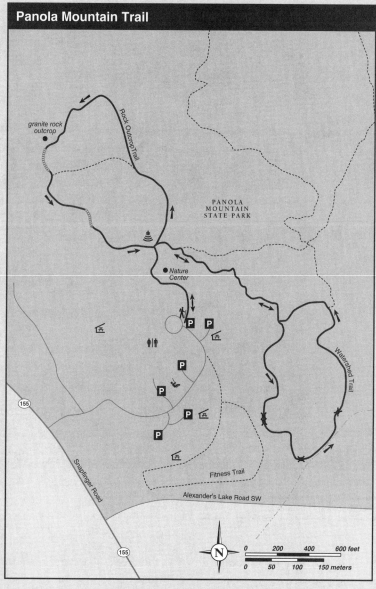

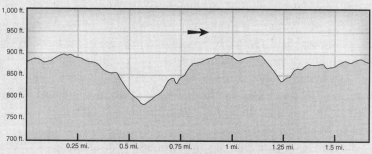

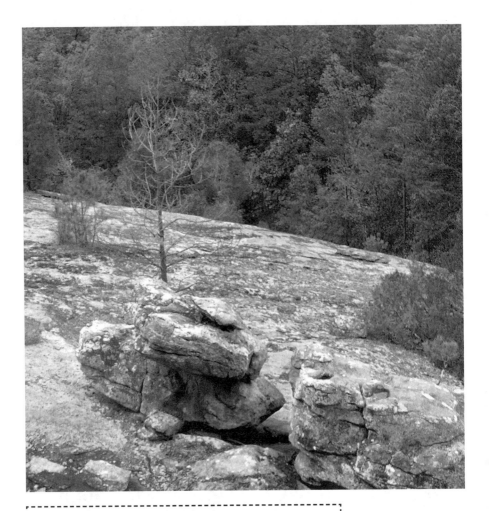

Lichens paint fantastic colors as they slowly do their work of making soil on the rocks at Panola Mountain.

streams that carry watershed runoff down to the creek, shaping the landscape as they go—the path crosses two of these on bridges. The first interpretive station leaves the trail to take hikers to a small gully created by erosion.

Stations 2 and 3 continue the hydrology lesson, but station 4 takes hikers out to a flat "pavement rock" formed by an exfoliation process, enhanced by the creek water. In addition, the interpretive stations introduce hikers to lichen, a plant that grows on exposed granite to create an environment where some plants, especially red moss, may follow. Cross another bridge and begin climbing back into the watershed of the stream. When the loop comes to a T-intersection at 0.8 mile, turn right to return to the trailhead.

At the trailhead, turn right again to follow Rock Outcrop Trail. This trail traverses a vastly different environment from that along the Watershed Trail, circling a low hill with surprising drop-offs to the right and a thicker forest to the left. The tree mix has also changed, with loblolly pine, sweet gum, black cherry, and hawthorn trees accenting white oaks on this yellow-blazed trail. The trail begins to descend when you see the first of several massive granite outcrops at 1.2 miles. Less than 0.1 mile later, this hike passes rock cairns; a single pole rail keeps visitors on the proper path. Please be mindful of the sensitive environment and stay on the trail. If you'd like to spend time on similar slabs, try the Arabia Mountain Trail (page 226), the Stone Mountain Loop (page 204), or the Stone Mountain Walk Up Trail (page 209). A small portion of this trail does traverse the granite.

After viewing the outcrops, continue to two boardwalks—one to the right, the other to the left—that take you to more trail interpretation. A small outdoor theater is on the left before you reach the trailhead kiosk.

If you decide to make the ranger-led trek to Panola Mountain, be certain to wear comfortable hiking shoes. The loop travels 3.5 miles to the largest exposed granite slab in the park and back again, and you'll stop frequently to discuss various topics.

NEARBY ACTIVITIES

Occupied mostly by baseball fields, **Heritage Park** (101 Lake Dow Rd., McDonough; 770-288-7300; **tinyurl.com/heritageparkga**) has not only a 0.9-mile multiuse path but also a heritage area that's worth the drive. A barn-shaped museum stands at the entrance to the village, which contains many historic buildings, a 1934 Old #7 steam locomotive, a covered bridge, and the Veterans Wall of Honor, dedicated in 2008. The park is open Monday–Friday, 8 a.m.–5 p.m.; the museum (free admission) is open Monday, Wednesday, and Friday, 10 a.m.–3 p.m., whenever county offices are also open. To get here, leave Panola Mountain and turn left on GA 155 South. After 13 miles, turn left on John Frank Ward Boulevard. Drive 0.33 mile and turn right on Lemon Street. At the next intersection, turn left on Keys Ferry Street/GA 81. Drive 1 mile and turn left on Lake Dow Road to enter the park, on your left.

54 PEACHTREE CITY CART PATH

KEY AT-A-GLANCE INFORMATION

LENGTH: 9.9 miles

CONFIGURATION: Loop

DIFFICULTY: Moderate

SCENERY: Lakeside views, forested wetlands, mansions

EXPOSURE: Mostly full sun, except near Flat Creek Nature Center

TRAFFIC: Heavy; multiuse trail includes access to electric golf carts

TRAIL SURFACE: Asphalt, some wood and compacted soil

WHEELCHAIR ACCESS: Yes

HIKING TIME: 5.5 hours

ACCESS: Daily, year-round, sunrise–sunset; free

MAPS: Available at Peachtree City Holiday Inn and many other area businesses; USGS *Tyrone*

MORE INFO: 770-487-7657; peachtree-city.org

FACILITIES: Restrooms in parks, including at Lake Kedron trailhead; picnic tables, some with grills; playgrounds along the hike

SPECIAL COMMENTS: Peachtree City is famous for its 90-mile network of multiuse paths for pedestrians, cyclists, and electric golf carts. Kids age 12 and older are permitted to drive carts in Peachtree City (visit the website above for details). The hike's strategically located parks with playgrounds are great for little ones.

DISTANCE: 18.2 miles from I-85 South/I-285 Southwest

GPS INFORMATION

N33° 25.385' W84° 34.161'

IN BRIEF

This hike explores Flat Creek, which creates Lake Peachtree, and a forested wetlands south of the dam. On the return trip, you visit city hall and cross GA 54 on an impressive pedestrian overpass.

DESCRIPTION

Embroiled in battles over integration, hardly anybody in Atlanta in the 1950s seemed to notice when bulldozers began sculpting a little corner of land 25 miles south of the city in rural Fayette County. The Phipps family (for whom Atlanta's Phipps Plaza shopping center is named) and its New York–based investment company, Bessemer Properties, purchased thousands of acres of farmland and began building streets, houses, and golf courses in a development called Peachtree City. The cart path was a logical extension of the concept and today affords visitors and residents almost 90 miles of multiuse paths.

Lake Kedron, where the hike begins, is a 235-acre reservoir owned by the Fayette County water system. The large public parking area connects to the Peachtree City cart path at the south end of the park, across Interlochen Drive. Initially climbing through a majority-pine (mostly loblolly) forest, commonly found south of Atlanta, the cart path

---

Directions

Take I-85 South to Exit 61/Senoia Road/GA 74 (Fairburn). At the end of the ramp, turn left on GA 74. Drive 7.4 miles to Peachtree Parkway and turn left at the light. Drive 1.8 miles to Fayette County's Lake Kedron Park and Reservoir, on your right. Enter the parking lot and continue to the far end.

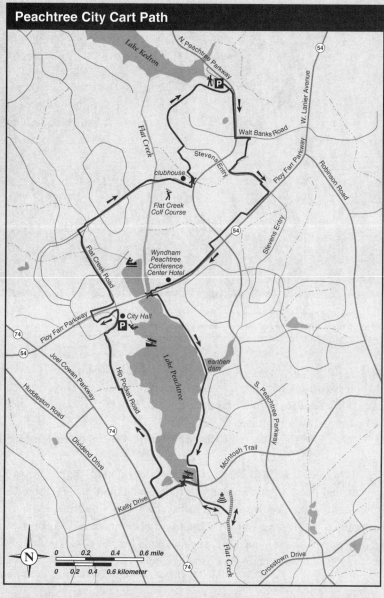

Peachtree City Cart Path

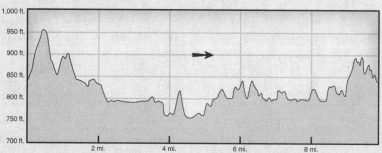

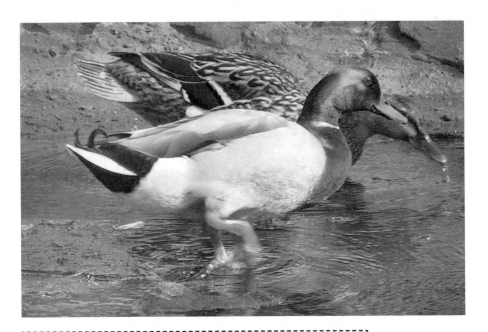

A pair of mallards dabble on underwater plants in a quiet stream along the trail.

parallels Peachtree Parkway as it climbs to Walt Banks Road, which it crosses at 0.4 mile before turning left. After crossing Peachtree Parkway, the cart path parallels Walt Banks Road to a four-way intersection, where it turns right before an unsigned road and begins an easy climb.

At 0.8 mile into the hike, the path turns right, crosses this unsigned road, and then turns left, running next to Stevens Entry road as it levels off. At GA 54, also known as Floy Farr Parkway, the cart path makes a hard right. Farr, a Tyrone banker, provided much of the funding for the development of Peachtree City, and he and his family were deeply involved in Fayette County politics.

Dropping to a three-way intersection, the trail comes to a T—turn right where a tunnel leads left. This path quickly curves left and abruptly comes out at a McDonald's, on the left. On the right is Peachtree Pointe Shopping Center. Walk to North Peachtree Parkway, cross the road, and continue straight, past a day-care center and a church. At the far end of the church parking lot, rejoin the cart path, turning left at 1.7 miles as you step onto the path, which almost immediately curves right.

Honeysuckle and Virginia creeper fill a white oak–loblolly pine forest as the trail drops into a vale adjacent to but beneath GA 54. Coming into full sun, the path drops into a gully formed by the road's embankment and a parking lot, before crossing the entrance to the Wyndham Peachtree Conference Center Hotel. After the hotel, the path drops and then quickly curves left before joining what appears to be a wide creek as it passes under Floy Farr Parkway. At 2.3 miles the path curves left again as Lake Peachtree suddenly opens before you in a scenic long-distance view down the lake. Continue a few feet to a four-way intersection—turn left. The cart path rises and curves left to a bridge for a better view of the lake. Return to the four-way intersection and go straight as the path follows the lakeshore, with upscale homes on the left. Asphalt paths to the left allow access to the lake from nearby roads.

The cart path jogs right and then left, at 2.8 miles. After the jog, you come to a fishing dock on the right, and the path crosses between two lakes on an earthen dam before reaching Battery Way Boat Ramp. At 3.2 miles the path curves right, continuing along the lakeshore as a couple of paths join from the left. The path turns right at a split rail fence and climbs away from the lake in an area with homes on either side. At 3.8 miles the cart path crosses a paved road, McIntosh Trail. Disregard a sign pointing left to the nature center, and continue along the cart path to a wooden boardwalk at 4.1 miles. Turn left at the boardwalk to cross a forested wetland, with a more diverse forest of sweet gum, black gum, water oak, and pignut hickory trees joining the standard hardwood mix.

Where the boardwalk ends, a compacted-soil trail explores a knoll with a garden of native plants. In this area are an amphitheater, city administration buildings, and a BMX track. Return to the cart path, cross it, and continue to the boardwalk on the other side. This section of the boardwalk explores the creek, curving south and running along the bank. Return to the cart path, turn left, cross McIntosh Trail, and then turn left again. At the bridge, Flat Creek flows out of Lake Peachtree as a spillway.

Follow the markings as the cart path crosses McIntosh Trail, continues a few yards, and crosses McIntosh again at 5.4 miles, this time at Hip Pocket Road. Over the next 1.3 miles, the trail closely follows this suburban road, occasionally sharing a well-marked track with vehicular traffic. At 6.5 miles Pebblepocket Park offers swings, slides, and other equipment, including a rock-climbing wall and picnic tables. Make the next right at Willow Bend, and on the right you'll see Memorial Park, dedicated to a local resident who was 17 when she died. Just beyond the park is a second playground; then the cart path enters a parking lot. Look on the far side for a bridge—cross it and turn left and then right; the cart path is directly in front of you. At City Hall the path turns right, along Floy Farr Parkway. A fountain at 6.8 miles makes a good rest stop.

Retrace your steps to Willow Bend, cross, and continue past a church on the left and an open space known as the Village Green on the right. Watch for the crossover bridge on the right, and head for it when the path reaches an intersection. After crossing, turn right at the four-way intersection. This path follows Floy Farr Parkway and then curves left, following Flat Creek Road until it crosses two streets in quick succession. At the T-intersection, turn right. The trail drops to Flat Creek, which has been developed into a golf course. As the path rises, watch for the impressive clubhouse on the left, across the street. After the golf course, the path turns left at a four-way intersection.

Entering full shade, the path comes to a bridge at 8.8 miles, across Flat Creek. On the right are some lovely cascades and falls as the creek comes out of

Lake Kedron. Turn around and take any of the first three paths to the left to return to Interlochen Drive. Turn left and follow the road around to Lake Kedron Park.

NEARBY ACTIVITIES

Farther south on GA 54 is tiny **Moreland, Georgia,** boyhood home of humorist Lewis Grizzard (*Elvis Is Dead and I Don't Feel So Good Myself*) and birthplace of Southern Gothic writer Erskine Caldwell (*God's Little Acre* and *Tobacco Road*). Typewriters, family photos, mementos, and manuscripts belonging to Grizzard are on display at the **Moreland Media Center,** inside the Moreland Hometown Heritage Museum on Moreland Square. Nearby on the square, at the corner of Main and Railroad Streets, is the **Erskine Caldwell Birthplace and Museum.** Hours for both museums are Thursday–Saturday, 10 a.m.–3 p.m.; admission for both is $15 adults, $12 seniors and military, $7.50 kids ages 6–17, and free for kids age 5 and younger. **God's Little Acre,** a community garden, is scheduled to open a living-farm-history exhibit in the spring of 2013. For more information, call 770-897-1890 or visit **morelandadventure.com.**

PIEDMONT NATIONAL
WILDLIFE REFUGE TRAILS

IN BRIEF

This hike combines the Red-Cockaded Wood-pecker and Allison Lake Trails to take you through a wilderness rich with wildlife.

DESCRIPTION

Our introduction to Piedmont National Wild-life Refuge was certainly thrilling. A black vul-ture with a wingspan as wide as the road led us to the trailhead, finally rising above the treeline and turning away from Allison Lake as we parked. Ringed in fieldstone, with a dark-brown roof, the trailhead kiosk contains extensive information on the creation and goals of Pied-mont NWR and the National Wildlife Refuge program in general. You'll also find information on the preservation of species native to the park, including the endangered red-cockaded woodpecker.

In 1939 President Franklin D. Roosevelt created Piedmont NWR by executive order. The land was substantially different from the way it now appears. Cleared and planted by settlers who grew cotton as their cash crop, the land was mostly abandoned by 1939

- -

Directions —————————————————▶

Take I-75 South to Exit 186/Juliette Road/Tift College Drive. Turn left on Juliette Road, at the end of the ramp. After crossing a bridge and passing through East Juliette, the road becomes Juliette–Round Oak Road. At 11.8 miles bear left at the PIEDMONT NATIONAL WILDLIFE REFUGE sign (the road to the right goes to Jarrell Plantation). In 5.3 miles turn left on a paved road, which is designated as GA 262 on maps but not on the road. After 0.8 mile, the road to the visitor center bears right and the road to the left continues to the trailhead, at 1.3 miles.

KEY AT-A-GLANCE INFORMATION

LENGTH: 3.8 miles

CONFIGURATION: Double loop

DIFFICULTY: Easy

SCENERY: Lakeside and creekside views, forested wetlands

EXPOSURE: Full sun in the vicinity of Allison Lake and the dam; mostly sunny on Red-Cockaded Woodpecker Trail; mostly shaded on Allison Lake Trail, except near the lakeshore

TRAFFIC: Light

TRAIL SURFACE: Compacted soil, gravel

WHEELCHAIR ACCESS: None

HIKING TIME: 2 hours

ACCESS: Daily, year-round, sunrise–sunset, except during big-game hunts; free

MAPS: Available at trailhead kiosk; USGS *Dames Ferry*

MORE INFO: 478-986-5441; fws.gov/piedmont

FACILITIES: Visitor center (open Monday–Friday, 8 a.m.–5 p.m., except on federal holidays)

SPECIAL COMMENTS: This is an excellent trail for bird-watchers and wildlife lovers, but beware of ticks and chiggers. More than 5 miles of walking trails and more than 50 miles of gravel refuge roads are open to vehicles most of the year.

DISTANCE: 71.0 miles from I-75 South/I-285 South

GPS INFORMATION

N33° 6.852' W83° 41.093'

718 Juliette Rd.
Round Oak, GA 31038

Piedmont National Wildlife Refuge Trails

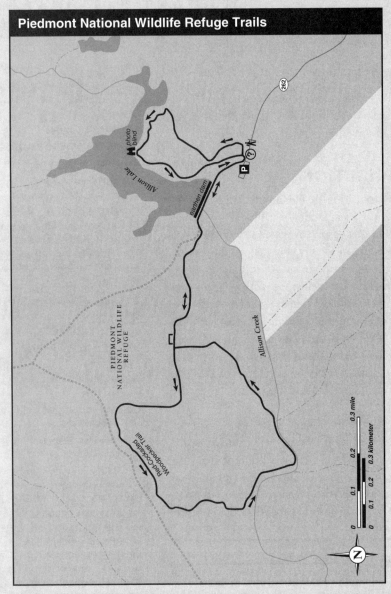

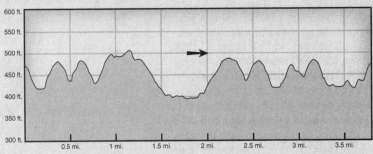

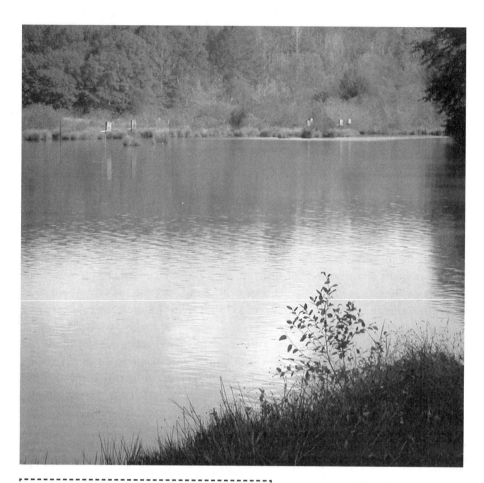

Duck houses provide a beneficial habitat at Allison Lake.

because of decreasing cotton prices, boll weevil infestations, and the Great Depression. The biggest problem facing the newly created refuge was erosion—the land was almost completely barren.

Today, thanks to more than 60 years of effective management by the U.S. Fish & Wildlife Service (FWS), as well as Mother Nature, the refuge is returning to a more pristine state. The symbol of this regeneration is the red-cockaded woodpecker. *Red* refers to a small patch of color on either side of the bird's head that appears during mating season and territorial battles. The woodpecker is black and white, its large white cheeks surrounded by a black cap and nape on either side of its head.

Both the Red-Cockaded Woodpecker (RCW) Trail and Allison Lake Wildlife Trail begin behind the kiosk. The RCW Trail heads left, making an easy descent through the woods to a gravel road. Turn right and continue descending to a well-marked left turn at Allison Lake, where the trail enters full sun and begins to cross the earthen dam that forms the lake. In the center of the dam, slanted cement sides lead to a flat, wide spillway—you must cross this to continue the hike, but you may find it impassable after a heavy rain, when the spillway has running water. Continue on the gravel road to the marked entrance to RCW Trail, on the left at 0.3 mile.

Almost immediately you enter a typical Southeastern shortleaf-pine second-growth forest, which is one of the woodpecker's habitats. Although this bird prefers mature pines infected with red heart fungus, it can be attracted to healthy younger-growth trees with a little help. The FWS produces habitat by using artificial inserts, essentially creating a cavity in the pine. The birds nest in these cavities carved in living trees; you'll easily spot the nests by the sap running from them. The woodpeckers are believed to use the sap to defend against predators such as the rat snake. Trees with inserts are marked with a white circle at the base.

A wooden bench at 0.6 mile marks the start of the RCW Trail's loop. Turn right and begin a descent to a wooden bridge over a small creek. After the creek, the trail bears right and rises to a small knob. On sunny summer days, the area has a number of butterflies, including the tiger swallowtail, viceroy, and zebra. At 1 mile, after the footpath curves left, a gravel road heads right. Just past the road, the trail begins climbing to its highest point.

An easy downhill extends over the next 0.6 mile. Just after beginning the descent, you'll reach a large field with a widely spread group of pines, clearly marked at the base with a ring of white paint. The cavities created by the FWS attract the woodpeckers and creatures that compete with them for similar nesting, such as the nocturnal flying squirrel. Just past the field, a rarely used road joins the path on the right.

As the trail begins to parallel a creek, the descent eases. Just before you cross the normally dry creek, watch for a red maple with evidence of yellow-bellied sapsuckers. In addition to the maple, this area of hardwoods includes tulip poplars, sweet gums, and a variety of oaks. Finally, at 1.8 miles, the trail reaches Allison Creek and a forested wetland. On one visit, we noted an active beaver den where the trail begins its climb back to the start of the loop. The trail also loses definition here, so follow the "well-worn trail" principle to return to the bench where the loop starts, at 2.3 miles. Turn right to return to the trailhead kiosk.

Allison Lake Wildlife Trail is often packed with all kinds of animals, from the common to the exotic. Bring your binoculars and be prepared to spend some quiet time in a blind when walking this trail, which begins behind the trailhead kiosk to the right. The trail is interpreted, so pick up a brochure at the kiosk. The numbers in the brochure correspond to those on signs bearing symbols that resemble a hiker's boot print. Unlike the RCW Trail, Allison Lake Wildlife Trail is mostly shaded, except for a portion by the lakeshore. At the start, shortleaf pines dominate, but as the trail descends the knob, the number of hardwoods increases.

Initially, the pathway descends, crossing a number of normally dry creek beds; then it rises to a knob. Descending the knob, the trail falls to the lake, eventually turning left and running parallel to but above the lakeshore. On the far side of the water, we once spotted deer and wild turkeys that were surprisingly close to one another. The plaintive call of the mourning dove and the rat-a-tat of a woodpecker added to the excitement.

Finally, on the approach to the lake, we realized that we were in for a treat. A kingfisher watched the water for fish. On the far side of the shore, a snowy egret waded among the grass, not bothering a line of turtles sunning on a submerged branch.

At 3.4 miles a blind for watching waterfowl juts into Allison Lake. Complete the loop to return to your car.

NEARBY ACTIVITIES

Not only does **The Whistle Stop Cafe** in Juliette (441 McCrackin St.; 478-992-8886; **thewhistlestopcafe.com**) serve delicious fried green tomatoes, but the building was also used as a location in *Fried Green Tomatoes,* the 1991 movie starring Jessica Tandy and Kathy Bates. **Jarrell Plantation** is a Georgia State Historic Site featuring an interpretive tour of an 18th-century estate (711 Jarrell Plantation Rd.; 478-986-5172; **gastateparks.org/jarrellplantation**). The plantation is open Thursday–Saturday, 9 a.m.–5 p.m., but is closed January 1, Thanksgiving, and December 25; admission is $4–$6.50.

56 PINE MOUNTAIN TRAIL: WOLFDEN LOOP

KEY AT-A-GLANCE INFORMATION

LENGTH: 6.5 miles

CONFIGURATION: Loop

DIFFICULTY: Moderate

SCENERY: Multiple waterfalls, long-distance view of Georgia's coastal plain from Beaver Pond Trail

EXPOSURE: Mostly shaded

TRAFFIC: Heavy from Roadside Park area to Wolf's Den, moderate elsewhere

TRAIL SURFACE: Compacted soil, rocky in places

WHEELCHAIR ACCESS: None

HIKING TIME: 4 hours

ACCESS: Daily, year-round, 7 a.m.–sunset, except for 2 days in early December and December 25; $5 state-park fee

MAPS: 2 maps available at park office ($4.50 for main map, $2.75 for kids' map; fees support the Pine Mountain Trail Association); USGS *Shiloh*

MORE INFO: 706-663-4858; gastateparks.org/fdroosevelt; pinemountaintrail.org

FACILITIES: None

SPECIAL COMMENTS: Native azaleas, dogwoods, rhododendrons, and mountain laurels bloom in April and May; central Georgia's leaves change well into November.

DISTANCE: 62.7 miles from I-85 South/I-285 Southwest

GPS INFORMATION

N32° 51.786' W84° 43.173'

IN BRIEF

Wolfden Loop explores waterfalls along Wolfden Branch and Cascade Branch of Cane Creek, then follows a ridge back.

DESCRIPTION

From the east end of the Rocky Point parking area, turn right and climb the steps to immediately enter a second-growth forest that was once part of a farm owned by Franklin D. Roosevelt. The land was donated to the state of Georgia after his death in 1945, at nearby Warm Springs; the state subsequently acquired additional land in the area and created Franklin Delano Roosevelt State Park, now the largest state park in the Georgia Department of Natural Resources system.

A scant 0.1 mile into the forest, the blue-blazed Pine Mountain Trail curves right and the white-blazed Beaver Pond Trail turns left—follow the Beaver Pond Trail. The valley to your right disappears, and a steep-sided 200-foot cliff replaces it as the trail follows the

---

Directions ————————————➤

Take I-85 South to Exit 41/GA 14/US 27 Alternate, and turn left at the end of the ramp. Drive on US 27A South for 35.1 miles in all, noting the following: at 21 miles the route loops around the courthouse in Greenville; in Warm Springs, US 27A is known as Spring Street; and at 31.6 miles you'll turn right on White House Parkway to continue on US 27A. Drive 3.5 miles to Pine Mountain Highway/GA 190 and turn right. Drive 1.9 miles to the Rocky Point parking area, on the left side of the road where the Pine Mountain Trail crosses the highway. (A second parking area, near the WJSP television tower on US 27, is often full on weekends.) Back into a space and then walk to the east side of the lot to begin the hike.

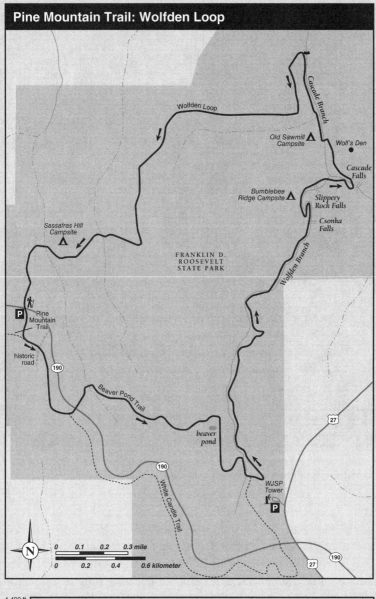

Pine Mountain Trail: Wolfden Loop

Wolfden Loop

Cascade Branch

Old Sawmill Campsite

Wolf's Den

Cascade Falls

Bumblebee Ridge Campsite

Slippery Rock Falls

Csonka Falls

Sassafras Hill Campsite

FRANKLIN D. ROOSEVELT STATE PARK

Wolfden Branch

Pine Mountain Trail

historic road

190

Beaver Pond Trail

beaver pond

190

White Candle Trail

27

WJSP Tower

N

0   0.1   0.2   0.3 mile

0   0.2   0.4   0.6 kilometer

27   190

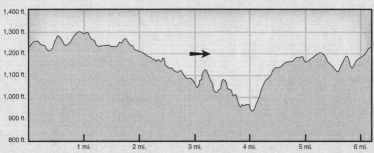

1,400 ft.
1,300 ft.
1,200 ft.
1,100 ft.
1,000 ft.
900 ft.
800 ft.

1 mi.   2 mi.   3 mi.   4 mi.   5 mi.   6 mi.

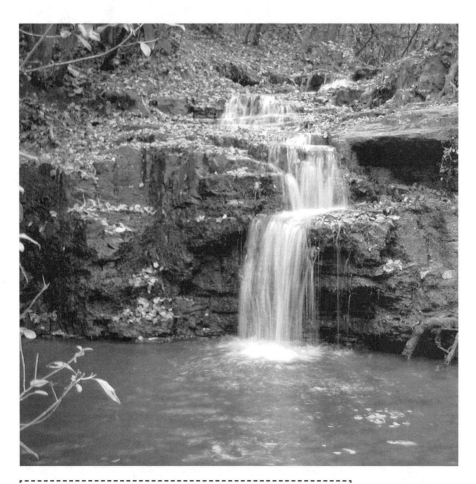

Water cascades gracefully over moss-covered rocks along the Wolfden Loop.

curve of the mountain to the right. You'll get a couple of long-distance scenic views into Georgia's coastal plain as you enter the semiarid conditions on this escarpment. On the south side of the mountain, sandy soil fills gaps in the rocky mountainside so that rainfall quickly evaporates, leaving little moisture for undergrowth. The rocky mountain prevents the trees from growing tall, and the landscape assumes a xeriscape appearance. This is the first and briefest of the three ecosystems through which the trail passes.

After crossing a historic road, the trail curves left and leaves the south-facing mountainside. Undergrowth and tree size start to increase, but watch for an area destroyed by a tornado that cut a wide swath through the forest. By the time the trail reaches GA 190, at 0.6 mile, the forest has returned to the transitional pine of the Georgia Piedmont. At almost 1 mile, the number of hardwoods begins to increase, marking the second ecosystem. Soil moisture is higher here, in part because of the higher humus content. Trees with full crowns moderate the heat of the sun, making the forest cooler. Point out to the kids in your group that there are many different types of trees, not just pines. One species worth noting is the chestnut oak, or American chestnut, which grows near the trail in this area. Watch for unusually large acorns that look like chestnuts; they range from 1 to 1.5 inches long, are about 1 inch around, and have leaves that grow up to 6 inches long, with crenate (rounded) edges.

After a short pine blowdown, watch on your left for the beaver pond that gives the trail its name. As the lake formed by the dam comes to an end, the White Candle Trail comes off to the right and the Beaver Pond Trail curves left, paralleling the Pine Mountain Trail to return to the start of the trail, near the WJSP-TV tower. At the registration mailbox and kiosk, the Beaver Pond Trail dead-ends into the Pine Mountain Trail. According to Jim Hall, board member of the Pine Mountain Trail Association, the site of FDR's farm is near this intersection. The farm encompassed most of the present-day park from this point to Dowdell's Knob.

Turn left and begin an easy descent along the most heavily traveled portion of the Wolfden Loop. Wolfden Branch, one of two streams that the trail explores, forms left of the trail, at the bottom of a gently sloping valley. After a 0.4-mile blowdown, the trail emerges at the top of a natural rock wall that drops some 15 feet immediately to the right of the trail. After the wall, the trail curves left and descends to Dry Falls, which normally flows only after a rain and marks the start of the third ecosystem. The stream plays a major role in adding moisture to the ecosystem. The soil, even that which is a significant distance from the stream, retains its moisture because of the high humus level. The full crown of trees and the north-facing position of the cove keep this area cooler than the adjacent ridgetops.

Mile marker 22 lies in a patch of mountain laurels that consumes the path, and Csonka Falls appears at 3 miles. Formed by a large, almost flat rock, the falls flows over the rock's lowest point to drop into a nearly circular pool of clear mountain water. At 0.3 mile after Csonka Falls, the trail becomes a muddy morass at the appropriately named Slippery Rock Falls. After the falls, the trail turns right and rises—watch for the double blaze indicating the turn. A short trail to Bumblebee Ridge campsite heads left at 3.5 miles. Wolfden Loop crosses the stream again and then climbs moderately up Cascade Branch. Just past mile marker 21, Cascade Falls comes into view.

One of FDR's favorite sites on his farm, Cascade Falls flows in from the right, dropping in a series of 10–15 cascades. The stream then turns and drops in three or four falls to a flat rock, culminating in a single 4-foot drop. Leaving the falls, the trail turns left and ascends the small handmade rock steps that lead to the Wolf's Den, a sheer rock wall with an overhang at the bottom. Climbing away from the Wolf's Den, the trail runs adjacent to a steep-sided drop on the left. Both tree size and the number of boulders begin to increase.

Once again the trail dips to Wolfden Branch, crosses it, and then rises to a rock formation commonly known as a fat man's squeeze. Old Sawmill campsite is down a short trail on the left. After this point, watch for Ferney, the tremendous

14-foot-circumference pine tree that is almost directly on the trail (other names for the massive tree are Big Pine and Old Pine). A dam on the right, at 4.2 miles, indicates that you're about to leave the cove.

As the footpath makes a lazy U-turn, it begins a moderate-to-difficult climb to the top of Hogback Mountain. Almost as soon as you begin this climb, the undergrowth and tree diversity lessen and the number of pine trees increases, but the forest is still mostly hardwood. Mile marker 20 marks a curve to the right where the climb eases significantly. At 5.5 miles the climb abates, having risen a total of 300 feet in 1.3 miles. From this point, the path falls and rises at an easy-to-moderate grade back to the Rocky Point parking area.

NEARBY ACTIVITIES

Warm Springs is rich with the history of our 32nd president. **Roosevelt's Little White House Historic Site** (401 Little White House Rd.) is open daily, 9 a.m.– 4:45 p.m., except January 1, Thanksgiving, and December 25; call 706-655-5870 or visit **gastateparks.org/littlewhitehouse** for more information. Gorgeous **Callaway Gardens** (17800 US 27; 800-225-5292; **callawaygardens.com**), spread over 13,000 acres in Pine Mountain, is noted for its luxury resort, golf course, and biking and hiking trails that run through extensive gardens, which include an enormous azalea display, a butterfly conservatory, and a marvelous free-flight birds-of-prey show.

SPREWELL BLUFF TRAIL

IN BRIEF

This trail in a Georgia wildlife-management area climbs to a high view of the Flint River, then follows the river past the base of Sprewell Bluff to a natural dam.

DESCRIPTION

Wide, clear, and fast-flowing at Sprewell Bluff, the Flint River begins as runoff from Hartsfield-Jackson Atlanta International Airport. This was the heart of Creek territory and near the homesite of Benjamin Hawkins, superintendent of Indian Affairs for the Southeast at the start of the 19th century. For more than 20 years, Hawkins represented the United States to the Creek Confederacy and supervised the representatives to the other American Indian nations. Hawkins is credited with the saying "God willing and the Creek don't rise," which had nothing to do with a stream overflowing its banks but the perception that the Creek people were warlike. Hawkins witnessed the devastation brought on by the war with the Red Sticks, a violent faction of the Creek tribe, in 1813 and 1814. In the same way that the Cherokees were forced west on the Trail of Tears, the Creeks were forcibly evicted from their homeland following the Treaty of Indian Springs (1825).

Directions

Take I-75 South to Exit 201/GA 36 (Barnesville). Turn right at the end of the ramp on Barnesville–Jackson Road/GA 36 West. Drive 29.8 miles to downtown Thomaston and bear slightly right on Main Street/GA 74. Drive 5.9 miles and turn left on South Old Alabama Road. Drive 3.9 miles and turn left on Sprewell Bluff Road. Drive 2.5 miles to the parking lot, on the bank of the Flint River.

KEY AT-A-GLANCE INFORMATION

LENGTH: 3.2 miles round-trip

CONFIGURATION: Out-and-back

DIFFICULTY: Easy except in the area of the double overlook, which is hard

SCENERY: Long-distance views of the Flint River

EXPOSURE: Full sun

TRAFFIC: Light

TRAIL SURFACE: Compacted soil

WHEELCHAIR ACCESS: None

HIKING TIME: 1.5 hours

ACCESS: Daily, year-round, 7 a.m.–sunset; Georgia Outdoor Recreation Pass required for visitors ages 16–64, $3.50/3 days or $19/year (buy at georgiawildlife.com /recreational-licenses; transaction fees may apply)

MAPS: USGS *Roland*

MORE INFO: 478-825-6354; gastateparks.org/sprewellbluff

FACILITIES: Restrooms; picnic tables and grills

SPECIAL COMMENTS: Mostly wide, with only a couple of steep sections, this is a great trail to enjoy with the family. In 2012 Sprewell Bluff changed from a state park to a state wildlife-management area.

DISTANCE: 79.2 miles from I-75 South/I-285 South

GPS INFORMATION

N32° 51.189' W84° 28.894'

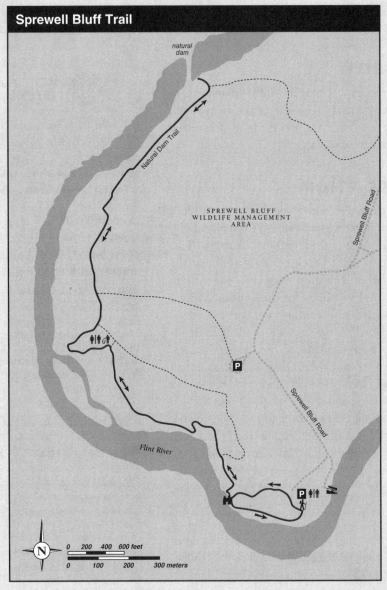

Sprewell Bluff Trail

natural dam

Natural Dam Trail

SPREWELL BLUFF
WILDLIFE MANAGEMENT
AREA

Sprewell Bluff Road

Sprewell Bluff Road

Flint River

P

P

N

| 0 | 200 | 400 | 600 feet |
| 0 | 100 | 200 | 300 meters |

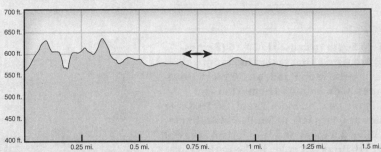

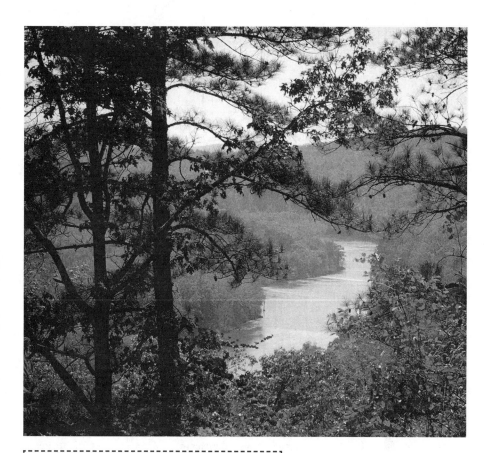

The Flint River, viewed from an overlook at Sprewell Bluff

From the parking area, look just in front of the treeline for the restrooms on the right. To the left of the structure is the trailhead, with a brown kiosk topped by a shingle roof. Beginning as a dirt road, the trail rises easily through an oak, maple, elm, and American beech forest. A path quickly comes off to the right—continue straight 0.4 mile, at which point double overlooks give you a stunning view of the Flint River basin and nearby watershed. As you come off the second overlook, the road splits. Bear left and the road follows a ridge to a moderately steep but short drop to the river's floodplain.

As you move farther from the rocky precipice, the floodplain widens and the diversity of the forest increases as river birch, dogwood, and ash trees join the other hardwoods. On the left, a number of trails lead down to the water for fishing. As the trail moves upriver, it begins to pull away from the Flint, and you can no longer hear the river at 0.7 mile. You come to a trailhead kiosk a short distance later. At the kiosk, a gravel road heads right and climbs into the Flint River watershed—continue around the curve to the left, which dips and then rises and curves right to reach a wooden restroom with a fiberglass roof.

As the trail turns left, it once again dips into a moist, boglike area of the floodplain of the Flint River, then rises to a low ridge and turns right. Less than 0.1 mile later, the trail bears right, turning inland to a three-way intersection at 0.9 mile. Turn left and cross a creek in a culvert through an oak, loblolly pine, and longleaf pine forest. After crossing the creek, the path turns left again and falls to a marshy area that may be difficult to cross after a heavy rain. Just beyond this, the trail joins the riverbank and turns right. As you approach the end of the trail, the sound of the water flowing over the natural dam becomes very loud.

Heading left at 1.5 miles, a side trail allows you to explore a sandy area and catch some good riverside views. Return to the main trail, turn left, and continue a few steps to a second viewing area with a better view of the dam, which is actually a series of rocks that seems to form a narrow shoal. The trail continues down to a clearly marked end just a few steps past the second viewing area. At this point, turn around and retrace your steps to the double overlook.

After the second overlook, watch for a trail that heads right and makes a moderate-to-difficult descent to the Flint River floodplain. Turn left and follow the riverbank. Sprewell Bluff is on the opposite side of the Flint River, rising 150 feet above the river. A number of rock outcrops are perched above the bank. The trail continues to a sign alerting hikers to the possibility of rapidly rising water. Return along the riverbank to your car.

NEARBY ACTIVITIES

One of the best-known and oldest attractions in Georgia is **Callaway Gardens** (17800 US 27; 800-225-5292; **callawaygardens.com**), 22 miles west of Sprewell Bluff Wildlife Management Area. In addition to a wide variety of accommodations and restaurants, the resort offers world-class golf and some surprisingly interesting attractions. As you leave Sprewell Bluff, turn left on Roland Road. At 2.1 miles, turn right on GA 36. Drive 12.1 miles to GA 41; then turn right and drive 5.7 miles, turning left on GA 190. In 11 miles, GA 354 heads right. Take this road 4 miles to the entrance to Callaway Gardens, on your left.

STARR'S MILL TRAIL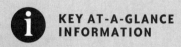

IN BRIEF

Explore Starr's Mill, the pond that powers the mill, and Whitewater Creek, and view a swamp at the north end of Starr's Millpond.

DESCRIPTION

Starr's Mill is the picturesque centerpiece of this 16-acre Fayette County park. Purchased by the county water system in February 1991, the park contains both Starr's Mill and Starr's Millpond, which the county intends to use as a water source as demand increases.

From the small gravel parking lot, walk toward the mill. Before the steps to the porch, you come to a ramp made of concrete blocks. Follow this down to Whitewater Creek, below the dam. When water levels are low, a small shoal extends almost entirely across the creek, affording a good vantage point for both the dam and the mill. Return to the mill's porch steps from the shoal. Built on aboveground pilings, the millworks were housed underneath the mill, but the grinding was done in the mill itself. A door on the river side of the mill allowed access to the millworks.

Many years ago, mills such as this were the focal points of rural areas nationwide. Farmers would bring their grains to be ground (or cracked, hence the term *cracker*). Mills were places to exchange political views and gossip and normally included a post office or

KEY AT-A-GLANCE INFORMATION

LENGTH: 1.5 miles round-trip

CONFIGURATION: Out-and-back

DIFFICULTY: Easy

SCENERY: Red mill and dam, river views

EXPOSURE: Full sun

TRAFFIC: Light

TRAIL SURFACE: Gravel road

WHEELCHAIR ACCESS: None

HIKING TIME: 45 minutes

ACCESS: Daily, year-round, sunrise–sunset; free

MAPS: USGS *Senoia*

MORE INFO: 770-461-1146; fayettecountyga.gov/water /recreation_activities.htm

FACILITIES: None

SPECIAL COMMENTS: No bodily contact with the water is allowed. Occasionally used as a filming location, the dark-red mill with a white porch and white trim was featured in the 2002 film *Sweet Home Alabama* as the glassworks shop of Reese Witherspoon's ex-husband (Josh Lucas).

DISTANCE: 25.9 miles from I-85 South/I-285 Southwest

Directions

Take I-85 to Exit 61/Senoia Road/GA 74 (Fairburn), and turn left. Drive 18.5 miles to GA 85 North and turn left. Drive 0.2 mile to the park entrance on Whitewater Way, a gravel road, and turn left. Follow the road around to the right to the parking area.

GPS INFORMATION

N33° 19.754' W84° 30.538'

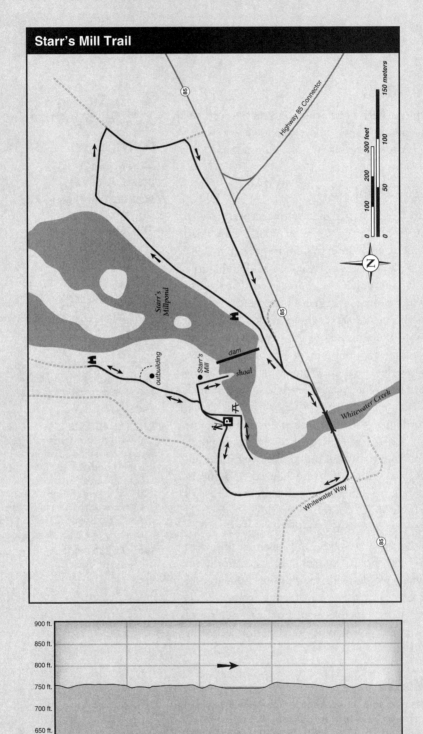

Starr's Mill Trail

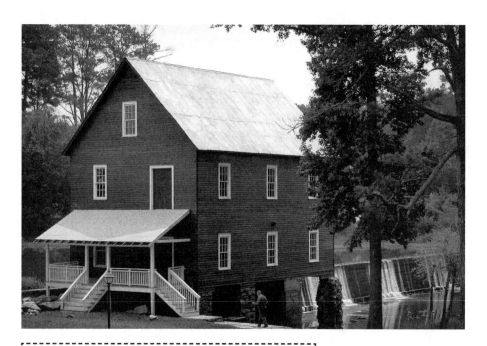

Historical Starr's Mill made an appearance in a hit Hollywood film.

small grocery store. Many times, towns would spring up around mills, as did the town of Starr's Mill.

Be careful climbing the steps to the mill's porch—even a casual inspection shows signs of rot. As you reach the top of the stairs, peek through the window for a look at the grinding apparatus in the center of the floor. Continue on and exit down the front of the porch, returning to the gravel road; turn right. Past the mill is an outbuilding, around which the road curves as it rises. Once around the building, follow the road to an intersection and turn left.

On your right is an extensive marshland that makes up the upper reaches of Starr's Millpond. In the distance you'll probably see at least a few of the larger common swamp birds, including egrets, herons, and mourning doves. As the road begins to rise, a NO TRESPASSING sign indicates the park boundary. Turn around and return to the intersection; then continue straight ahead. As the road curves right, it returns to the lakeshore.

Fishing is a popular pastime at this pond, and anglers normally park at least a couple of cars along the road. The clear land at the water's edge offers an excellent view of the entire lake. During late fall and early spring, migratory birds, especially geese, visit the pond. Return on the gravel road to the Starr's Mill parking lot. From the lot, walk past the picnic tables down to the river's edge and follow it, walking away from the mill.

Looking down Whitewater Creek, notice the luxuriant growth along the banks. These vegetated borders are known as riparian zones, their full, lush growth indicative of both a healthy river and clean water. The plants hold the banks in place, even during high water, and provide nesting grounds for amphibians and insects and shelter for small animals. As you walk along the river, it suddenly turns 90 degrees and flows toward the bridge over GA 85. At this long-distance view, notice that the creek's riparian zones continue as far as the eye can see.

Return to the gravel road and follow it as it curves left to the entrance of the park at Whitewater Way. Turn left, continue to GA 85, and turn left again. Walk over the bridge across Whitewater Creek and turn left down a dirt driveway.

Continue walking along the creek side, toward the dam. After heavy rainfalls, the volume of water flowing over the dam enhances photographs of the mill. Once past the dam, you'll see the lake, and on windless days the mill reflects in the millpond. Photographers should get here before sunrise to capture the mill in the morning light. Mid-November is especially beautiful, thanks to the autumn colors of the maple trees behind the mill.

As you walk along the lakeshore, the path reaches the low rise that forms the swamp and becomes overgrown. Turn right and continue to the road embankment; then turn right again to return to the driveway. Climb to GA 85, turn right, and return to the parking lot on Whitewater Way.

NEARBY ACTIVITIES

Dauset Trails Nature Center in Jackson (360 Mt. Vernon Church Rd.; 770-775-6798; **dausettrails.com/trails.htm**) encompasses more than 20 miles of hiking and mountain biking trails. The center is open Monday–Saturday, 9 a.m.–5 p.m. and Sunday, noon–5 p.m.; admission is free.

SWEETWATER HISTORY (RED) AND EAST SIDE (YELLOW) TRAILS

IN BRIEF

The Red, or History, Trail follows an old road through the historic city of New Manchester to Sweetwater Mill and then continues to an overlook of Sweetwater Creek's falls. The Yellow (East Side) Trail crosses the river and climbs into the watershed before returning along the river.

DESCRIPTION

After purchasing this land in 1845, former Georgia governor Charles McDonald began construction on Sweetwater Manufacturing Company in 1846. He began producing thread, yarn, and cloth three years later; his textile mill was taller than any building in nearby Atlanta when it was completed. In 1857 Sweetwater was reorganized as the New Manchester Manufacturing Company, the name it retained until it was destroyed by Union troops on July 9, 1864.

From the trailhead kiosk at the east end of the parking lot, the Red, or History, Trail descends gradually to Sweetwater Creek, turning right at 0.15 mile and following the curves of the bank of Sweetwater Creek. The trail is a wide, level gravel road through a forest of American beeches, white oaks, loblolly pines, and sweet gums. Watch for a large square indentation on the right and an

KEY AT-A-GLANCE INFORMATION

LENGTH: 5.1 miles

CONFIGURATION: Double loop

DIFFICULTY: Moderate except for the section between Sweetwater Mill and the falls, which is hard

SCENERY: Scenic views of Sweetwater Creek, falls, historic mill

EXPOSURE: Full sun–partial shade along the riverbanks, mostly shaded elsewhere

TRAFFIC: Heavy on the trail to the mill, moderate elsewhere

TRAIL SURFACE: Compacted soil

WHEELCHAIR ACCESS: None

HIKING TIME: 4 hours

ACCESS: Visitor-center hours: daily, year-round, 9 a.m.–5 p.m.; park hours: daily, year-round, 7 a.m.–sunset; $5 state-park fee

MAPS: Available at visitor center; USGS *Austell, Ben Hill, Campbellton, Mableton*

MORE INFO: 770-732-5871; gastateparks.org/sweetwatercreek

FACILITIES: Restrooms, picnic areas, pavilions

SPECIAL COMMENTS: Sweetwater Creek is one of the largest tributaries of the Chattahoochee River. The confluence of these two waterways is only a couple of miles from the mill.

DISTANCE: 11.8 miles from I-20 West/I-285 West

Directions

Take I-20 West to Exit 41/Lee Road, and turn left. Drive 1 mile and turn left on Cedar Terrace Road. Drive 0.8 mile and turn left on Mt. Vernon Road. Drive 0.3 mile and turn left on Factory Shoals Road. Drive 0.6 mile to the parking lot.

GPS INFORMATION

N33° 45.201' W84° 37.708'

Sweetwater History (Red) and East Side (Yellow) Trails

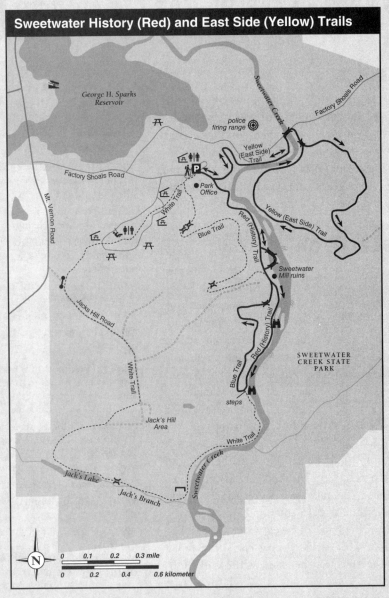

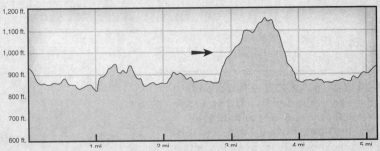

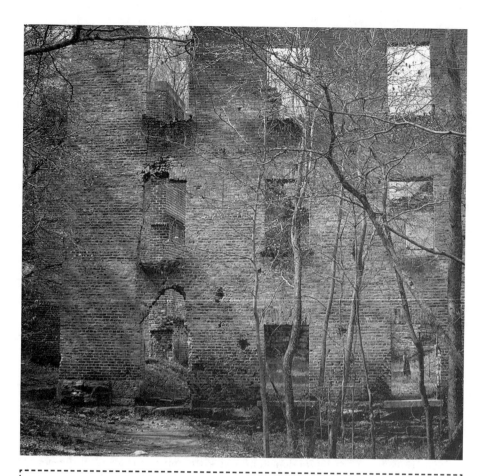

The historic New Manchester Manufacturing Company textile-mill ruins, on the banks of Sweetwater Creek, can be seen from the Red and the Blue Trails. These haunting five-story ruins are all that remain of New Manchester, a mid-19th-century mill town that was destroyed during the Civil War.

interpretive sign on the left that tells the story of New Manchester. Here Nathaniel Humphries ran the company store, which contained a post office and possibly a shoe-manufacturing operation during the Civil War. On the left is the start of the millrace that ends at Sweetwater Manufacturing. Almost immediately, a wooden bridge allows you to cross the millrace and explore what is now an artificial island. Return to the main trail and continue left. At the end of the island, the spillway is now used to divert the water from the mill in an attempt to preserve it.

On the left, at 0.6 mile, a wooden walkway before the mill gives you an up-close look at the power room of Sweetwater Mill. Notice that the old bed of the millrace makes a 90-degree turn between the platform and the closest end of the building. Water from Sweetwater Creek coursing through the millrace followed this curve into the power room, where it would turn a wheel to generate

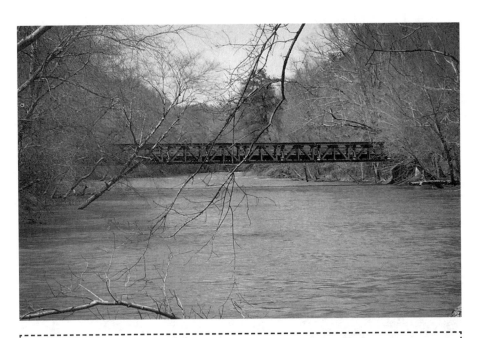

power. Machinery in the middle room wove the thread, yarn, and fabric, which was stored at the far end of the building to be transported to Atlanta.

The Blue Trail continues straight, but the Red Trail turns left after passing the mill and descends a set of wooden steps, quickly coming to the end of the boardwalk. From this point to Sweetwater Falls, we consider the trail difficult because it involves multiple trail-narrowing rock outcrops, and the trail is rocky and heavily rooted. A chain railing carries hikers across a particularly difficult area at 0.8 mile, after which you reach a wooden bridge and an overlook. Just over a mile into the hike, a series of rock outcrops narrows the path. As the trail curves right, into a cove, a massive 25-foot boulder seems to block the way, but wooden steps allow trekkers to scale the rock.

Hikers making it to the top of the rock are rewarded with an excellent view from the first of two platforms over the next 0.1 mile. Continue to the second platform for a superb view of Sweetwater Falls. As you leave the platform, climb the steps straight ahead and follow the Blue Trail to return to the mill. At the mill, take the Red Trail to return to the trailhead. Just before the starting point, watch for a side trail on the right with a yellow blaze and a brown hiking sign. Turn right onto the Yellow, or East Side, Trail.

The Yellow Trail begins an easy descent into a river valley, making a U-turn near a paved park road and running alongside a creek to a wooden bridge. Turn right, cross a small wooden bridge, and briefly follow the riverbank to a bridge across Sweetwater Creek. Built in 2012, it replaced a 1950s-vintage bridge that was washed away by floodwaters in 2009. An antebellum structure, known as Ferguson's Bridge, spanned Sweetwater Creek in about the same place and was used to haul bricks and lumber for the mill from the far side of the creek.

After crossing the bridge, walk down the steps to the right. The footpath winds along the creek bank and comes to a wooden bridge. Shortly after the bridge, 2.8 miles into the hike, turn left on the Yellow, or East Side, Trail and begin an extended climb into the watershed of Sweetwater Creek. Over the next 0.8 mile the trail rises some 300 feet in full sun. Watch for a yellow-topped post on the left and three consecutively blazed trees. The signs are in place to ensure that you don't turn on the historic road, which heads left. Continue straight on the Yellow Trail to a right turn marked by a double blaze.

Still climbing, the Yellow Trail turns left at 3.4 miles, and a scenic view comes less than 0.1 mile later, after a marked right turn. As the trail continues around to the right, it comes to a bench and then bears left, beginning to run along a creek bed as it descends. In an area of rock outcrops and cascades, the trail rock-hops across the stream, crossing back onto a bridge a little later. Reaching the river-bank, the trail curves right and easily climbs back to the loop's start. Retrace your steps to Ferguson's Bridge, and turn left after the crossing. Following the bank of the river, the trail returns you to the bridge near the start of the Yellow Trail.

NEARBY ACTIVITIES

Inside Sweetwater Creek State Park, **George H. Sparks Reservoir** (770-732-5871; **gastateparks.org/sweetwatercreek**) is a great place to take the kids fishing for bream, crappie, catfish, and the occasional bass. The Georgia Department of Natural Resources, which manages the 215-acre reservoir, has added brush along the banks to make them fish-friendly. You can also rent an electric-powered boat for an off-shore adventure.

60 SWEETWATER NONGAME WILDLIFE TRAILS

KEY AT-A-GLANCE INFORMATION

LENGTH: 5.1 miles

CONFIGURATION: Loop

DIFFICULTY: Moderate

SCENERY: Creekside views, long-distance views into a river gorge, lake, remains of a cotton mill, waterfalls

EXPOSURE: Mostly shaded except during the first mile and in the vicinity of the river

TRAFFIC: Moderate, except in the vicinity of the cotton mill and falls, where it is heavy

TRAIL SURFACE: Gravel, historic roads, compacted soil

WHEELCHAIR ACCESS: None

HIKING TIME: 3 hours

ACCESS: Visitor-center hours: daily, year-round, 9 a.m.–5 p.m.; park hours: daily, year-round, 7 a.m.–sunset; $5 state-park fee

MAPS: Available at visitor center; USGS *Austell, Ben Hill, Campbellton, Mableton*

MORE INFO: 770-732-5871; gastateparks.org/sweetwatercreek

FACILITIES: Restrooms, picnic tables with grills

SPECIAL COMMENTS: Arrive early in the morning to see the most wildlife.

DISTANCE: 11.8 miles from I-20 West/I-285 West

GPS INFORMATION

N33° 45.200' W84° 37.709'

IN BRIEF

This deep-woods experience is only a few minutes west of downtown Atlanta. Hikers on the nongame wildlife trails frequently see deer, wild turkeys, and other large animals.

DESCRIPTION

The Sweetwater nongame wildlife trails, also known as the White and Blue Trails, begin as a gravel road, on the right side of the visitor center as you face the building. Almost immediately, the return loop joins the trail from the left. Over the first 1.3 miles, the well-marked treadway follows gravel roads and occasionally enters the woods. Within the picnic area, the White Trail crosses two paved roads, quickly reentering the forest each time, and then becomes a gravel road at 0.6 mile. At a three-way intersection, the trail bears left at 0.8 mile. For no apparent reason, the trail jogs left and then turns almost immediately right, into the woods, at 1.2 miles. It returns to a dirt road a little farther into the hike. At the top of a knoll, the trail turns right at a four-way intersection, follows the ridge 0.3 mile, and then turns right again and begins a dramatic easy-to-moderate descent into the Sweetwater Creek valley.

Almost immediately, the valley on the right drops off, the sides become steep, and the area is filled with a diverse second-growth oak–American beech forest. As the road follows the

----

Directions ⟶

Take I-20 West to Exit 41/Lee Road, and turn left. Drive 1 mile and turn left on Cedar Terrace Road. Drive 0.8 mile and turn left on Mt. Vernon Road. Drive 0.3 mile and turn left on Factory Shoals Road. Drive 0.6 mile to the parking lot.

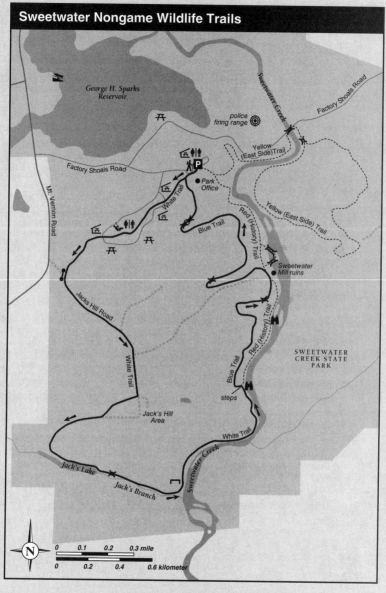

Sweetwater Nongame Wildlife Trails

George H. Sparks
Reservoir

police
firing range

Sweetwater Creek

Factory Shoals Road

Yellow (East Side) Trail

Factory Shoals Road

Mt. Vernon Road

White Trail

Park
Office

Blue Trail

Red (History) Trail

Yellow (East Side) Trail

Sweetwater
Mill ruins

Jacks Hill Road

White Trail

Red (History) Trail

SWEETWATER
CREEK STATE
PARK

Blue Trail

steps

Jack's Hill
Area

White Trail

Jack's Lake

Sweetwater Creek

Jack's Branch

N

| 0 | 0.1 | 0.2 | 0.3 mile |

| 0 | 0.2 | 0.4 | 0.6 kilometer |

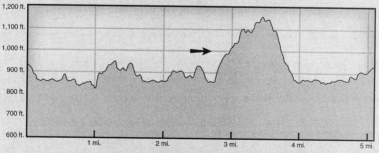

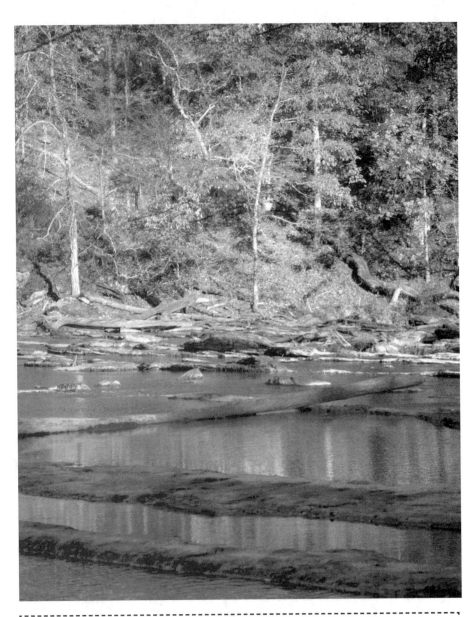

Charming Sweetwater Creek reflects flaming fall colors in the late-afternoon light. With its Class III–IV rapids, the creek is a popular rafting and kayaking destination.

curve of the mountain to the left, a scenic view opens to your right—a lake formed by a dammed creek. The trail continues to wrap around the mountain, still descending as it begins to parallel the lakeshore. After the pathway levels, it turns right and begins crossing an earthen dam to a set of long wooden steps on the left; these will carry you down to a streamside trail. Before descending these steps, spend a few minutes watching for large waterfowl that visit the lake. The path traverses moist,

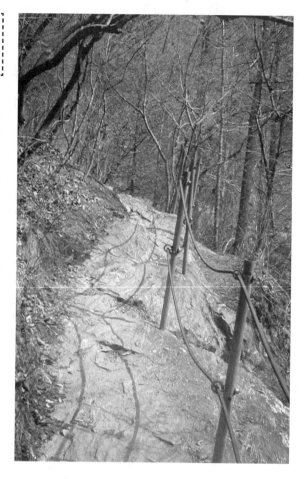

fern-covered soil and then reaches a double bridge at 2 miles.

After the bridge, the trail follows a historic road past a massive granite boulder that signifies a change: the number of rock outcrops begins to increase, as do the number and size of boulders in the creek bed. Near 2.4 miles the treadway bears left and comes out at a park bench that faces the normally loud Sweetwater Creek, which at this point is completing a rapid descent—a 60-foot drop in just over 0.5 mile—through the fractured and sheared rock of the Brevard Fault zone. The trail briefly joins Sweetwater Creek before it moves slightly inland and up, climbing a massive rock outcrop along the creek, where the water crashes over a series of boulders. After climbing around the outcrop, the trail returns to run along the creek bank, offering good long-distance views into the gorge formed by the hills on either side of the creek. Step across a rivulet at 2.7 miles and then climb the wooden steps at 3 miles for an excellent view of the falls, where the river tumbles through a series of cascades.

After the steps, the White Trail crosses a rocky area and a bridge; then it reaches a T-intersection with the Blue Trail at a second set of stairs. Turn right and descend to the overlook that marks the end of both the Red Trail (see previous hike) and the Blue Trail. Once again you'll find good scenic views into the gorge that was formed over eons by Sweetwater Creek. From the overlook, turn around and begin climbing the steps, passing the White Trail on your left and making your way to the top of a small hill. Still in a diverse hardwood forest, the Blue Trail turns right and then hugs the curve of the hill as the creek comes into view some 100 feet below.

Almost entirely in the forest, the Blue Trail is a significantly different pathway from the White Trail. At 3.5 miles the Blue Trail curves sharply inland, exploring a lush cove and tributary of Sweetwater Creek. Watch the trail closely as it joins one of the many historic roads that crosscut these once-populated hills. The trail makes a U-turn deep in the cove, and the footpath leaves the road. As you approach the gorge of Sweetwater Creek, the trail curves left, falling gently to the remains of a three-story brick textile mill that was once the tallest building in the Atlanta area. Sweetwater Manufacturing began production in 1849. Eventually, New Manchester Manufacturing was formed, and Sweetwater became a part of that larger operation. In 1864 the Union cavalry captured the mill and burned it to the ground. For more information on the mill at New Manchester, see the preceding hike profile.

As you leave the mill, turn right—the Red and Blue Trails immediately split. Follow the Blue Trail to the left as it rises and moves inland, once again following a gravel road deep into a forested cove. At 4.2 miles, the road makes a U-turn in the cove and returns to a winter view of the creek on the right 0.2 mile later. Paralleling the river but running well away from it, the trail slowly curves left until it makes a hard left on a gravel road at 4.7 miles. This roadway carries you into another cove, turning right to leave the road, crossing a bridge, and turning right again, until the trail reaches the visitor center.

NEARBY ACTIVITIES

The kids—and the adults, for that matter—might enjoy a trip to **Six Flags Over Georgia** after this hike. The park's specialty is roller-coaster-style rides, beginning with the traditional Great American Scream Machine and the Georgia Cyclone. Other coasters have more-contemporary themes. The Goliath is a "hypercoaster," which means that it's built for speed and air time. Thunder River and Splash Water Falls are fun water rides. After you leave Sweetwater Creek, drive 2 miles east on I-20 to Exit 46/Six Flags Drive, and follow the signs. Hours and admission vary according to the season; for more information, call 770-948-9290 or visit **sixflags.com/overgeorgia**.

APPENDIX A:
HIKING STORES

BASS PRO SHOPS
basspro.com
5900 Sugarloaf Pkwy.
Lawrenceville, GA 30043
678-847-5500

BARGAIN BARN
bargainbarn.com
3622 Camp Rd.
Jasper, GA 30143
706-253-WHOA (9462)
877-337-WHOA

DICK'S SPORTING GOODS
dickssportinggoods.com

ALPHARETTA
North Point Mall
6440 North Point Pkwy.
Alpharetta, GA 30022
770-521-1195

ATLANTA
Lenox Marketplace
3535 Peachtree Rd. NE
Atlanta, GA 30326
404-267-0200

BUFORD
Mall of Georgia
3333 Buford Dr.
Buford, GA 30519
678-482-1200

CANTON
Canton Marketplace
1810 Cumming Hwy.
Canton, GA 30114
770-345-1218

CUMMING
Cumming Town Center
2145 Marketplace Blvd.
Cumming, GA 30040
770-292-9834

KENNESAW
Town Center Commons
691 Ernest W. Barrett Pkwy.
Kennesaw, GA 30144
770-281-0200

NORCROSS
Peachtree Square
6050 Peachtree Pkwy., Ste. 450
Norcross, GA 30092
770-613-0077

HIGH COUNTRY OUTFITTERS
highcountryoutfitters.com

ATLANTA
Buckhead
3906-B Roswell Rd. NE
Atlanta, GA 30342
404-814-0999

MARIETTA
The Avenue East Cobb
4475 Roswell Rd., Ste. 1120
Marietta, GA 30062
770-321-4780

MOUNTAIN CROSSINGS AT WALASI-YI
mountaincrossings.com
9710 Gainesville Hwy.
Blairsville, GA 30512
706-745-6095

APPENDIX A:
HIKING STORES (CONT'D.)

**NORTH GEORGIA
MOUNTAIN OUTFITTERS**
hikenorthgeorgia.com
583 Highland Crossing, Ste. 230
East Ellijay, GA 30540
706-698-HIKE (4453)

REI
rei.com

ATLANTA

Buckhead/Brookhaven
1800 Northeast Expy. NE
Atlanta, GA 30329
404-633-6508

BUFORD

Mall of Georgia
1600 Mall of Georgia Blvd., Ste. 800
Buford, GA 30519
770-831-0676

KENNESAW

Target Plaza
740 Ernest W. Barrett Pkwy., Ste. 450
Kennesaw, GA 30144
770-425-4480

PERIMETER CENTER

Perimeter Square West
1165 Perimeter Center W., Ste. 200
Atlanta, GA 30338
770-901-9200

THE OUTSIDE WORLD
theoutsideworld.net
471 Quill Dr.
Dawsonville, GA 30534
706-265-4500

APPENDIX B:
HIKING CLUBS

ATLANTA OUTDOOR CLUB
atlantaoutdoorclub.com

ATLANTA SINGLE HIKERS
atlantasinglehikers.com

BENTON MACKAYE TRAIL ASSOCIATION
bmta.org

GEORGIA APPALACHIAN TRAIL CLUB
404-494-0968
georgia-atclub.org

PINE MOUNTAIN TRAIL ASSOCIATION
706-569-0497 *(evenings only)*
pinemountaintrail.org

INDEX

DEAR CUSTOMERS AND FRIENDS,

SUPPORTING YOUR INTEREST IN OUTDOOR ADVENTURE, travel, and an active lifestyle is central to our operations, from the authors we choose to the locations we detail to the way we design our books. Menasha Ridge Press was incorporated in 1982 by a group of veteran outdoorsmen and professional outfitters. For many years now, we've specialized in creating books that benefit the outdoors enthusiast.

Almost immediately, Menasha Ridge Press earned a reputation for revolutionizing outdoors- and travel-guidebook publishing. For such activities as canoeing, kayaking, hiking, backpacking, and mountain biking, we established new standards of quality that transformed the whole genre, resulting in outdoor-recreation guides of great sophistication and solid content. Menasha Ridge continues to be outdoor publishing's greatest innovator.

The folks at Menasha Ridge Press are as at home on a white-water river or mountain trail as they are editing a manuscript. The books we build for you are the best they can be, because we're responding to your needs. Plus, we use and depend on them ourselves.

We look forward to seeing you on the river or the trail. If you'd like to contact us directly, join in at www.trekalong.com or visit us at www.menasharidge.com. We thank you for your interest in our books and the natural world around us all.

SAFE TRAVELS,

Bob Sehlinger

BOB SEHLINGER
PUBLISHER